Endocrine Pathology

Other books in this series:

Neuropathology

Gastrointestinal and Liver Pathology

Head and Neck Pathology

Breast Pathology

Other books coming soon in this series:

Dermatopathology

Bone and Soft Tissue Pathology

Genitourinary Pathology

Hematopathology

Gynecologic Pathology

Fine Needle Aspiration Cytology

Pulmonary Pathology

Endocrine Pathology

A Volume in the Series
Foundations in Diagnostic Pathology

Edited by

Lester DR Thompson, MD, FASCP
Department of Pathology
Southern California Permanente Medical Group
Woodland Hills Medical Center
Woodland Hills, California

Series Editor

John R Goldblum, MD, FCAP, FASCP, FACG
Chairman, Department of Anatomical Pathology
The Cleveland Clinic Foundation
Cleveland Clinic Lerner College of Medicine
Case Western Reserve University
Cleveland, Ohio

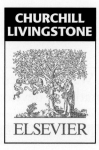

CHURCHILL
LIVINGSTONE

ELSEVIER

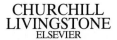

CHURCHILL LIVINGSTONE
An imprint of Elsevier Inc.

ENDOCRINE PATHOLOGY
© 2006, Elsevier Inc. All rights reserved.

ISBN-13: 978-0-443-06685-6
ISBN-10: 0-443-06685-X

NOTICE

Medical knowledge is constantly changing. Standard safety precautions must be followed, but as new research and clinical experience broaden our knowledge, changes in treatment and drug therapy may become necessary or appropriate. Readers are advised to check the most current product information provided by the manufacturer of each drug to be administered to verify the recommended dose, the method and duration of administration, and contraindications. It is the responsibility of the practitioner, relying on experience and knowledge of the patient, to determine dosages and the best treatment for each individual patient. Neither the Publisher nor the author assume any liability for any injury and/or damage to persons or property arising from this publication.

The Publisher

First published 2006

British Library Cataloguing in Publication Data
A catalogue record for this book is available from the British Library

Library of Congress Cataloging in Publication Data
A catalog record for this book is available from the Library of Congress

Commissioning Editor: Belinda Kuhn
Project Development Manager: Karen Carter
Project Manager: Cheryl Brant
Design Manager: Louis Forgione
Marketing Manager(s) (UK/USA): Lisa Damico/Clara Tombs

Printed in China

Last digit is the print number: 9   8   7   6   5   4   3   2   1

Working together to grow
libraries in developing countries

www.elsevier.com | www.bookaid.org | www.sabre.org

ELSEVIER   BOOK AID International   Sabre Foundation

To all students
Every What of Illumination
Needs the Why of Intelligence

Contributors

Carol Adair, MD
Associate Clinical Professor
Department of Pathology
Uniformed Services University of Health Sciences
Bethesda, MD;
Residency Program Director
Department of Pathology
Walter Reed Army Medical Center
Washington, DC

Jason C Fowler, PA (ASCP)
Clinical Instructor
Department of Pathology
West Virginia University School of Medicine
Morgantown, WV

Clara S Heffess, MD
Chief, Endocrine Division
Department of Endocrine and Otorhinolaryngic – Head
and Neck Pathology
Armed Forces Institute of Pathology
Washington, DC

Jennifer Hunt, MD, MEd
Head, Section of Surgical Pathology
Director, Head and Neck and Endocrine Pathology
Director, AP Molecular Diagnostics Unit
Cleveland Clinic Foundation,
Cleveland, OH

Paul Komminoth, MD, MEd
Professor of Pathology
University of Zurich
Chief, Institute of Pathology
Kantonsspital Baden AG
Baden
Switzerland

Ronald R de Krijger, MD, PhD
Josefine Nefkens Institute
Department of Pathology
Erasmus MC – University Medical Center Rotterdam
Rotterdam
The Netherlands

Leslie H Sobin, MD
Chief, Division of Gastrointestinal Pathology
Department of Gastrointestinal and Hepatic Pathology
Armed Forces Institute of Pathology
Washington, DC

Lester DR Thompson, MD
Consultant Pathologist
Southern California Permanente Medical Group
Woodland Hills, CA

Jacqueline A Wieneke, MD
Chief, Division of Otorhinolaryngic – Head and Neck
Pathology
Department of Endocrine and Otorhinolaryngic – Head
and Neck Pathology
Armed Forces Institute of Pathology
Washington, DC

Foreword

The study and practice of anatomic pathology are both exciting and overwhelming. Surgical pathology, with all of the subspecialties it encompasses, and cytopathology have become increasingly complex and sophisticated, and it is not possible for any individual to master the skills and knowledge required to perform all of these tasks at the highest level. Simply being able to make a correct diagnosis is challenging enough, but the standard of care has far surpassed merely providing a diagnosis. Pathologists are now asked to provide large amounts of ancillary information, both diagnostic and prognostic, often on small amounts of tissue, a task that can be daunting even to the most experienced pathologist.

Although large general surgical pathology textbooks are useful resources, they by necessity could not possibly cover many of the aspects that pathologists need to know and include in their reports. As such, the concept behind Foundation in Diagnostic Pathology was born. This series is designed to cover the major areas of surgical and cytopathology, and each edition is focused on one major topic. The goal of every book in this series is to provide the essential information that any pathologist, whether general or subspecialized, in training or in practice, would find useful in the evaluation of virtually any type of specimen encountered.

Dr Lester Thompson, a renowned and prolific head and neck and endocrine pathologist, formerly of the Armed Forces Institute of Pathology and currently at the Southern California Permanente Medical Group, Woodland Hills, California, has edited a state-of-the art book on the essentials of endocrine pathology. General surgical pathologists encounter these specimens with some regularity, especially specimens derived from the thyroid gland, an area of great challenge to most surgical pathologists. Although most pathologists evaluate parathyroid, adrenal and pituitary gland specimens much less frequently, the problems encountered when evaluating these specimens are shared by all, and this comprehensive text addresses these issues in an easy-to-understand and thorough manner.

Dr Thompson has gathered a small group of contributors (in addition to himself) who are undoubtedly at the top of this field, including Drs Carol Adair, Jacqueline Wieneke, Ronald de Krijger, Paul Kommonith, Clara Heffess, Leslie Sobin and Jennifer Hunt. The organization and clarity in writing style make this book exceedingly user-friendly and of practical use for day-to-day sign out. There are innumerable tables that concisely summarize the essentials of the information presented in the text, and the photomicrographs are of uniformly high quality.

This book is organized into thirteen chapters and three appendices, including a review of the TNM classification and consensus reporting of endocrine tumors. There are separate chapters that provide thorough overviews of non-neoplastic, benign and malignant neoplasms of the thyroid gland, parathyroid gland, adrenal gland, pituitary gland and paraganglia system. The appendices are similarly comprehensive and include a review of the anatomy, embryology and histology of the endocrine system, as well as a discussion pertaining to intraoperative consultation and grossing techniques.

I am truly grateful to Dr Thompson and all of the contributors who put forth a tremendous effort to allow this book to come to fruition. It is truly an outstanding addition to the Foundations in Diagnostic Pathology series, and I sincerely hope you enjoy this volume of the series as much as I did.

JOHN R GOLDBLUM, MD

Throughout the centuries, man's fascination with healing the sick or wounded has been at the forefront of scientific endeavours. These decades of study have yielded nearly insurmountable catalogues of information. However, it is the provenance of the modern surgical pathologist to precisely scrutinize this data, parse the meanings of disease, and attempt to clarify all that one 'sees' into a cogent diagnosis which will guide clinical treatment. It is towards this end that the outstanding pathologist must strive.

The pages which follow will, through a highly templated format, allow for the acquisition of a compendium of knowledge as it relates to diseases of the endocrine organs. Selected disorders of the thyroid gland, parathyroid glands, pituitary gland, adrenal glands and paraganglia will be presented in a fashion which allows for quick cross referencing and comparison. As a branch of medicine, pathology is essentially a study of the abnormal function of the body. While pathologists are experts at microscopic interpretation of diseases, they too must apply their 'microscopic' knowledge to guide other clinicians and scientists in their management of the afflicted patient. While the 'clinical' disease may be identical, the causes are separate and unique: granulomatous inflammation caused by fungal infection or metastatic squamous cell carcinoma. Through a keen and discerning eye, the pathologist is able to fuse the clinical, radiographic, laboratory, macroscopic, microscopic, histochemical, immunohistochemical, ultrastructural, and molecular results into a coherent and reasoned whole. This information can then be used to be a 'physician's physician', ultimately leading to the correct patient management.

It is the intense aspiration of this editor that the information found within this primer on pathology will provide the information necessary to achieve this goal.

Lester DR Thompson, MD, FASCP

Acknowledgments

The road to success is paved with how much you contribute rather than how much you achieve. Contribution, however, requires superb material, an agreeable work environment, time for reflection and deliberation, and most importantly, affable colleagues. To that end, I would like to show my appreciation and acknowledge those who have contributed to this milestone. So many people have contributed to my life professionally and privately, that I have selected only a few whose support contributed directly to this work.

- My Parents, Dawn and Ronald Thompson who saw potential in my brother and I, and gave up all they knew and held dear in South Africa to start again in the United States in order to allow us to attend American medical schools.
- My Brother, Dr Glynn M Thompson, for always being ahead of me to guide the way, sometimes laying down his own ambitions so that I could achieve mine.
- Dr Clara S Heffess for having the temerity to tell me 'You are wrong', and yet still to be a close friend and confidant, always saying 'No', and yet doing what was asked immediately.
- Dr Francis H Gannon for providing for my spiritual sanity. His weekly prayer meeting was a constant in a turbulent world. Even though he said 'Just say no', he still supported me when I said 'Yes'.
- Saving the best for last, my wife, Pamela 'Sweet P' Thompson, with whom all things become possible. Her generous spirit, kind heart, ferocious loyalty, unflagging devotion, and tireless love gave me the energy to complete this project. On a practical note, her computer programming expertise that organized the book, templated and structured the chapters, color corrected the images, systematically arranged countless illustrations, scanned transparencies, backed up files, and helped with data management is of incalculable value!

I also acknowledge the superb illustrations of Trisha Haszel. Many gave professional assistance at Elsevier, but I would like to specifically thank Karen Carter (Development Manager), Cheryl Brant (Project Manager), and Belinda Kuhn (Commissioning Editor) for their constant editorial assistance and guidance, and Natasha Andjelkovic for her original support. Thanks to Dr John Goldblum for positing the original request.

Although axiomatic, the responsibility for any errors, omissions or deviation from current orthodoxy is mine alone!

Lester DR Thompson, MD, FASCP

Acknowledgment

Contents

1

Non-neoplastic Lesions of the Thyroid Gland

Carol Adair

THYROGLOSSAL DUCT CYST

Persistence of the tract which represents the migratory path of the thyroid anlage from the foregut (foramen cecum) to its normal position in the midline neck can give rise to fistulous tracts, sinuses or cysts anywhere along the tract. Thyroglossal duct cysts represent the most common midline mass in children, but may also be found in adults and in the elderly.

CLINICAL FEATURES

Thyroglossal duct anomalies are found in about 7% of adults. Approximately two-thirds present as cysts and one-third are fistulas. Fistulas or sinus tracts usually reflect secondary trauma or infection. Occurring equally in the genders, two thirds are diagnosed in children or young adults. Approximately 75% of thyroglossal duct cysts are found in the midline of the neck, at or immediately below the hyoid bone. Other locations include intralingual (2%), suprahyoid or submental (25%), and suprasternal (13%). Slightly off midline may be seen.

Most patients discover an asymptomatic midline mass on their own (Figure 1-1), although sometimes there is pain, a draining sinus or fistula, or dysphagia. The cysts may fluctuate in size, especially if infected. Thyroglossal duct cysts move vertically with swallowing or protrusion of the tongue.

PATHOLOGIC FEATURES

GROSS FINDINGS

The surgical specimen usually consists of the thyroglossal duct cyst, measuring up to 4 cm, as well as the fibrous tract extending to the foramen cecum and

---

THYROGLOSSAL DUCT CYST
DISEASE FACT SHEET

Definition
▸ A persistent tract representing the embryologic migratory path of the thyroid anlage in the anterior neck

Incidence and Location
▸ Approximately 7% of adults
▸ 75% in anterior midline of neck, at or immediately below hyoid bone with intralingual, suprahyoid (submental), suprasternal comprising the remainder

Morbidity and Mortality
▸ May become secondarily infected
▸ Thyroid carcinoma, usually papillary type, develops in 1% of cases; associated with favorable prognosis

Gender, Race and Age Distribution
▸ Equal gender distribution
▸ Most common in children or young adults

Clinical Features
▸ Asymptomatic midline neck mass
▸ Draining sinus or fistula and pain, if infected

Prognosis and Therapy
▸ 4–6% recurrence rate with Sistrunk procedure
▸ Preferred treatment is Sistrunk procedure

THYROGLOSSAL DUCT CYST
PATHOLOGIC FEATURES

Gross Findings
▸ Cyst filled with mucoid or purulent material
▸ Fibrous tract from area of foramen cecum to hyoid bone
▸ One-third present as fistulas, usually due to infection
▸ Solid areas sampled to exclude neoplasm

Microscopic Findings
▸ Cyst lined by respiratory or squamous epithelium
▸ If infected, granulation tissue may replace epithelium
▸ Fibrosis and chronic inflammation in cyst wall
▸ Thyroid tissue identified in up to two-thirds of cases
▸ If carcinoma is present, 90% are papillary type

Fine Needle Aspiration
▸ Thick mucoid or purulent material, sparsely cellular with inflammatory material the rule

Pathologic Differential Diagnosis
▸ Epidermoid cysts, degenerated adenomatoid nodules

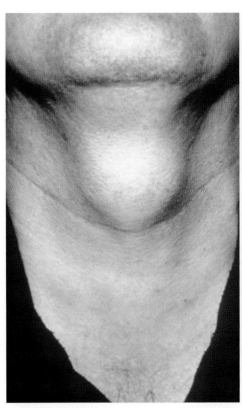
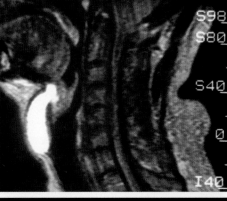
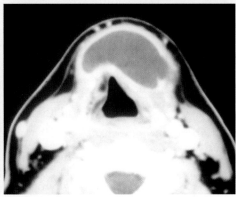

FIGURE 1-1

Left: A mass in the midline, encompassing the hyoid bone, which moves with swallowing. Right upper: A MRI showing a bright signal of the fluid filled thyroglossal duct cyst as it extends from the foramen cecum. Right lower: A CT image showing a large fluid filled cyst anterior to the larynx. Note a slight 'shift' to the left of midline.

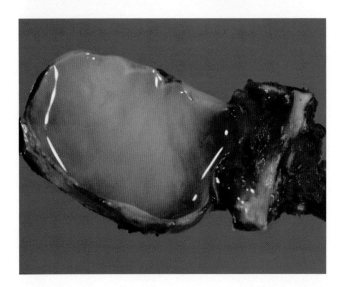

FIGURE 1-2

This thyroglossal duct cyst is from a Sistrunk procedure and includes the cyst, the tract of the thyroglossal duct and the mid-section of the hyoid bone.

the central one to two centimeters of the hyoid bone (Figure 1-2). The cyst may contain clear mucoid fluid or, if infected, purulent material. Solid or firm areas should be carefully sampled to exclude an associated neoplasm.

MICROSCOPIC FINDINGS

The thyroglossal duct cyst is normally lined by respiratory epithelium, but squamous metaplasia is

extremely common (Figures 1-3 and 1-4). If the cyst has been infected, the lining epithelium may be replaced by granulation tissue, sometimes with granulomatous elements such as foamy histiocytes and multinucleated giant cells (Figure 1-4). Fibrosis and chronic inflammation are common in the cyst wall. Thyroid tissue is not invariably present, but is found in up to two-thirds of cases with careful examination.

The associated thyroid tissue may harbor any inflammatory, hyperplastic, or neoplastic alteration that can be seen in the normal follicular epithelial component of the thyroid gland. Up to 1% of thyroglossal duct cysts will have an associated carcinoma, with papillary carcinoma representing about 90% of cases. Thyroglossal duct cysts in elderly patients are much more likely to harbor malignancies. No examples of medullary carcinoma are documented, presumably due to the different embryologic origin of the C-cells of the thyroid from the ultimobranchial body.

ANCILLARY STUDIES

FINE NEEDLE ASPIRATION

Fine needle aspiration is not widely used in the diagnosis of thyroglossal duct cyst because of the limited cytologic findings, but it is useful in documenting other lesions which may form midline neck masses. Aspirates consist of thick mucoid or purulent material and are sparsely cellular; inflammatory cells tend to outnumber the benign squamous or respiratory epithelial cells.

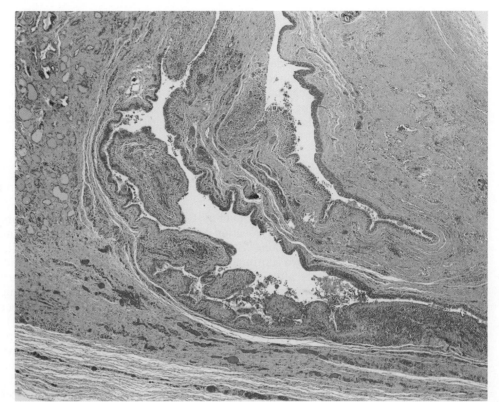

FIGURE 1-3

Thyroglossal duct cyst. The cyst is lined by epithelium and is surrounded by fibrous tissue with chronic inflammation and a small amount of thyroid tissue.

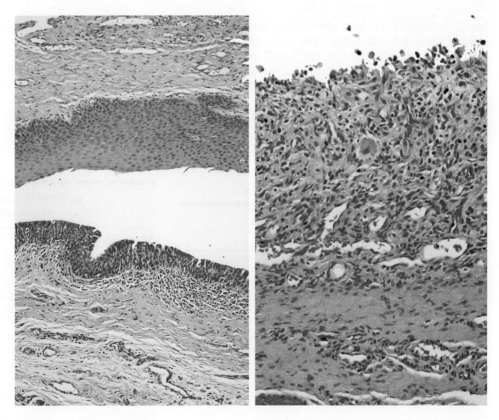

FIGURE 1-4

Left: The cyst lining may be either respiratory type (lower) or squamous epithelium (upper). Right: Infection may cause denudation of the epithelial lining, which is replaced by granulation tissue.

DIFFERENTIAL DIAGNOSIS

Epidermoid cysts of the thyroid or degenerated cystic adenomatoid nodules may be considered in the differential diagnosis; but the midline location and respiratory and/or squamous epithelial lining are key elements in making the diagnosis of thyroglossal duct cyst.

PROGNOSIS AND THERAPY

The preferred treatment for a thyroglossal duct cyst is the Sistrunk procedure, which requires resection of the entire tract of the thyroglossal duct, along with the cyst or fistula and the central one or two centimeters of the hyoid bone. The recurrence rate after this procedure is 4–6%; if the hyoid bone segment is not removed, the recurrence rate increases above 25%. Well-differentiated thyroid carcinoma arising in a thyroglossal duct cyst has an excellent prognosis with the Sistrunk procedure. Total thyroidectomy is not usually required, except in high risk patients.

ULTIMOBRANCHIAL BODY REMNANTS

Small remnants of the ultimobranchial apparatus, known as 'solid cell nests', are associated with the embryologic development of the C-cell population of the thyroid. They are encountered as an incidental finding, usually in the posterior medial and posterior lateral lobes, but never in the isthmus.

CLINICAL FEATURES

Solid cell nests are of no clinical significance, but are fairly common. They are identified in about 25% of thyroid resection specimens; their discovery is largely related to the generosity of sampling of 'normal' thyroid tissue.

PATHOLOGIC FEATURES

Ultimobranchial remnants are quite small, most measuring no more than 0.1 mm. They are represented by a cluster of small epithelial nests or a small lobulated structure, and may be solid or partially cystic (Figure 1-5). The epithelial cells are small and ovoid to polygonal, with slightly elongated nuclei. The chromatin is finely granular and evenly dispersed. A longitudinal nuclear groove is often present (Figure 1-6). The overall histologic pattern is very similar to immature squamous metaplasia, but keratinization and intercellular bridges are not visible. Occasional cells with clear cytoplasm may be scattered through the epithelium; degenerative changes are thought to account for the occasional presence of mucicarmine-positive material in ultimobranchial remnants.

ANCILLARY STUDIES

Although immunohistochemical studies are certainly not necessary for making a diagnosis, occasionally staining with chromogranin, synaptophysin, calcitonin, and carcinoembryonic antigen suggest a developmental relationship with C-cells.

**ULTIMOBRANCHIAL BODY REMNANTS
DISEASE FACT SHEET**

Definition
▸ Small remnant of the ultimobranchial apparatus, associated with development of thyroid C-cells

Incidence and Location
▸ Incidental finding in about 25% of thyroid specimens
▸ Postero-medial and lateral area of lobes; *never* in isthmus

Clinical Features
▸ Patients present with unrelated thyroid nodule(s)

Prognosis and Therapy
▸ No clinical significance

**ULTIMOBRANCHIAL BODY REMNANTS
PATHOLOGIC FEATURES**

Microscopic Findings
▸ Small nests or lobulated aggregates of polygonal epithelial cells, usually about 0.1 mm
▸ Some examples are partially cystic
▸ No keratinization or intercellular bridges
▸ Nuclei ovoid, with evenly distributed chromatin, and frequent longitudinal nuclear groove
▸ Occasional clear cells and mucoid material may be seen

Immunohistochemical Results
▸ May stain with chromogranin, synaptophysin, calcitonin, carcinoembryonic antigen (small size limits study)

Pathologic Differential Diagnosis
▸ Squamous metaplasia, incidental papillary thyroid carcinoma

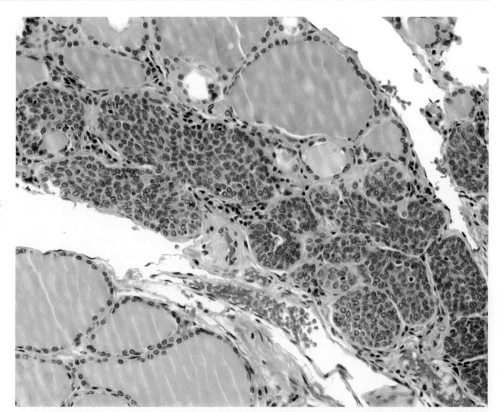

FIGURE 1-5

This ultimobranchial body remnant is a solid cell nest, adjacent to normal thyroid parenchyma, and is an incidental finding.

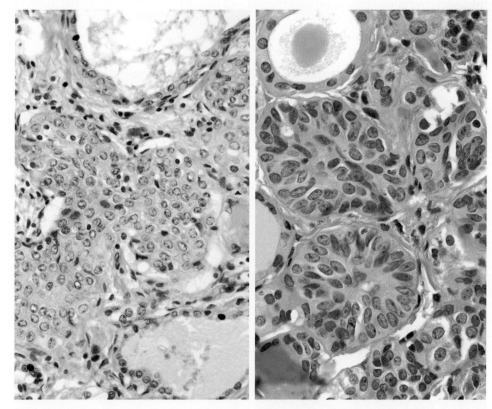

FIGURE 1-6

Left: The ultimobranchial body epithelium is reminiscent of immature squamous metaplasia. Note the lack of keratinization and intercellular bridges. Right: The nuclei are ovoid, often with a longitudinal groove. Note the thyroid follicle at the top as a point of comparison.

DIFFERENTIAL DIAGNOSIS

Ultimobranchial remnants are sometimes mistaken for incidental microscopic papillary carcinomas. Although nuclear grooves are frequent in ultimobranchial remnants, these lesions lack the other nuclear features of papillary carcinoma as well as an adjacent stromal desmoplastic reaction.

While not necessarily within the differential diagnosis, endodermally derived tissues may be encountered in the thyroid gland, including thymic tissue, parathyroid gland (Figure 1-7), and salivary gland tissue. These 'inclusions' are usually of no clinical significance, typically representing incidental findings in surgical resection specimens. Thymic tissue retains its lobulated appearance, has small cystic islands of squamous epithelium (Hassall's corpuscles) with an abundant lymphoid component which may be mistaken for lymphocytic thyroiditis or a lymph node. Parathyroid tissue, particularly if it is hyperplasic or neoplastic, can be difficult to distinguish from a cellular adenomatoid nodule or follicular thyroid neoplasm. Oxyphilic change makes separation a challenge. Parathyroid cells are usually smaller than follicular epithelial cells, and the nuclei are very small, round, and hyperchromatic, with rather coarse chromatin that suggests a neuroendocrine cell type. A cytologic preparation (particularly a 'scrape prep') is especially useful in the differential diagnosis of parathyroid versus thyroid nodules; they are highly recommended in all intraoperative consultations on parathyroid and thyroid lesions.

PROGNOSIS AND THERAPY

No therapy is necessary as this is an incidental finding.

BLACK THYROID

Administration of minocycline and related tetracycline antibiotics is associated with accumulation of brown to black pigment in the thyroid, resulting in dark discoloration of the gland, the so-called 'black thyroid'. The pigment is thought to include lipofuscin and melanin-like compounds. The mechanism of pigment deposition is not completely clear, but possible factors include degradation products of the drug combined to lipofuscin, drug alteration of tyrosine metabolism, or lysosomal dysfunction associated with drug-lipofuscin complexes.

CLINICAL FEATURES

The minocycline-associated changes in the thyroid, while striking in gross appearance, are of no clinical significance to the patient. Usually, the history is unknown at the time of surgery or pathology examination. The patient may relate a history of acne or

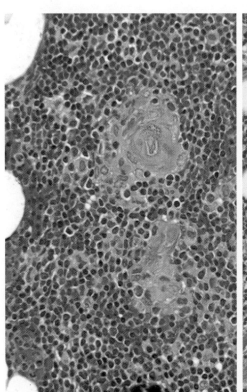
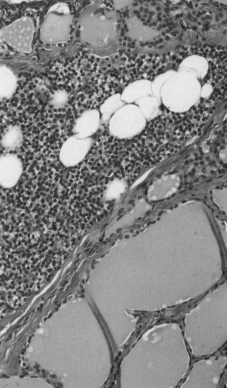

FIGURE 1-7

Thymic (left) and parathyroid tissue (right) can be found within the thyroid gland. These are normal elements without any tissue reaction.

BLACK THYROID
DISEASE FACT SHEET

Definition
▸ Dark discoloration of the thyroid gland due to accumulation of brown-black pigment in follicular cells and colloid, associated with use of minocycline and other tetracycline antibiotics

Incidence and Location
▸ Unknown, dependent on medication utilization

Clinical Features
▸ Incidental finding in nodules removed for another reason
▸ Thyroid function normal unless there is underlying thyroid disease
▸ History of acne or infection treated with minocycline or related tetracycline may be reported

Prognosis and Therapy
▸ Excellent (no clinical significance)

BLACK THYROID
PATHOLOGIC FEATURES

Gross Findings
▸ Gland is black or dark brown
▸ Neoplasms may not take up pigment

Microscopic Findings
▸ Granular, dark brown to black pigment in follicular epithelial cells, and to lesser degree, in colloid
▸ Pigment may or may not be seen in nodular lesions

Ancillary Studies
▸ Pigment stains with Fontana stain, lipofuscin stain, PAS
▸ Prussian blue stain (for iron) is negative
▸ Follicular epithelial cells with have nuclear hyperchromatism and nuclear chromatin clumping; pigment may be mistaken for hemosiderin laden macrophages on FNA material

Pathologic Differential Diagnosis
▸ Hemochromatosis, ochronosis and ceroid storage disease

---

an infection which was treated with minocycline or another tetracycline. Discoloration of the teeth may be noted on examination. Thyroid function is normal, unless there are other underlying reasons for thyroid dysfunction.

PATHOLOGIC FEATURES

GROSS FINDINGS

The thyroid is not enlarged and lacks nodules, unless a nodular goiter or other co-existing abnormality is present. The gland is diffusely dark brown to jet black, suggesting the specimen has been inked.

MICROSCOPIC FINDINGS

Granular dark brown to black pigment is seen in the follicular epithelial cells as well as in the colloid (Figure 1-8). If adenomatoid nodules or thyroid neoplasms are present they may or may not demonstrate the pigment accumulation in the same way as the normal thyroid tissue, although neoplasms tend not to take up the pigment.

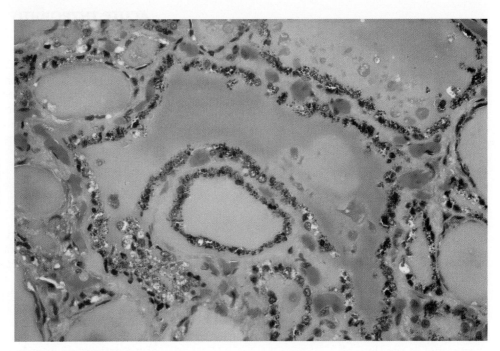

FIGURE 1-8
The follicular epithelial cells contain cytoplasmic granules of brown-black pigment. The pigment is seen to a lesser degree within the colloid.

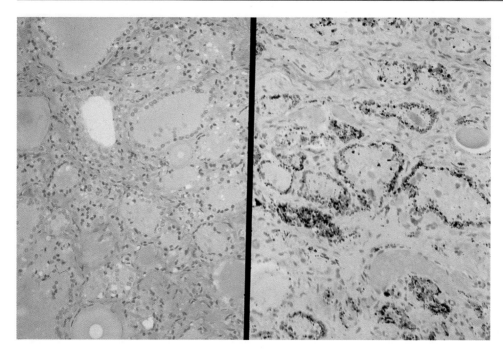

FIGURE 1-9

The Prussian blue stain for iron, left, is negative; the black granules are positive with the Fontana Masson stain, right. (With permission, Wenig BM, Heffess CS, Adair CF. Atlas of Endocrine Pathology, WB Saunders: Philadelphia, 1997.)

ANCILLARY STUDIES

HISTOCHEMICAL STUDIES

Traditional histochemical stains, such as PAS, lipofuscin stains, and the argentaffin stain (Fontana) highlight the pigment. The iron stain (Prussian blue) is negative (Figure 1-9).

FINE NEEDLE ASPIRATION

In aspiration cytology specimens, the degenerative changes in follicular epithelial cells found in black thyroid glands can cause nuclear hyperchromatism and chromatin clumping. Pigment present in follicular epithelial cells in fine-needle aspirates can also be mistaken for hemosiderin-laden macrophages.

DIFFERENTIAL DIAGNOSIS

Rarely a diagnostic dilemma, hemochromatosis is associated with iron accumulation in the parenchyma, yielding a deep brown when severe. The iron stain readily makes the distinction with black thyroid, and, of course, the clinical setting of hemochromatosis is helpful. Ochronosis and ceroid storage diseases are exceptional in the thyroid.

PROGNOSIS AND THERAPY

Black thyroid is a benign incidental finding which requires no specific treatment. It is usually discovered during thyroidectomy for other reasons or during autopsy.

ACUTE THYROIDITIS

Acute inflammation with a neutrophilic inflammatory infiltrate in the thyroid parenchyma is rare; it may be associated with either a localized or systemic infection due to bacterial, fungal or viral agents such as rubella and cytomegalovirus. Predisposing factors include neck trauma or immunosuppression.

CLINICAL FEATURES

Most examples of acute thyroiditis represent secondary involvement due to generalized sepsis or spread from an adjacent head and neck site of infection, such as suppurative pharyngitis. Patients usually are febrile, and complain of chills, malaise, and pain and swelling of the anterior neck. Dysphagia or hoarseness may also be noted. While most patients are euthyroid, occasional patients demonstrate clinical and laboratory evidence of hyperthyroidism or hypothyroidism.

**ACUTE THYROIDITIS
DISEASE FACT SHEET**

Definition

▶ Acute inflammation of the thyroid parenchyma, associated with a local or systemic viral, bacterial, or fungal infection

---

Incidence and Location

▶ Rare
▶ Most cases associated with immunosuppression or trauma

Morbidity and Mortality

▶ Part of generalized sepsis or spread from traumatic entry

Clinical Features

▶ Most cases due to generalized sepsis or extension from an adjacent head and neck site
▶ Fever, chills, malaise, pain, swelling of anterior neck
▶ Dysphagia or hoarseness occasionally
▶ Most patients are euthyroid; occasionally hypo- or hyperthyroid

---

Prognosis and Therapy

▶ Prognosis related to underlying condition
▶ Cultures to determine causative agent
▶ Aggressive antibiotic or anti-fungal therapy with surgery reserved for abscess drainage or injury debridement

---

PATHOLOGIC FEATURES

GROSS FINDINGS

The thyroid is seldom removed for acute thyroiditis; a specimen is usually submitted as part of an incision and drainage of an abscess or debridement following neck trauma. The gland is erythematous and soft, and may contain pockets of purulent exudate or areas of necrosis.

MICROSCOPIC FINDINGS

The key feature is the presence of polymorphonuclear leukocytes infiltrating the thyroid parenchyma. Microabscesses, foci of necrosis (Figure 1-10), and vasculitis may be seen. Identification of a causative organism may be possible with histochemical stains such as tissue gram stains, Gomori's methenamine silver or PAS stains for fungi, or mycobacterial stains. Immunosuppressed patients may develop an acute rather than the typical granulomatous infectious thyroiditis in response

---

**ACUTE THYROIDITIS
PATHOLOGIC FEATURES**

Gross Findings

▶ Thyroid erythematous, soft, with pockets of purulent exudate or necrosis

---

Microscopic Findings

▶ Infiltration of parenchyma by neutrophils
▶ Microabscesses, foci of necrosis, vasculitis common
▶ Organisms may be identified on histology in some cases

Pathologic Differential Diagnosis

▶ Subacute (granulomatous) thyroiditis

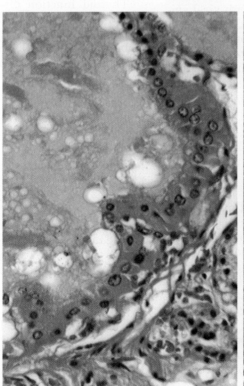
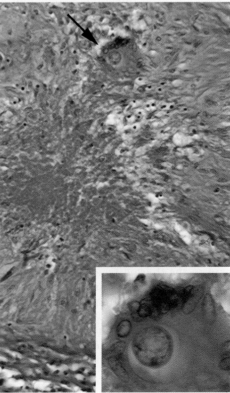

FIGURE 1-10
Left: The thyroid follicular epithelium is oncocytic with organisms identified within the colloid. Right: Coccidiomycosis organisms are identified in a background of necrosis in this case of acute thyroiditis.

to fungal or mycobacterial organisms. Tissue cultures are invaluable in identifying the organism and in determining its sensitivity to antibiotic therapy.

DIFFERENTIAL DIAGNOSIS

Subacute (granulomatous thyroiditis), also has a neutrophilic infiltrate, but it is folliculocentric with accompanying histiocytes, lymphocytes, and multinucleated giant cells. No infectious agent is identified.

PROGNOSIS AND THERAPY

The prognosis is favorable in the absence of underlying predisposing factors such as immunosuppressive states or extensive neck trauma that may carry their own risk of poor outcome. Appropriate treatment requires identification of the infectious agent, preferably by culture, and initiation of effective antibiotic therapy. If abscesses or areas of infarction are present, surgical incision and drainage or debridement may be necessary.

GRANULOMATOUS THYROIDITIS

Also known as de Quervain's disease or subacute thyroiditis, granulomatous thyroiditis is a self-limited inflammatory disorder widely thought to be related to a systemic viral infection. Association with viral epidemics such as mumps, influenza, Coxsackie adenovirus, and measles has been reported. Although seasonal variation has been noted in the past, some recent studies show only a modest increase in cases in the spring and summer. An autoimmune component is also postulated due to the presence of thyroidal autoantibodies in some patients.

CLINICAL FEATURES

The annual incidence in the US is estimated to 5 per 100 000 population. Women are more commonly affected than men, with a female : male ratio of 3.5 : 1. The mean age of onset is in the fifth decade (range, 14 to 87 years). The most common presenting symptom is pain in the thyroid region, sometimes radiating to the jaw. Other complaints include dysphagia, 'sore throat', low-grade fever, arthralgia, myalgia, tremor, excessive sweating, and weight loss.

Physical examination typically reveals pain on palpation of the thyroid. The entire gland is usually involved; however, the changes may be localized to one lobe or to a distinct nodule.

GRANULOMATOUS THYROIDITIS
DISEASE FACT SHEET

Definition
- Self-limited inflammatory disorder thought to be related to systemic viral illness and possible autoimmune factors
- Also called deQuervain's thyroiditis, subacute thyroiditis

Incidence and Location
- About 5/100 000 population/year
- Seasonal increase in spring and summer may occur

Gender, Race and Age Distribution
- Female >> Male (3.5 : 1)
- Peak in fifth decade (range, 14–87 years)

Clinical Features
- Pain in the thyroid region, tender to palpation
- Other complaints include dysphagia, 'sore throat', fever, arthralgia, myalgia, tremor, excessive sweating, weight loss
- Entire gland usually involved, but may be localized
- Thyroid function varies: hyperthyroidism may occur early; hypothyroidism may develop in mid-phase
- Most patients euthyroid after resolution

Prognosis and Therapy
- Usually self-limiting disease which resolves in months, although may recur (years after initial disease)
- 5% remain hypothyroid
- Treatment includes aspirin, non-steroidal anti-inflammatory drugs, steroids, and beta-blocking agents if hyperthyroidism present

---

Thyroid function often varies with disease activity. In the early phase patients may be hyperthyroid due to destruction of follicles and release of thyroglobulin. Serum TSH is suppressed, total and free T4 and T3 are elevated, and radioactive iodine uptake is decreased. With disease progression, thyroid epithelium is destroyed, resulting in hypothyroidism. Most patients regain normal thyroid function after resolution of the disease.

PATHOLOGIC FEATURES

GROSS FINDINGS

The rare resection (surgery is unnecessary) specimen of the thyroid shows asymmetric enlargement, vague nodularity and a somewhat firm consistency.

MICROSCOPIC FINDINGS

The findings are usually seen throughout the gland. The inflammatory infiltrate is distributed in a relatively nodular fashion and includes lymphocytes, plasma cells, foamy histiocytes, epithelioid histiocytes, multinucleated giant cells, and neutrophils (Figure 1-11). A variable

GRANULOMATOUS THYROIDITIS PATHOLOGIC FEATURES

Gross Findings

▶ Rarely removed, but shows asymmetrically enlarged, firm, vaguely nodular gland

Microscopic Findings

▶ Nodular, but whole gland affected
▶ *Early stage:* follicle-centered with groups of follicles disrupted by lymphohistiocytic infiltrate with neutrophils aggregated in follicle lumens
▶ *Late stage:* multinucleated giant cells more prominent and neutrophils absent, with extensive destruction of follicular epithelium, obscuring follicle-centered disease
▶ *Resolution:* follicular regeneration, little fibrosis remains

Fine Needle Aspiration

▶ Aggregates of lymphocytes, histiocytes, plasma cells, multinucleated giant cells
▶ Neutrophils may be prominent in early phase
▶ Giant cells may contain colloid fragments
▶ Colloid and follicular epithelial cells usually scant

Pathologic Differential Diagnosis

▶ Sarcoidosis, mycobacterial or fungal granulomatous infection, palpation thyroiditis

background of fibrosis is also present. In the hyperthyroid phase of the disease, the inflammatory process is centered on the follicle. A group of follicles is surrounded and disrupted by a lymphohistiocytic infiltrate; aggregates of neutrophils within the follicle lumens are very characteristic of this phase (Figure 1-12). Multinucleated giant cells, often containing engulfed colloid, become more prominent in the hypothyroid phase. The inflammatory infiltrate is largely composed of lymphocytes, plasma cells, and histiocytes during this phase (Figure 1-13). Much of the follicular epithelium has been destroyed, making it less obvious that the process was centered on the thyroid follicle. With time, the gland recovers, with regeneration of the follicles and, in most cases, with resolution of the fibrosis and inflammatory infiltrate.

ANCILLARY STUDIES

In most patients the diagnosis of granulomatous thyroiditis can be made on clinical evidence alone. Occasionally fine needle aspiration may be requested, particularly in the minority of patients without thyroid pain. The aspirate contains a mixed inflammatory infiltrate, including lymphocytes, plasma cells, foamy and epithelioid histiocytes, and multinucleated giant cells (Figures 1-14 and 1-15); neutrophils are seen in the early phase of the disease. Follicular cells vary in number with the phase of disease; early phase aspirates

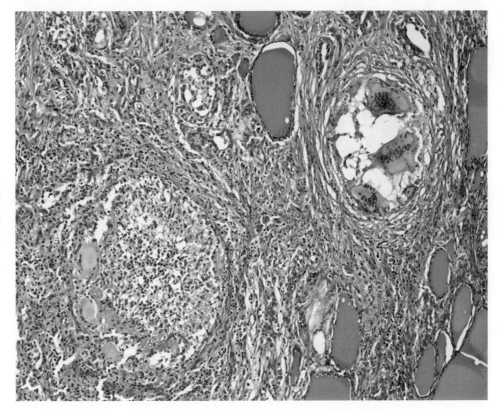

FIGURE 1-11

The thyroid is affected by nodules of a follicle-centered inflammatory infiltrate including lymphocytes, plasma cells, histiocytes, giant cells, and neutrophils. The follicles are destroyed by the process.

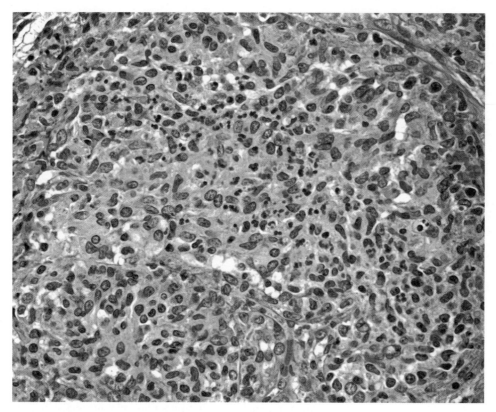

FIGURE 1-12

The destroyed follicle contains an admixture of histiocytes and lymphocytes with neutrophils, characteristic for the early phase of the disease.

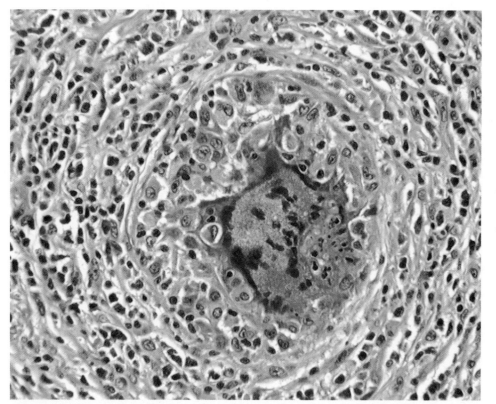

FIGURE 1-13

The follicular epithelium is replaced by a layer of histiocytes with a large giant cell, more prominent in the later phases of the process.

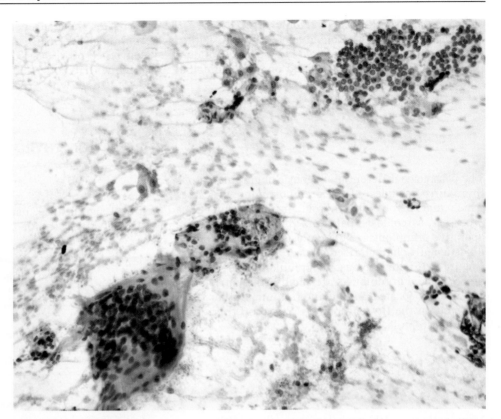

FIGURE 1-14

A fine needle aspiration demonstrates a sheet of benign follicular epithelium with a mixed inflammatory infiltrate which includes lymphocytes, histiocytes, and multinucleated giant cells (alcohol fixed).

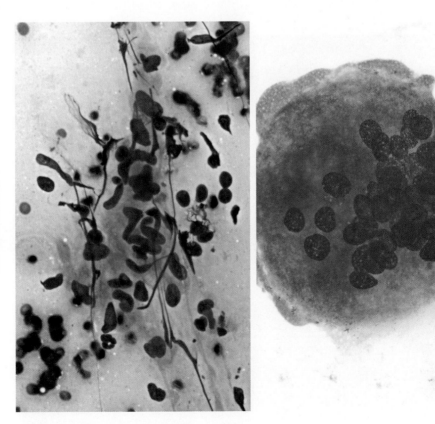

FIGURE 1-15

Left: Aggregates of epithelioid histiocytes suggest the granulomatous nature of this process. Right: A multinucleated giant cell. While typical of this type of granulomatous thyroiditis, giant cells are not specific as they may be seen in adenomatoid nodules, lymphocytic thyroiditis, and papillary thyroid carcinoma (air dried).

often contain small sheets of follicular cells or isolated cells (Figure 1-14). Colloid may be present within small acinar groups or as isolated fragments. Abundant thin colloid, seen in normal gland or in adenomatoid nodules, is not present.

DIFFERENTIAL DIAGNOSIS

The pathologic differential diagnosis of granulomatous thyroiditis includes other granulomatous processes which may involve the thyroid, including infectious processes, sarcoidosis, palpation thyroiditis, and postoperative granulomas. Tuberculosis or fungal thyroiditis is usually characterized by necrotizing granulomas (Figure 1-16), in contrast to granulomatous thyroiditis. Sarcoidal granulomas are small and compact, and are usually located in the interstitium, rather than centered on the thyroid follicles. Palpation thyroiditis lacks neutrophils.

PROGNOSIS AND THERAPY

Most patients with granulomatous thyroiditis experience a self-limiting disease which resolves within several months. Treatment modalities include aspirin, nonsteroidal anti-inflammatory drugs, prednisone (for more severe symptoms), and, if thyrotoxicosis

is present, beta-adrenergic blocking agents such as propranolol. A small number of patients experience recurrence of disease years after the initial episode. Permanent hypothyroidism occurs in approximately 5% of patient with granulomatous thyroiditis.

PALPATION THYROIDITIS

Palpation thyroiditis is an incidental finding of no clinical significance, usually found in thyroid glands removed surgically for other reasons. It is thought to

---

PALPATION THYROIDITIS
DISEASE FACT SHEET

Definition
▶ Microscopic granulomatous foci, follicle centered, seen as an incidental finding in resected thyroid gland thought to result from rupture of follicles due to palpation

Clinical Features
▶ The palpation thyroiditis is of no clinical significance
▶ Patients almost always have a thyroid nodule(s)
▶ Palpation thyroiditis may be very prominent in 'completion thyroidectomy' specimens
▶ Serum thyroglobulin not elevated

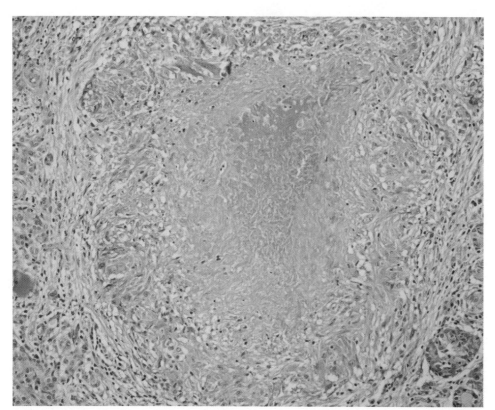

FIGURE 1-16

The patient has disseminated tuberculosis has extensive granulomatous inflammation in the thyroid. The central necrosis distinguished these granulomas from those seen in subacute thyroiditis, palpation thyroiditis, and sarcoidosis.

result from the traumatic rupture of follicles caused by vigorous palpation of the gland preoperatively. Occasionally, martial arts blows to the thyroid may have a similar finding. The lesions are tiny granulomatous foci, centered on thyroid follicles.

CLINICAL FEATURES

Clinical findings in patients who have palpation thyroiditis histologically are not directly related to the palpation thyroiditis. Most patients have a palpable nodule (over 80%), which may represent a thyroid neoplasm, an adenomatoid nodule, or thyroiditis. Thyroid function is normal unless related to the nodule or underlying thyroid disease. Serum thyroglobulin is not elevated.

PATHOLOGIC FEATURES

GROSS FINDINGS

There are no gross findings related directly to the palpation thyroiditis. The thyroid usually contains a nodule which prompted the vigorous palpation and subsequent surgery.

MICROSCOPIC FINDINGS

Lesions of palpation thyroiditis are widely scattered throughout the gland, usually involving only a single follicle, or, at most, a few adjacent follicles (Figure 1-17). The affected follicle contains mononuclear histiocytes with foamy pale cytoplasm, an occasional multinucleated histiocyte, and a few lymphocytes (Figure 1-18). Most of the tiny granulomas are located within follicles, but they may also be found adjacent to a ruptured follicle. There is minimal fibrous response to these lesions. No acute inflammatory cells or necrosis is present.

**PALPATION THYROIDITIS
PATHOLOGIC FEATURES**

Microscopic Findings
▸ Lesions are usually widely scattered throughout the gland and are small
▸ Lesions centered on one or a few adjacent follicles
▸ Follicle contains aggregates of foamy histiocytes, a few lymphocytes, and occasional multinucleated giant cells.
▸ No neutrophils

Pathologic Differential Diagnosis
▸ Subacute thyroiditis, sarcoidosis, infections

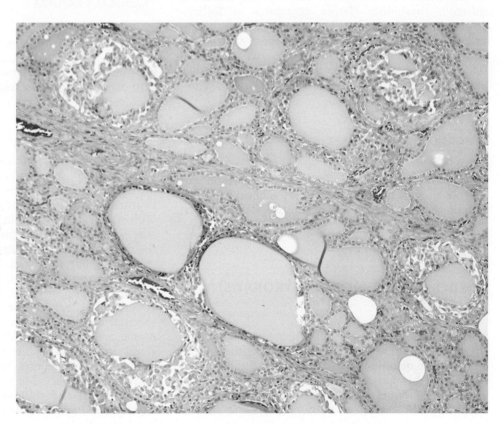

FIGURE 1-17
Scattered foci of palpation thyroiditis are centered on a few follicles in each location.

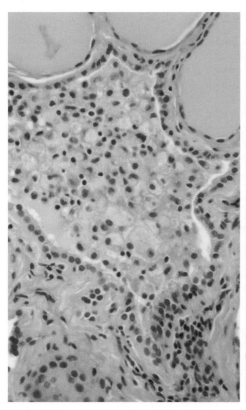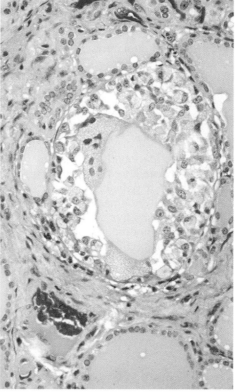

FIGURE 1-18

Left: Early palpation thyroiditis with foamy histiocytes colonizing the follicles. Right: More fully developed lesions have mononuclear histiocytes and lymphocytes, with occasional multinucleated giant cells.

DIFFERENTIAL DIAGNOSIS

The differential diagnosis includes the other causes of granulomatous change in the thyroid, including subacute thyroiditis (larger aggregates of follicle-centered granulomas, with neutrophils and histiocytes), sarcoidosis (tight, small, compact granulomas within the interstitium), and tuberculosis and fungal infections (destructive granulomas with possible necrosis).

PROGNOSIS AND THERAPY

The patient's outcome is not affected by the presence or absence of palpation thyroiditis, but is entirely dependent on the nature of the abnormality which prompted the surgery.

REIDEL DISEASE (REIDEL THYROIDITIS)

Riedel thyroiditis is a rare fibrosing form of chronic thyroiditis without a known etiology, although an autoimmune disorder is postulated. The thyroid gland is replaced by dense fibrous tissue, often extending beyond the thyroid gland to involve the soft tissues of the neck; in some cases a similar process is seen in other sites, such as the retroperitoneum, mediastinum, eyes, hepatobiliary tree, and pancreas.

CLINICAL FEATURES

Riedel thyroiditis is noted in <0.3% of thyroidectomy specimens. The disease is much more common in women (F : M = 5 : 1 ratio). There is a peak in the fifth decade, although a wide range of 23 to 77 years is documented. Nearly one third of patients with Riedel thyroiditis develop another fibrosing disorder within a ten year period. These idiopathic fibrosclerotic diseases include retroperitoneal fibrosis, sclerosing cholangitis, mediastinal fibrosis, orbital pseudotumor, pulmonary fibrosis, subcutaneous fibrosclerosis, fibrous parotitis, diffuse pancreatic fibrosis, Dupuytren's contractures, Peyronie's disease, among others. Patients present with a firm goiter (thyroid enlargement), often associated with pressure symptoms such as discomfort in the anterior neck, dysphagia, dyspnea, or stridor. The infiltrative nature of the disease may cause damage to the recurrent laryngeal nerve (vocal cord paralysis and hoarseness) or to the sympathetic trunk (Horner syndrome). Advanced fibrosis in the neck may produce vascular compromise such as superior vena cava syndrome, or hypoparathyroidism secondary to parathyroid gland destruction. While most patients are euthyroid at the time of diagnosis, up to 40% develop hypothyroidism over a period of ten years. Although variable, thyroglobulin and thyroid peroxidase antibodies are slightly elevated in up to two thirds of patients. The

REIDEL DISEASE
DISEASE FACT SHEET

Definition
▸ Rare fibrosing form of chronic thyroiditis with extensive replacement of thyroid parenchyma by dense fibrosis

Incidence and Location
▸ <0.3% of thyroidectomy specimens
▸ Fibrosing disorder may also affect retroperitoneum, lung, mediastinum, biliary tree, pancreas, kidney, subcutis

Morbidity and Mortality
▸ Vascular compromise, recurrent laryngeal nerve damage, hypoparathyroidism

Gender, Race and Age Distribution
▸ Female >> Male (5:1)
▸ Peak in fifth decade (range, 23–77 years).

Clinical Features
▸ Most present with very firm goiter
▸ Symptoms include dysphagia, hoarseness, stridor, Horner's syndrome, fever, neck pain
▸ Most euthyroid at diagnosis
▸ Mass may be mistaken for malignant neoplasm

Prognosis and Therapy
▸ Benign, self-limited disease
▸ About one-third develop another fibrosing disorder within 10 years
▸ 40% develop hypothyroidism over ten years
▸ Poor outcome is associated with fibrosis in other organs
▸ Corticosteroid and tamoxifen useful in control or reversal of disease
▸ Surgery may be necessary for symptoms of compression

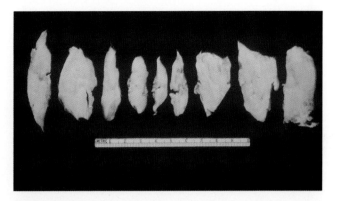

FIGURE 1-19
The thyroid gland in Riedel thyroiditis is pale and woody; the surgical border of the gland is quite ragged following a difficult dissection resulting from extrathyroidal extension of the fibrosing process. (With permission, Wenig BM, Heffess CS, Adair CF. Atlas of Endocrine Pathology, WB Saunders: Philadelphia, 1997.)

REIDEL DISEASE
PATHOLOGIC FEATURES

Gross Findings
▸ Diffuse enlargement of thyroid with adherence to strap muscle and perithyroidal soft tissue
▸ Surgical margins 'ragged' due to difficult dissection
▸ Cut surface white, with a woody texture

Microscopic Findings
▸ Extends into soft tissue without a specific interface
▸ Extensive fibrosis predominates over inflammatory infiltrate
▸ Patchy infiltrate of lymphocytes, plasma cells, monocytes, neutrophils, and occasional eosinophils
▸ Rare, peripheral entrapped thyroid follicles
▸ 'Occlusive phlebitis' with small to medium sized veins infiltrated by inflammatory cells with thickened walls and myxoid change

Fine Needle Aspiration
▸ Paucicellular to acellular aspirates
▸ Scant material with atypical spindle cells is misleading

Pathologic Differential Diagnosis
▸ Undifferentiated thyroid carcinoma, diffuse sclerosing variant of papillary carcinoma, solitary fibrous tumor, fibrous variant of Hashimoto thyroiditis, Hodgkin lymphoma, sarcoma

concurrence of other thyroid autoimmune diseases, as mentioned above, will, of course, affect the laboratory profile.

RADIOLOGIC FEATURES

Ultrasound, computed tomography, and radioactive iodine scanning are not particularly useful in diagnosing Riedel thyroiditis. However, magnetic resonance imaging demonstrates homogeneous hypointensity on both T1 and T2 weighted images, findings distinct from the all other forms of thyroiditis and thyroid neoplasia.

PATHOLOGIC FEATURES

GROSS FINDINGS

The thyroid is usually diffusely abnormal without normal tissue; rarely will only one lobe be affected.

The gland is pale tan to white, with a woody consistency. The surgical margins of the specimen are typically ragged due to extension of the fibrosing process into perithyroidal soft tissue (Figure 1-19). Remnants of strap muscle may be adherent to the gland's surface.

MICROSCOPIC FINDINGS

There is a distinctive fibroinflammatory process extensively involving the gland, extending into the

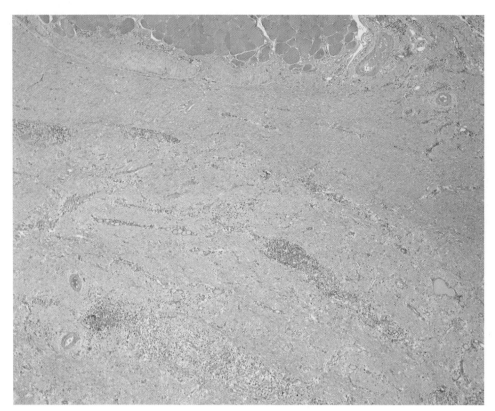

FIGURE 1-20

A low-power view of Riedel thyroiditis demonstrates the dense fibrosis obscuring the architecture of the thyroid and extending into the perithyroidal soft tissue. Note the skeletal muscle at the upper edge.

perithyroidal soft tissue and strap muscles (Figure 1-20). The interface between thyroid gland and soft tissue of the neck is lost. The fibrosis typically predominates over the inflammatory infiltrate, which consists of patchy aggregates of lymphocytes, plasma cells, monocytes, neutrophils, and eosinophils (Figure 1-21). Giant cells, granulomas, and germinal centers are not present. If residual thyroid tissue is present, rare entrapped follicles may be identified in the sclerotic periphery (Figure 1-22). Oxyphilic follicular epithelial metaplasia is absent. A characteristic vascular alteration, 'occlusive phlebitis' (Figure 1-23), is pathognomonic of Riedel thyroiditis. Small and medium-sized veins are infiltrated by a sparse infiltrate of lymphocytes and plasma cells. The vessel walls are thickened, often with myxoid change.

ANCILLARY STUDIES

IMMUNOHISTOCHEMICAL RESULTS

Immunohistochemical studies are not necessary for the diagnosis. However, it is of interest that T-cells predominate in Riedel thyroiditis, in contrast to the fibrous variant of Hashimoto thyroiditis in which B-cells predominate.

FINE NEEDLE ASPIRATION

Fine needle aspiration is typically unsuccessful, with paucicellular to acellular aspirates due to the densely fibrotic gland. The scant material may, in fact, be misleading. Rare atypical spindle cells, sometimes with intranuclear cytoplasmic intrusions, should not be over interpreted as anaplastic carcinoma.

DIFFERENTIAL DIAGNOSIS

Riedel thyroiditis must be separated from undifferentiated carcinoma, solitary fibrous tumor, fibrous variant of Hashimoto's thyroiditis, diffuse sclerosing variant of papillary carcinoma, Hodgkin lymphoma, and sarcoma. The paucicellular variant of undifferentiated thyroid carcinoma includes areas of infarction or necrosis, highly atypical spindle or epithelioid cells with a high mitotic rate, and at least focal positive staining for cytokeratin. Solitary fibrous tumor is circumscribed and lacks the inflammatory infiltrate of thyroiditis. Immunohistochemical studies for CD34, CD99, and bcl-2 are positive. The diffuse sclerosing variant of papillary carcinoma demonstrates numerous psammoma bodies, lymphocytic thyroiditis, and areas of tumor with the diagnostic nuclear features of papillary carcinoma. Hodgkin lymphoma (nodular sclerosis type) should have Reed-Sternberg cells and lacunar cells positive for CD15 and/or CD30 and an appropriate background of inflammatory elements. Sarcomas will have cytologic atypia, necrosis, and mitotic figures.

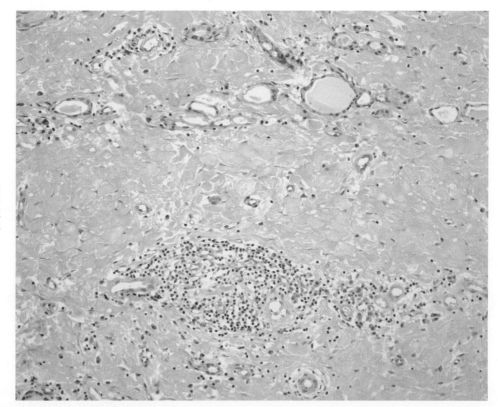

FIGURE 1-21

The lobular pattern of the thyroid has been destroyed by the fibro-inflammatory process in Riedel thyroiditis. Only scattered residual follicles remain in this gland.

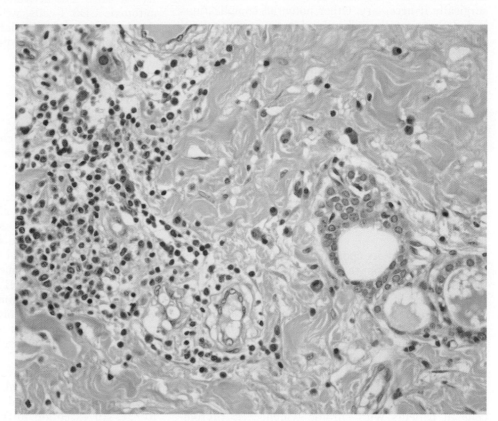

FIGURE 1-22

The inflammatory infiltrate in Riedel thyroiditis includes lymphocytes, plasma cells, and occasional eosino-phils. Note the atrophic appearance of the follicular epithelium.

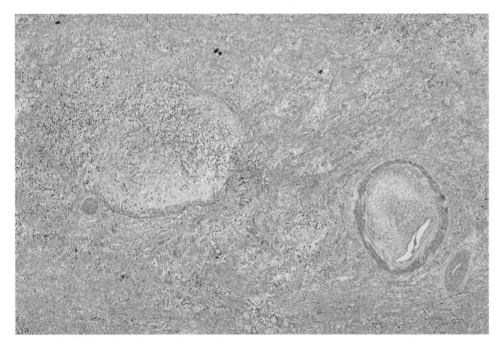

FIGURE 1-23
'Occlusive phlebitis' is characteristic of Riedel thyroiditis. Several small and medium-sized veins demonstrate thickening of the vessel walls with myxoid degeneration and a chronic inflammatory infiltrate.

PROGNOSIS AND THERAPY

Riedel thyroiditis is a benign, and often self-limiting, disease. The chief morbidity is related to hypothyroidism, since the local effects of the goiter can be addressed surgically if necessary. Other potential complications include hypoparathyroidism and nerve injury related either to the disease or to the difficulty of surgery in these patients. In those individuals with multifocal systemic fibrosclerosis, other organ systems may be affected by life threatening disease. Corticosteroid therapy has been successful in the majority of patients in controlling disease progression or in complete or partial reversal of symptoms.

CHRONIC LYMPHOCYTIC THYROIDITIS (HASHIMOTO'S THYROIDITIS)

Widely known by its eponym, Hashimoto thyroiditis, chronic lymphocytic thyroiditis (previously struma lymphomatosa) is an autoimmune chronic inflammatory disorder of the thyroid associated with diffuse enlargement of the gland and several thyroid autoantibodies. A fibrous variant is associated with marked fibrosclerosis and atrophy of the thyroid epithelium. The mechanism of autoimmunity is not clearly understood; however, expression of major histocompatibility complex class II proteins, HLA-DR, HLA-DP, and HLA-DQ, are expressed by the follicular epithelial cells in patients with chronic lymphocytic thyroiditis; these proteins are necessary for presentation of antigen to CD4 T-cells. The activated helper T-cells, in turn, stimulate autoreactive B-cells to be recruited into the thyroid where they secrete autoantibodies. The key target antigens for this autoimmune reaction are thyroglobulin, thyroid peroxidase, and the thyrotropin receptor. Thyrotropin receptor antibodies may contribute to hypothyroidism by blocking the binding capacity for TSH. The activated helper T-cells also recruit cytotoxic CD8 T-cells, which may be responsible for the destruction of follicular epithelial cells, which ultimately leads to hypothyroidism in many patients.

CLINICAL FEATURES

The actual incidence of chronic lymphocytic thyroiditis is difficult to determine as many cases are subclinical. Whereas some degree of lymphocytic thyroiditis is present in autopsy series in 40–45% of women and in 20% of men, high titers of anti-thyroid peroxidase antibodies are found in about 1% of the population (increasing with age) to suggest an approximate incidence. A familial association is seen, while there is also an increased incidence in individuals with Down's syndrome, Turner's syndrome, and familial Alzheimer's disease. HLA-DR3 and HLA-DR5 have been linked to the disease. Other autoimmune diseases may be found in patients with Hashimoto thyroiditis, including pernicious anemia, diabetes mellitus, Addison's disease, Graves' disease, chronic active hepatitis, and Sjögren's syndrome.

Hashimoto thyroiditis can be found over a wide age range, though with a peak in middle age. Women are much more often affected, with a female:male ratio of 5–7:1. An exception to this is the fibrous variant of Hashimoto thyroiditis, which is more common in older males. The risk of the disease seems highest in countries with the highest iodine intake (United States and

Definition
▶ An autoimmune chronic inflammatory disorder of the thyroid associated with diffuse enlargement and thyroid autoantibodies

Incidence and Location
▶ Incidence difficult to determine due to high number of subclinical cases, although about 1% of population has anti-thyroid antibodies
▶ Familial cases well documented

Morbidity and Mortality
▶ Chief morbidity due to hypothyroidism
▶ Increased risk of thyroid lymphoma (up to 80-fold increase)

Gender, Race and Age Distribution
▶ Female >> Male (5–7:1), except for fibrous variant
▶ Highest incidence in US and Japan related to high iodine intake
▶ Peak in middle age (mean, 59 years), but wide age range

Clinical Features
▶ Diffusely enlarged, nontender gland
▶ Enlargement usually gradual
▶ Hypothyroidism common, but rarely hyperthyroidism
▶ Other associated autoimmune disorders

Laboratory Findings
▶ Serum thyroid antibodies are elevated (various types)

Prognosis and Therapy
▶ Increased incidence of thyroid lymphoma
▶ Thyroxin replacement for hypothyroidism and antithyroid drugs for Hashitoxicosis
▶ Surgery if symptomatic or for suspicious nodules

Japan). Furthermore, amiodarone and lithium are associated with an increased risk of both hypothyroidism and development of thyroid autoantibodies.

Patients with lymphocytic thyroiditis have a gradual, diffuse enlargement of a firm, nontender thyroid gland, usually two to three times the normal weight. Occasionally patients with the fibrous variant of Hashimoto thyroiditis have rapid enlargement of the gland; however, this finding should raise the suspicion of thyroid lymphoma in a patient with a history of autoimmune thyroiditis.

Hypothyroidism is common, but not invariably present at the time of presentation. Rare patients present with hyperthyroidism, known as Hashitoxicosis. Laboratory evidence of Graves' disease may or may not be present; the histologic features in such cases are identical to other cases of chronic lymphocytic thyroiditis.

Laboratory assessment requires testing for serum thyroid antibodies (antithyroglobulin, antithyroid microsomal antibodies, anti-thyroid peroxidase antibodies), although antithyroglobulin is less commonly elevated and is least useful. In population studies 50–75% of

subjects with positive thyroid antibodies are euthyroid; 25–50% have subclinical hypothyroidism; and 5–10% have overt hypothyroidism. Thyrotropin assay is routine in suspected Hashimoto thyroiditis, in order to assess for hypothyroidism. Severe hypothyroidism is commonly associated with the fibrous variant of the disease.

Juvenile Hashimoto thyroiditis, usually seen in adolescents and young adults, may present with hypothyroidism or hyperthyroidism; the patients often have a strong family history of thyroid disease. Some patients also have hypoadrenalism (Schmidt's syndrome), hypoparathyroidism, diabetes mellitus, or hypogonadism.

RADIOLOGIC FEATURES

Radiologic imaging is not necessary in the diagnosis of autoimmune thyroiditis, and may, in fact, be misleading. Radioactive iodine uptake is usually normal or increased in Hashimoto thyroiditis, suggesting Graves' disease, even in patients with hypothyroidism.

PATHOLOGIC FEATURES

GROSS FINDINGS

Thyroidectomy is often performed because of a thyroid nodule (Figure 1-24). The gland is diffusely

Gross Findings
▶ Diffusely enlarged gland, may be lobulated or nodular
▶ Pale white cut surface resembles lymphoid tissue
▶ Nodules or fibrous bands common in long-standing disease

Microscopic Findings
▶ Diffuse, dense lymphoplasmacytic infiltrate, often with well-developed germinal centers
▶ Follicular atrophy with decrease in colloid
▶ Oxyphilic, or 'Hürthle' cell metaplasia (follicular cells with intensely granular eosinophilic cytoplasm)
▶ Squamous metaplasia is common
▶ Fibrous variant shows dense lymphoid infiltrate, extensive fibrosis and minimal residual follicular epithelium

Fine Needle Aspiration
▶ Mixed, polymorphic lymphoplasmacytic infiltrate
▶ Occasional multinucleated giant cells and histiocytes
▶ Oxyphilic epithelial cells in small clusters and sheets
▶ Scant colloid in most cases

Pathologic Differential Diagnosis
▶ Papillary thyroid carcinoma, extranodal marginal zone B-cell lymphoma, Riedel thyroiditis, non-specific lymphocytic thyroiditis

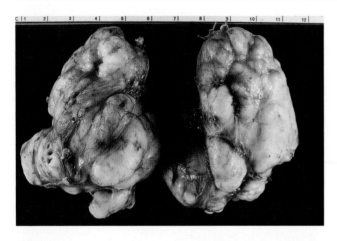

FIGURE 1-24

The thyroid is enlarged, with a lobulated appearance in lymphocytic thyroiditis. The pale white tan color reflects the dense lymphoid infiltrate.

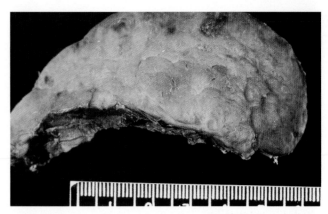

FIGURE 1-26

The extensive fibrosis seen in the fibrous variant of Hashimoto thyroiditis results in a firm nodular gland with a pattern reminiscent of hepatic cirrhosis. (With permission, Wenig BM, Heffess CS, Adair CF. Atlas of Endocrine Pathology, WB Saunders: Philadelphia, 1997.)

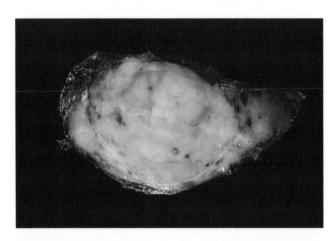

FIGURE 1-25

The cut surface of lymphocytic thyroiditis bears a striking resemblance to lymph nodal tissue.

enlarged and pale gray to white, with a consistency of lymphoid tissue (Figure 1-25). If the disease is long-standing it may contain distinct nodules and bands of fibrous tissue. The fibrous variant is very firm and fibrotic, with a multinodular cut surface resembling cirrhosis of the liver (Figure 1-26).

MICROSCOPIC FINDINGS

The histologic features of classic Hashimoto thyroiditis include diffuse and rather dense infiltration of the gland, predominantly by small lymphocytes, but often with germinal centers as well; plasma cells, histiocytes, and, sometimes, giant cells may be present. At low power the lobular pattern of the thyroid is preserved (Figure 1-27). The lymphocytic infiltrate is usually confined to the thyroid, but rarely extends into the adjacent soft

tissue. The appearance of the follicular epithelium may vary from area to area, with some follicles remaining intact. The hallmark of Hashimoto thyroid, however, is follicular atrophy accompanied by oxyphilic metaplasia of the follicular epithelial cells (Figures 1-28 and 1-29). The follicles may be small, with scant colloid, or they may be destroyed, leaving small islands of oxyphilic epithelium surrounded by an intense lymphoid infiltrate or areas of fibrosis (Figure 1-30). The oxyphilic ('Hürthle') cells are strikingly different from normal follicular epithelial cells. The nuclei are enlarged, often with irregular nuclear contours, vesicular chromatin and grooving which may be confused with that of papillary carcinoma (Figure 1-31). Prominent eosinophilic nucleoli are frequently observed. The cytoplasm of the oxyphilic cells is abundant, eosinophilic, and very granular. Squamous metaplasia is common in the atrophic follicular epithelium (Figure 1-32), particularly in more advanced cases and in the fibrous variant. Squamous or respiratory epithelial-lined cysts are occasionally present, and, if unusually large, may suggest a branchial cleft anomaly ('lymphoepithelial cysts').

The fibrous variant of Hashimoto thyroiditis, also known as 'advanced lymphocytic thyroiditis', represents approximately 10% of cases. A lobular pattern is still evident from the distribution of the lymphoid infiltrate around the severely atrophic follicles. Fibrosis dominates the histologic picture; it has a dense keloidal appearance (Figures 1-33 and 1-34). The atrophic variant ('fibrous atrophy') has more extreme follicular atrophy with small glands (often less than 5 g), most likely the end stage of the disease process. Long-standing Hashimoto thyroiditis tends to become nodular. The nodules have a pushing border, as seen in adenomatoid nodules; however, they are frequently quite cellular.

The juvenile form has the lymphocytic infiltrate, but tends to have minimal follicular atrophy and oxyphilic metaplasia.

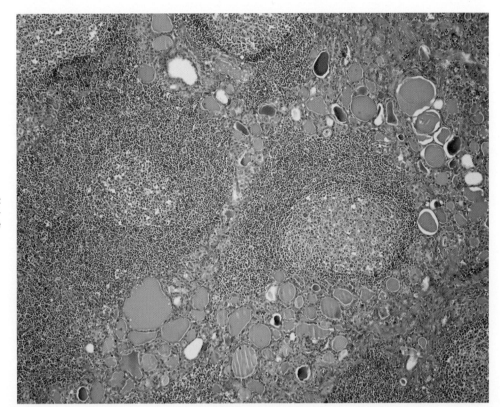

FIGURE 1-27

There is a dense, diffuse chronic inflammatory infiltrate with germinal centers. Note the atrophy of the thyroid follicles.

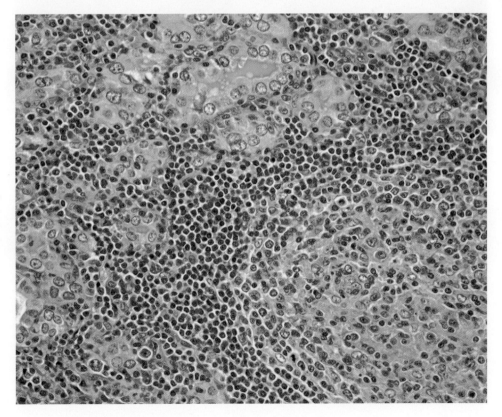

FIGURE 1-28

The key histologic features include a dense lymphocytic infiltration of the gland, atrophy of the follicular epithelial component, and oxyphilic change in the follicular epithelial cells.

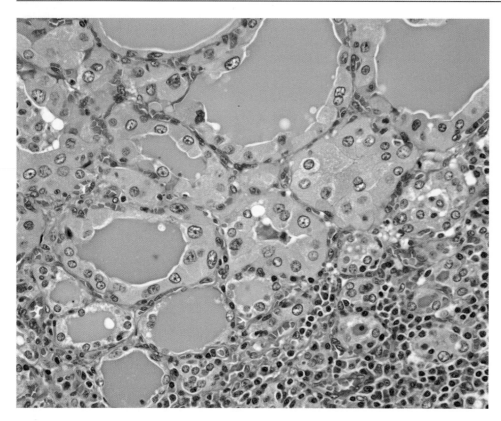

FIGURE 1-29

The cytologic features of fully developed oxyphilia include abundant granular eosinophilic cytoplasm, nuclear enlargement, prominent eosinophilic nucleoli, and irregularities of chromatin distribution and nuclear contour.

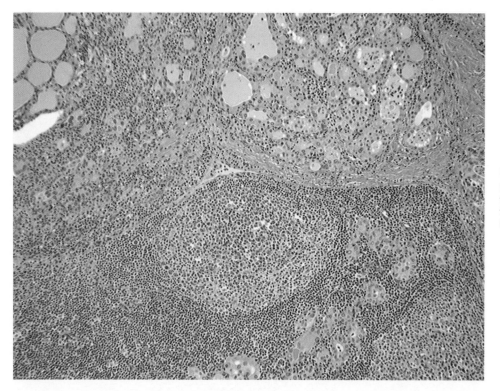

FIGURE 1-30

Bands of fibrosis separate the thyroid into small nodules. Note the isolated oncocytic cells in the lymphoid stroma.

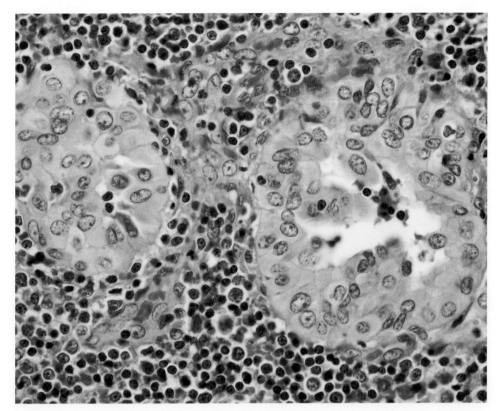

FIGURE 1-31
Oxyphilic cells may have rather striking nuclear atypia, with features which overlap with papillary thyroid carcinoma.

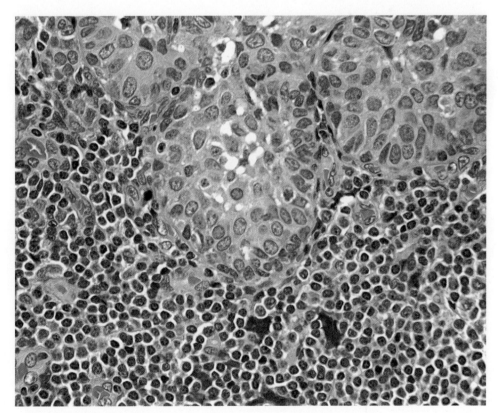

FIGURE 1-32
Squamous metaplasia of the epithelium in association with lymphocytic thyroiditis.

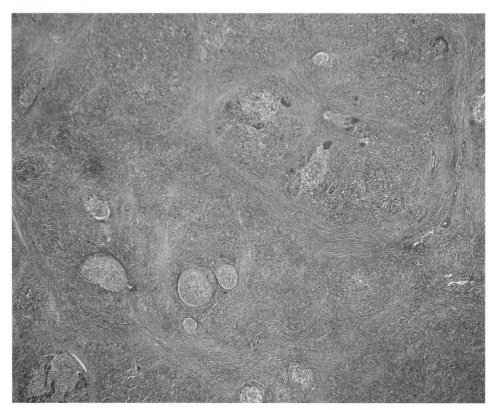

FIGURE 1-33

Extreme follicular atrophy and dense bands of fibrosis are clearly seen at low power. Note that the lobular pattern of the thyroid is still suggested by the distribution of the inflammation and residual follicular epithelium.

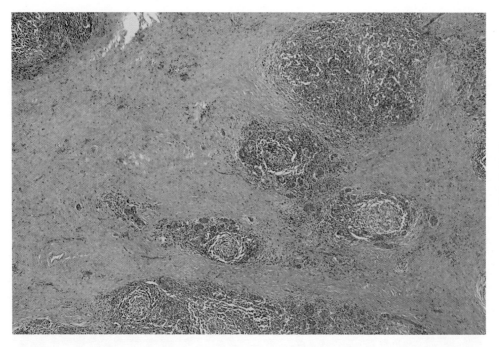

FIGURE 1-34

Little remains of the thyroid parenchyma, small islands of epithelium are found among the patches of chronic inflammation.

ANCILLARY STUDIES

IMMUNOHISTOCHEMICAL RESULTS

Immunohistochemical studies are rarely necessary for making the diagnosis of Hashimoto thyroiditis; however, if extranodal lymphoma is a diagnostic concern, particularly in the patient with rapid enlargement of the thyroid, they may be helpful in excluding malignancy. If lymphoma is suspected, it is prudent to reserve fresh tissue for flow cytometric immunophenotyping.

The infiltrate in Hashimoto thyroiditis demonstrates a mixed B and T-cell population, which includes CD20, CD3, CD4, and CD8 positive cells. The plasma cells in the background are polyclonal for immunoglobulin heavy and light chains.

FINE NEEDLE ASPIRATION

The cellular features of Hashimoto thyroiditis include a mixed, polymorphic lymphoplasmacytic infiltrate, with a spectrum lymphoid cells from small round lymphocytes to the activated cells found in germinal centers (Figure 1-35). Histiocytes and the occasional multinucleated giant cell may be seen. Colloid is usually sparse in well-developed Hashimoto thyroiditis. The follicular epithelium is usually scant, found in small flat sheets or as single cells. The cytoplasm is very granular and oxyphilic (Figure 1-36). The nuclei of the epithelial cells may be enlarged, have vesicular or 'pale' chromatin, and irregular nuclear contours. Oxyphilic cells are probably the most significant pitfall in thyroid aspiration cytology, but a sheet-like architecture, lack of syncytial cell groups, the intense oxyphilia of the follicular cell cytoplasm, and the background lymphoid cells should be helpful in distinguishing thyroiditis from papillary carcinoma. Cellular adenomatoid nodules may be indistinguishable from an oxyphilic follicular neoplasm by cytology alone; examination of the periphery of the nodule histologically is necessary to make that distinction.

DIFFERENTIAL DIAGNOSIS

Extranodal marginal zone B-cell lymphoma ('MALT' lymphoma), papillary carcinoma, Riedel thyroiditis, and non-specific inflammation are differential considerations. There is an increased risk of MALT lymphoma in lymphocytic thyroiditis patients (up to 80-fold). Rapid enlargement of the gland, a diffuse, sheet-like effacement of the thyroid parenchyma, lymphoepithelial lesions, and supporting immunohistochemistry and/or flow cytometry will help to make the diagnosis of lymphoma. Nuclear irregularities can be pronounced in the follicular epithelial cells near lymphocytic thyroiditis. However, the oxyphilic change in multiple foci and a lack of architectural features and an infiltrative pattern should make the separate possible. Riedel thyroiditis has a diffuse pattern of effacement by fibrosis and has vasculitis. Lymphocytic thyroiditis, which is typically patchy in its distribution within the gland, and which lacks the clinical and laboratory features of an autoimmune thyroid disorder. It is frequently encountered as an incidental finding in thyroids resected for other reasons.

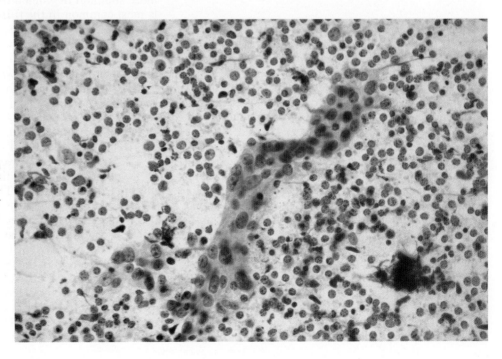

FIGURE 1-35

A fine needle aspiration yields a dense infiltrate with a polymorphous lymphoplasmacytic population with oncocytic follicular epithelium (Papanicolaou stained).

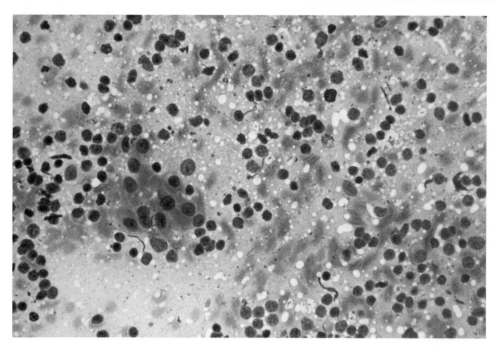

FIGURE 1-36
The oxyphilic follicular cells may be scant in number. They are usually seen as small sheets of polygonal cells with abundant granular, blue cytoplasm (Diff-Quick preparation).

PROGNOSIS AND THERAPY

Treatment depends on the clinical manifestations in a given patient. Those with hypothyroidism require thyroxin replacement, usually lifelong, while those presenting with hyperthyroidism are treated accordingly. Surgery may be recommended if the thyroid enlargement is symptomatic or if suspicious nodules develop. The increased incidence of lymphoma, usually an extranodal marginal zone B-cell lymphoma although transformation to a diffuse large B-cell lymphoma occurs, suggests lifelong monitoring to exclude this development.

DIFFUSE HYPERPLASIA (GRAVES' DISEASE)

Widely known by its eponym, Graves' disease is an autoimmune condition of the thyroid which results in diffuse hyperplasia with excess thyroid hormone production unchecked by the normal feedback loop between the pituitary gland and the thyroid. The immune abnormality is mediated by antibodies to the thyrotropin receptor found on follicular epithelial cells. The most specific antibody, known as thyroid-stimulating immunoglobulin (TSI), when bound to the thyrotropin receptor, mimics the action of pituitary thyrotropin, stimulating the follicular epithelium to produce hormone. Other antibodies are often present in Graves' disease, including thyroid growth-stimulating immunoglobulin, which is associated with thyrocyte proliferation, and TSH-binding antibodies, which may either inhibit or stimulate TSH activity. The clinical effect of this autoimmune process is thyrotoxicosis, accompanied by diffuse thyroid enlargement and an infiltrative ophthalmopathy, and a spectrum of systemic effects of thyroid hormone excess.

CLINICAL FEATURES

Graves' disease is the most common cause of spontaneous hyperthyroidism, representing up to 80% of all cases. The incidence is approximately 0.5–1% of the population, with a slightly higher incidence in areas of particularly high iodine intake. It is five to ten times more common in women than in men. Graves' disease is most common in the third and fourth decades. Men, however, tend to develop Graves' disease at an older age, often with a more severe form of thyrotoxicosis.

Genetic factors play a role, with familial clustering common. However, while susceptibility has been associated with polymorphisms within the HLA region (particularly DR3) and in the CTLA-4 gene (cytotoxic T-lymphocyte-associated gene), environmental factors (infections, stress, gonadal steroid hormones) are also involved in the etiology of this disease.

The symptoms of Graves' disease reflect the effect of thyrotoxicosis and of the autoimmune process on multiple organ systems. The spectrum of complaints includes weight loss, heat intolerance, fatigue, weakness, palpitations, dyspnea on exertion, stridor due to tracheal compression, hoarseness, chest pain, dysphagia, oligomenorrhea, hair loss or change in hair texture, a 'gritty' sensation in the eyes, proptosis, conjunctivitis, memory loss, poor attention span, emotional lability, muscle weakness, and irritability or agitation. Physical findings include localized myxedema (particularly pretibial, and most often in females), hair loss, a wide-eyed stare or proptotic appearance (Figure 1-37), irrita-

DIFFUSE HYPERPLASIA (GRAVE'S DISEASE)
DISEASE FACT SHEET

Definition

▸ An autoimmune process which results in clinical hyperthyroidism and histologic diffuse hyperplasia of the follicular epithelium

Incidence and Location

▸ Incidence 0.5–1% worldwide
▸ Somewhat higher incidence in areas with highest iodine intake
▸ Responsible for 80% of cases of hyperthyroidism

Morbidity and Mortality

▸ Thyroid storm with hypertension and cardiac disease

Gender, Race and Age Distribution

▸ Female >> Male (5–10 : 1)
▸ Peak in third and fourth decades

Clinical Features

▸ Greatest risk factor is positive family history (with susceptibility associated with polymorphisms in HLA DR3 and CTLA-4 gene)
▸ Thyrotoxicosis has affect on multiple organ systems
▸ Common symptoms include weight loss, heat intolerance, fatigue, weakness, palpitations, dyspnea on exertion, stridor due to compression, hoarseness, chest pain, tremor, oligomenorrhea, amenorrhea, hair loss, change in hair texture, conjunctival irritation, proptosis, poor attention span, emotional lability, agitation
▸ Physical findings including localized myxedema (especially pretibial), hair loss, wide-eyed stare or proptosis, keratoconjunctivitis, lid lag, diplopia, tachycardia, hyperactive reflexes
▸ Thyroid usually diffusely enlarged although sometimes nodular
▸ 'Apathetic hyperthyroidism' in elderly shows atrial fibrillation, weight loss, worsening cardiac disease, tremor

Laboratory Findings

▸ T3 and T4 elevated
▸ TSH markedly suppressed
▸ Thyroid antibodies (especially thyroid stimulating immunoglobulin) present
▸ RAIU increased

Prognosis and Therapy

▸ Overall prognosis is excellent, although thyroid storm is a life-threatening exacerbation requiring rapid antithyroid drug therapy
▸ When thyroid carcinomas are present, they may behave more aggressively due to thyroid stimulating antibodies
▸ Drug failure (up to 40%) requires surgery or radiation
▸ Permanent hypothyroidism can be a complication
▸ Therapy includes antithyroid drugs, radioactive iodine and surgery

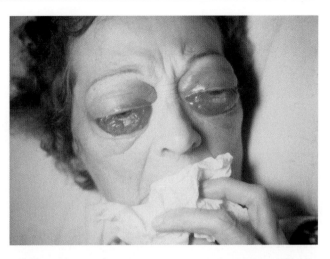

FIGURE 1-37
One of the most striking features of diffuse hyperplasia is a proptotic wide-eyed stare, keratoconjunctivitis, and limited movement of the extraocular muscles. In this very advanced case the enlarged extraocular muscles are visible. (With permission, Wenig BM, Heffess CS, Adair CF. Atlas of Endocrine Pathology, WB Saunders: Philadelphia, 1997.)

acterized by development of nodules. Elderly patients may show few of the classic signs and symptoms mentioned above ('apathetic hyperthyroidism'). The diagnosis should be considered in patients with new onset atrial fibrillation, unexplained weight loss, worsening cardiovascular disease, and new onset of tremor. A life-threatening exacerbation of thyrotoxicosis, 'thyroid storm', is usually precipitated by surgery, infection, or trauma, and is characterized by central nervous system agitation or depression and high fever.

Laboratory evaluation of the patient with Graves' disease is essential. The serum thyroid hormone level, represented by free T4 or T3, is elevated; only about 5% of cases are caused by T3 thyrotoxicosis. Serum TSH is markedly suppressed. Anti-thyroidal antibodies are detected.

RADIOLOGIC FEATURES

Radioactive iodine scans demonstrate a diffuse increase in uptake within the thyroid; however, this is not a specific finding and is not necessary for establishing the diagnosis of Graves' disease.

PATHOLOGIC FEATURES

GROSS FINDINGS

The thyroid gland is diffusely and symmetrically enlarged and beefy red (Figure 1-38). The cut surface gives an impression of hypervascularity. Average weights range from 50–150 g. If the patient has been treated or

tive keratoconjunctivitis, lid lag, diplopia, tachycardia, smooth, warm and velvety skin, and hyperactive reflexes. The thyroid is diffusely enlarged; a bruit may be appreciated over the thyroid area. Nodules may be present in the thyroid, suggesting the possibility of Plummer's disease (toxic multinodular goiter or a toxic adenoma). Long-standing or treated Graves' disease is often char-

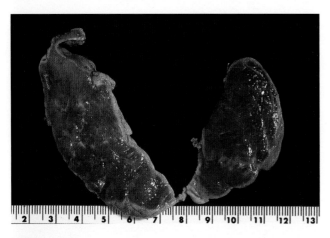

FIGURE 1-38

This thyroidectomy specimen from a child with hyperthyroidism is enlarged and hyperemic, with a 'beefy red appearance'. (With permission, Wenig BM, Heffess CS, Adair CF. Atlas of Endocrine Pathology, WB Saunders: Philadelphia, 1997.)

DIFFUSE HYPERPLASIA (GRAVE'S DISEASE) PATHOLOGIC FEATURES

Gross Findings

▶ Diffuse thyroid enlargement with beefy red gland
▶ Average weights range from 50–150 g
▶ Treatment may result in nodules and prominent fibrosis

Microscopic Findings

▶ Highly cellular gland with little colloid
▶ Hyperplastic, redundant follicular epithelium with papillary infoldings; follicle lumens stellate
▶ Follicular cells columnar, with eosinophilic granular cytoplasm
▶ Follicular cell nuclei round and only slightly enlarged and are basally oriented
▶ If colloid present, scalloping is seen (small vacuoles along apical border of epithelial cells)
▶ Accentuation of lobular pattern of gland, with increased fibrosis in interlobular septae
▶ Patchy lymphocytic infiltrate
▶ After treatment follicles regain colloid; mild hyperplastic changes persist
▶ Following radioactive iodine gland may become nodular, with increased fibrosis and atypia of follicular epithelial cells

Fine Needle Aspiration

▶ Highly cellular smears
▶ Minimal or no colloid
▶ Sheets of follicular epithelial cells
▶ Follicular cells have abundant granular cytoplasm ('flame cells'), nuclei with compact chromatin

Pathologic Differential Diagnosis

▶ Papillary carcinoma, toxic nodular goiter (Plummer's disease), Hashimoto thyroiditis

---

if the Graves' disease is long standing or 'burnt-out', the gland may contain multiple nodules or patches of fibrosis.

MICROSCOPIC FINDINGS

The low-power appearance of the gland is remarkable for accentuation of the normal lobular pattern of the thyroid. This is due to increased fibrous tissue in the interlobular septae (Figure 1-39). A patchy lymphocytic infiltrate is present in the perifollicular stroma; the density varies from case to case: it is sparse in some patients, but conspicuous, with germinal centers, in others, related to the autoimmune nature of the underlying process.

An important microscopic feature of Graves' disease is the diffuse nature of the pathologic findings: *the entire gland is affected*. The thyroid follicles are lined by columnar epithelial cells with basally located round nuclei with relatively dense chromatin; the cytoplasm is granular and eosinophilic. The hyperplastic follicular epithelium forms infoldings into the lumen of the follicle, producing a stellate outline (Figure 1-40). These infoldings may resemble papillae, and must not be mistaken for evidence of papillary carcinoma (Figure 1-41). Vacuoles are noted along the apical aspect of the follicular cells, giving the colloid a 'scalloped' appearance.

In cases of *treated* Graves' disease the histologic appearance depends on the type and duration of treatment. Potassium iodide causes involution, with follicular cells reverting to their normal cuboidal or flattened appearance, alternating with areas retaining some of the features of hyperplasia (Figure 1-42). Radioactive iodine therapy may produce a nodular gland, with nodules which are often quite cellular and may exhibit striking nuclear atypia (Figure 1-43). The periphery of such nodules should be scrutinized for evidence of capsular or vascular invasion that would identify them as follicular carcinomas. Fibrosis and areas of follicular atrophy are frequently present (Figure 1-44).

ANCILLARY STUDIES

IMMUNOHISTOCHEMICAL RESULTS

Immunohistochemical studies are not required for the diagnosis of Graves' disease, but HLA-DR positivity is typically demonstrable in the follicular epithelial cells as well as in the lymphoid cells.

FINE NEEDLE ASPIRATION

Cytologic examination of diffuse hyperplasia (Graves' disease) is treacherous, and seldom attempted in patients with active clinical disease. However, FNA may be requested in two settings:

• A patient with a nodule, in order to exclude malignancy; and

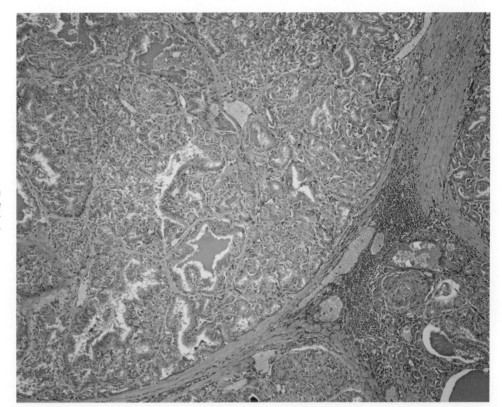

FIGURE 1-39

The gland is intensely cellular, with little colloid. Note the prominence of the somewhat fibrotic interlobular septae, which are usually unapparent in a normal thyroid gland.

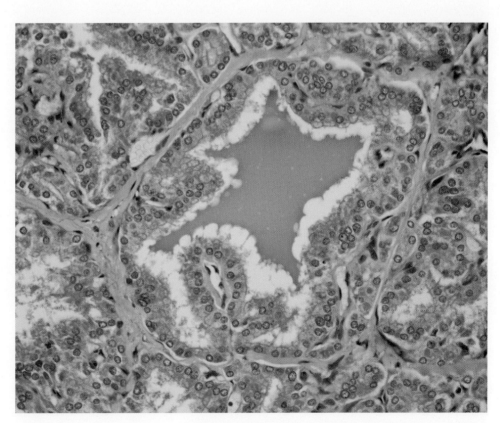

FIGURE 1-40

The hyperplastic epithelium is redundant, giving the follicle lumen a stellate outline.

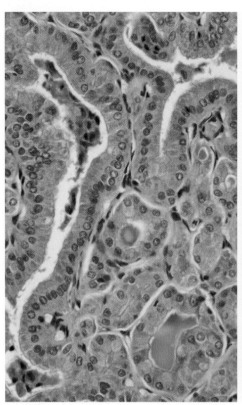 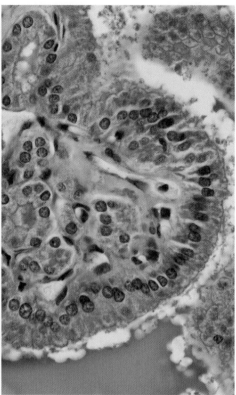

FIGURE 1-41
Papillary structures are present in some of the hyperplastic follicles, with nuclei which are hyperchromatic and basally located.

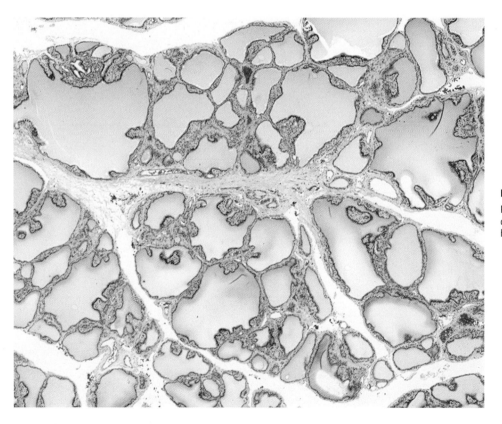

FIGURE 1-42
Partial involution with increased colloid, but still showing focal hyperplastic changes.

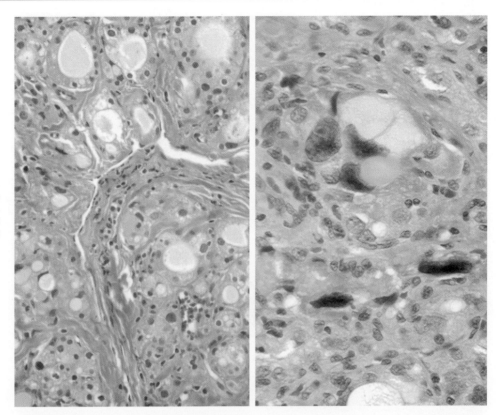

FIGURE 1-43

Left: The gland still demonstrates some degree of hyperplastic change, though reaccumulation of colloid is apparent. Right: Nuclear atypia is prominent in this example.

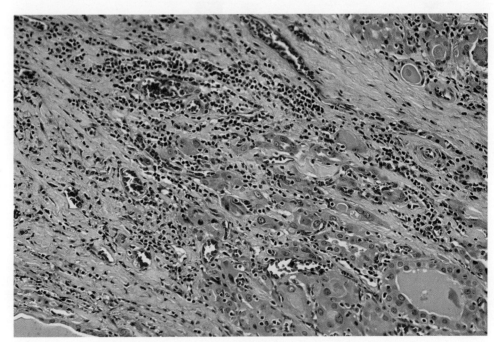

FIGURE 1-44

Extensive fibrosis with follicular atrophy may be observed between nodular areas in some patients.

- A patient with treated Graves' disease who has developed a nodule, or nodules, months to years after treatment.

In the patient with active disease the aspirate is typically extremely cellular, consisting of columnar cells with round nuclei with dense chromatin. The cyto-plasm is usually intensely granular ('flame cells'), suggesting oxyphilia on both Romanovsky and Papanicolaou stained-smears (Figures 1-45 and 1-46). If the clinical information regarding Graves' disease is not provided, a follicular neoplasm is almost invariably favored. Because of the degree of cellularity inherent

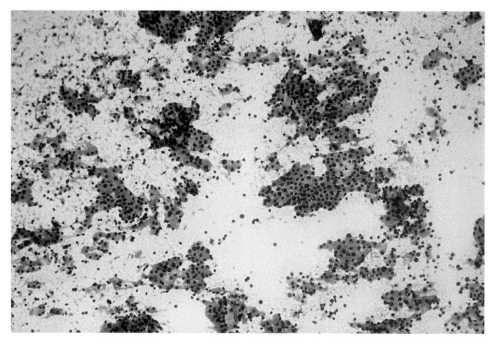

FIGURE 1-45
Fine needle aspiration yields a very cellular sample, with minimal colloid in a patient with active disease and a somewhat nodular gland (Diff-Quick stain).

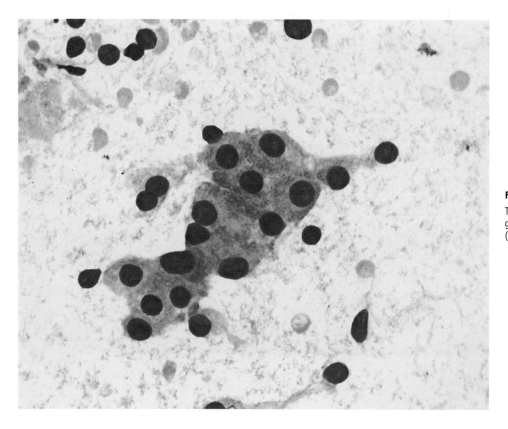

FIGURE 1-46
The epithelial cells have abundant granular (oxyphilic) cytoplasm (Diff-Quick stain).

in this setting, fine needle aspiration is useful only in excluding papillary thyroid carcinoma, and not a follicular neoplasm.

The patient with Graves' disease treated remotely with radioactive iodine or medical therapy, who presents with a nodular gland, is similarly problematic. Cellular adenomatoid nodules are common in these patients; they cannot be distinguished cytologically from follicular neoplasms. The presence of nuclear atypia, which may be bizarre in some instances, should not prompt a diagnosis of malignancy. Fine needle aspiration biopsy is useful, again, in excluding papillary thyroid carcinoma in this setting.

DIFFERENTIAL DIAGNOSIS

Sometimes Graves' disease is mistaken for papillary carcinoma. Findings which may suggest that diagnosis include papillary infoldings of the hyperplastic follicular epithelium, sometimes with small fibrovascular cores, and the rare occurrence of true psammoma bodies in Graves' disease. Much more common, dystrophic calcifications and inspissated colloid aggregates should be distinguished from psammoma bodies. The small, round, basally-oriented nuclei, with preserved nuclear polarity, and dense chromatin pattern seen in Graves' disease are quite different from the nuclei of papillary thyroid carcinoma, which are enlarged and overlapping, with irregular contours and fine, evenly distributed 'powdery' chromatin.

Other causes of hyperthyroidism may be clinically confused with Graves' disease, but they are usually readily distinguished by gross and histologic examination. Hashimoto's thyroiditis may present with thyrotoxicosis. It is distinguished from Graves' disease by the density of the lymphoid infiltrate (often with germinal centers), striking epithelial oxyphilia, and areas of follicular atrophy. Toxic nodular goiters contain multiple nodules, some of which display hyperplastic changes similar to the diffuse changes which are characteristic of Graves' disease. In treated Graves' disease, cellular nodules are impossible to separate from follicular neoplasms. A follicular carcinoma is based on capsular invasion and/or vascular invasion, features not seen on FNA preparations.

PROGNOSIS AND THERAPY

The overall prognosis is excellent. Thyroid storm is a life-threatening exacerbation of thyrotoxicosis with severe central nervous system and cardiac manifestations; it requires rapid treatment, usually with antithyroid drugs for initial control. Incidental papillary carcinomas may be identified and if a follicular carcinoma is identified, there may be a more aggressive behavior under the influence of thyroid-

stimulating immunoglobulin and thyroid growth-stimulating immunoglobulin.

The three chief treatment options for Graves' disease are antithyroid drugs, radioactive iodine, and surgery. Medical therapy includes iodine and iodine-containing compounds (decrease storage of organic iodine and thyroxin secretion) and beta blockers (propranolol, thiocyanate and perchlorate compounds) that inhibit iodine transport. A 40 % failure rate forces these patients to consider radioactive iodine or surgery. Radioactive iodine therapy is the most popular treatment modality among endocrinologists in North America. It is very effective in controlling Graves' disease, but at the cost of permanent hypothyroidism in over one third of patients, requiring life-long medical replacement therapy. Surgery is a rapid and efficient method of treating Graves' disease. The usually approach is subtotal thyroidectomy, leaving a remnant of thyroid behind. Recurrence of hyperthyroidism in such patients is approximately 15 %, with an up to 50 % rate of hypothyroidism. Surgery is preferred in patients with a suspicious or malignant nodule, in those with severe ophthalmopathy, and in children.

ADENOMATOID NODULE (NODULAR GOITER)

The common multinodular goiter represents diffuse enlargement of the thyroid with varying degrees of nodularity. The 'building block' of multinodular goiter is the adenomatoid nodule. Similar nodules may be seen in long-standing or treated Graves' disease and in Hashimoto thyroiditis.

A variety of factors are involved in the development of multinodular goiters; most are associated with some impairment of thyroid hormone production. The response is increased secretion of TSH, which stimulates proliferation of the follicular epithelium and increased thyroglobulin production in a compensatory process, with increased thyroid mass and hormone-producing capacity. In iodine deficient areas of the world, multinodular goiters at one time affected over half of adolescent girls; this was essentially reversed by iodine supplementation. Excess iodine intake, including iodine containing medications, or other goitrogens, can also induce multinodular goiter by interfering with efficient organification of iodine in the production of thyroid hormone. A genetic component may play a role in multinodular goiter development.

CLINICAL FEATURES

Adenomatoid nodules are common, found in about 10 % of autopsies (up to 50 % if microscopic nodules are included), but clinically detectable nodules are found in less than 5 % of individuals. Most patients are

ADENOMATOID NODULE (NODULAR GOITER) DISEASE FACT SHEET

Definition

▶ Diffuse enlargement of the thyroid with varying degrees of nodularity, usually associated with some impairment of thyroid hormone production and increased TSH secretion

Incidence and Location

▶ Clinically detectable nodules found in <5% of patients
▶ Highest incidence in areas with iodine deficient diets; may also occur with excess iodine intake

Gender, Race and Age Distribution

▶ Female >>> Male (8:1)
▶ Wide age range, although usually adults

Clinical Features

▶ One or more thyroid nodules usually discovered by patient or health care provider
▶ Most patients are euthyroid
▶ A dominant nodule may be mistaken clinically for a thyroid neoplasm
▶ Tracheal compression or dysphagia may develop with large nodules

Prognosis and Therapy

▶ Multinodular goiters are usually treated for cosmetic or comfort reasons
▶ Thyroxin therapy is often used to suppress nodules
▶ Surgery is typically chosen for cosmetic reasons, or for a dominant nodule that may be suspicious for neoplasm
▶ Radioactive iodine ablation for poor surgical candidates, toxic nodules
▶ Hypothyroidism may develop, especially after surgical or radioactive iodine therapy

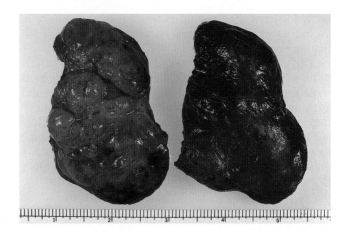

FIGURE 1-47
This thyroid lobe is very large, with many gelatinous fleshy nodules bulging from the cut surface.

ADENOMATOID NODULE (NODULAR GOITER) PATHOLOGIC FEATURES

Gross Findings

▶ Enlarged gland with multiple nodules of variable size
▶ May be gelatinous with colloid exuding from cut surface
▶ Degenerative changes include hemorrhage, central scars, fibrous pseudocapsules, cystic change, calcification, and metaplastic bone formation
▶ Sample periphery for histologic sections

Microscopic Findings

▶ Nodules lack a capsule, but have a pushing border that merges with the surrounding follicles or may have a 'pseudocapsule'
▶ Hemorrhage common, with hemosiderin-laden macrophages and cystic change
▶ Most nodules contain large follicles distended with colloid
▶ The lining epithelium of flattened and inconspicuous epithelial cells may demonstrate prominent oxyphilic change
▶ Cellular nodules with increased cellularity (solid, microfollicular) and little colloid
▶ Papillary fronds may be dominant, but with round, basally oriented nuclei

Fine Needle Aspiration

▶ Usually low cellularity and abundant, thin colloid, often with scratches, waves, or cracks
▶ Sheets of follicular epithelium with small, round, dense nuclei arranged in a 'honeycomb pattern'
▶ Hemosiderin-laden macrophages if degeneration is present
▶ Cellular nodules have high cellularity and scant colloid, difficult to distinguish from follicular neoplasm

Pathologic Differential Diagnosis

▶ Papillary carcinoma, follicular neoplasm, metastatic thyroid carcinoma versus parasitic nodule

euthyroid; however, a few patients develop hyperthyroidism, a condition known as 'toxic nodular goiter', or Plummer's disease.

Adenomatoid nodules are more common in women, by a ratio of eight to one. They occur over a very wide age range, but tend to come to attention in adulthood. Nodules often become noticeable during pregnancy. Patients present with one or more nodules, or the nodule is discovered by a health care provider. The nodules are usually multiple, but one may be dominant and suggest a solitary nodule. Nodules which attain a large size may produce symptoms due to compression of adjacent structures (dysphagia, hoarseness, stridor). Radiologic studies are not usually necessary, although ultrasound may demonstrate the multiplicity and heterogeneous appearance of nodules.

PATHOLOGIC FEATURES

GROSS FINDINGS

The thyroid is diffusely enlarged and nodular (Figure 1-47). The weight of the gland is quite variable, up to

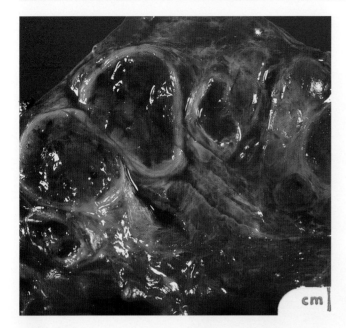

FIGURE 1-48
Multiple adenomatoid nodules which are all very similar, but heterogeneity is more often the rule.

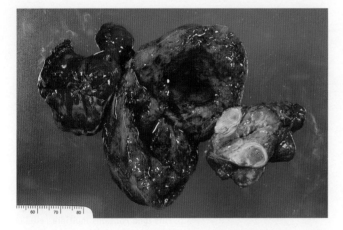

FIGURE 1-49
This gland illustrates a spectrum of adenomatoid nodules, including one with cystic degeneration and another with fibrosis. Nodules with a 'capsule' should be carefully examined histologically to exclude a carcinoma.

several hundred grams or more. Sectioning may reveal nodules that are similar in texture, with a fleshy gelatinous surface; colloid made exude from the cut surface on scraping with a scalpel blade (Figure 1-48), while other glands are characterized by the heterogeneity of their nodules (Figure 1-49). Nodules may demonstrate hemorrhage in the form of central hematomas or areas of organization with brown patches representing hemosiderin deposits. Cystic degeneration is common, particularly in larger nodules or following fine needle aspiration, which may go on to develop thick fibrous pseudocapsules. Fibrous scars may be seen in some nodules; degenerated nodules are often calcified, and may require decalcification prior to histologic processing.

Necrosis, if present, is usually central and confluent due to vascular insufficiency. Sections from the periphery of nodules are more useful than those from the center of the lesion. It is always prudent to remember that a multinodular goiter can easily harbor a thyroid neoplasm among its nodules. Therefore, nodules with capsules or pseudocapsules should be generously sampled, concentrating on the periphery or 'capsule' of the lesion to exclude carcinoma (papillary or follicular carcinoma).

MICROSCOPIC FINDINGS

In addition to the large macroscopic nodules selected for histologic assessment one usually finds small areas of insipient nodularity scattered through the grossly unremarkable portions of the thyroid. They are seen as small groupings of enlarged follicles which stand out among the normal background follicles.

The histologic features of adenomatoid nodules are as heterogeneous as the gross findings. Most adenomatoid nodules are composed of enlarged follicles distended with colloid, lined by flattened follicular epithelial cells (Figure 1-50). Some adenomatoid nodules are more cellular, sometimes appearing solid, with minimal colloid (Figure 1-51). The cytologic appearance varies, including oxyphilic cells (common) and clear cells (occasionally). It is important to realize that oxyphilic cells may exhibit some of the nuclear features of papillary carcinoma, including nuclear enlargement, vesicular chromatin, and irregular nuclear contours, but these are set in the architecture of a nodule (Figure 1-52).

Some adenomatoid nodules, usually those with cystic change, develop papillary structures (Figure 1-53). The cells lining these papillae, unlike papillary carcinoma, usually have small round nuclei with dense chromatin; the polarity of the cells is maintained, with the nuclei aligned evenly at the base of the epithelium. Hemosiderin pigment may be seen in the cytoplasm of these cells.

Hemorrhage and cystic degeneration often go hand in hand (Figure 1-54). Hemosiderin may be seen deposited in granulation tissue or fibrous scar tissue in areas of degeneration. Hemosiderin-laden macrophages are often seen in the cystic areas and in adjacent parenchyma. In areas of marked hemorrhage small granules of hemosiderin may be present in the cytoplasm of follicular cells, giving them a red-brown appearance. A chronic inflammatory infiltrate may be present. A variety of metaplastic changes may be seen, including squamous, cartilaginous, and osseous metaplasia.

A phenomenon which occasionally causes confusion, particularly during frozen section examination, is the parasitic nodule (Figure 1-55). This represents a nodule of thyroid tissue which has become separated from the thyroid gland, often demonstrating either adenomatoid nodules or nodular Hashimoto thyroiditis. The attachment to the thyroid is by an inconspicuous cord of fibrous tissue, often overlooked intraoperatively. The histologic appearance is usually that of an adenomatoid nodule; however, in cases associated with a dense lymphocytic infiltrate, they may resemble lymph node, especially when submitted as such during intraoperative

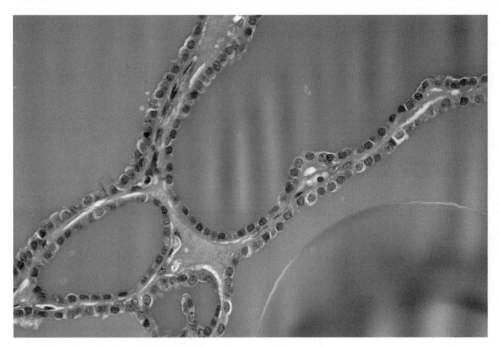

FIGURE 1-50
The classic adenomatoid nodule is composed of large follicles distended with colloid and lined by flattened follicular epithelium.

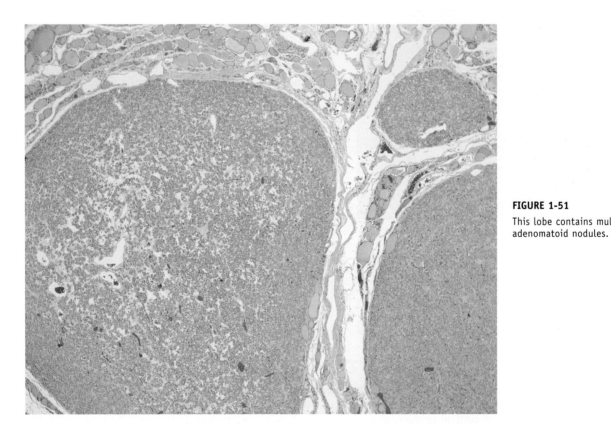

FIGURE 1-51
This lobe contains multiple cellular adenomatoid nodules.

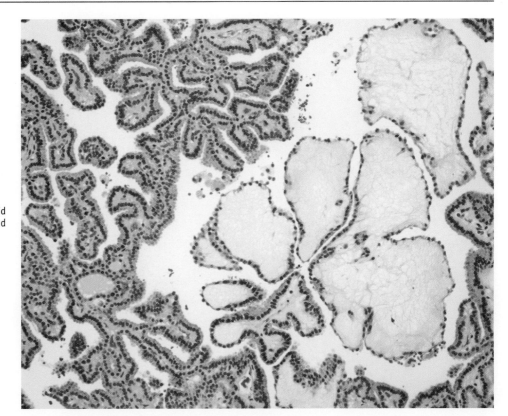

FIGURE 1-52

Papillary structures in adenomatoid nodules may be edematous and bulbous or fine and arborizing.

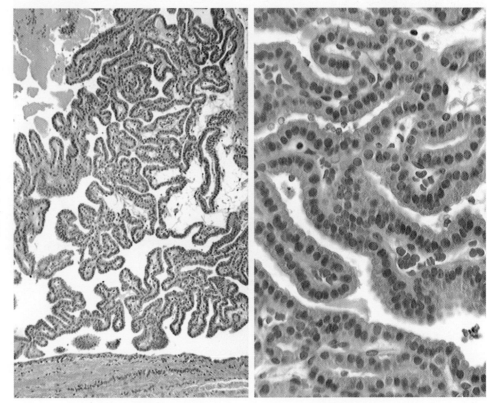

FIGURE 1-53

Left: This cystic adenomatoid nodule has a striking papillary architectural pattern. Right: The epithelium demonstrates small, round nuclei with well-preserved basal orientation and no loss of polarity.

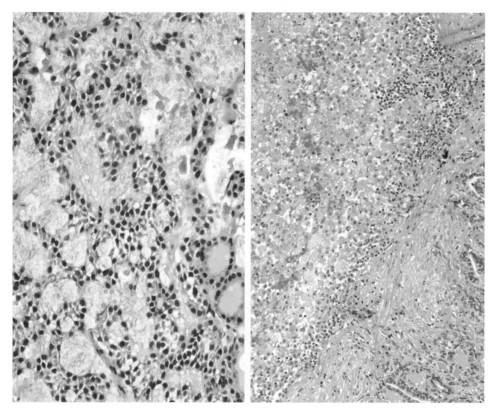

FIGURE 1-54
Left: Myxoid degeneration can sometimes be seen in adenomatoid nodules. Right: Hemorrhage and hemosiderin laden macrophages with reactive fibrosis in a degenerated adenomatoid nodule.

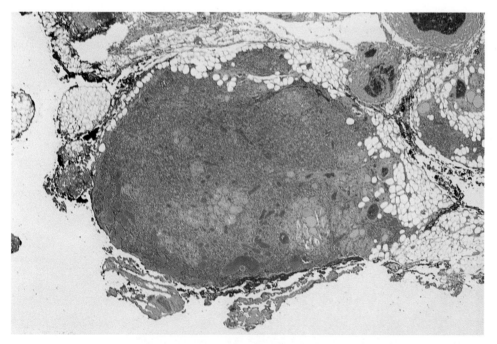

FIGURE 1-55
This patient had a multinodular goiter with a background of lymphocytic thyroiditis. Small fragments of inflamed thyroid epithelium, detached from the gland, may resemble lymph nodes intraoperatively and histologically.

assessment. As parasitic nodules lack the structures of a lymph node (subcapsular sinus, sinusoids, etc), the misdiagnosis of metastatic papillary carcinoma in a lymph node can be averted.

ANCILLARY STUDIES

The cytologic features of the usual adenomatoid nodule include abundant, usually thin, colloid and relatively low cellularity with hemosiderin laden macrophages (Figure 1-56). The follicular epithelial cells from the large follicles ruptured by the aspiration process are usually found as large flat sheets, with evenly spaced, round nuclei, in a honeycomb pattern. The nuclei of the follicular cells have dense chromatin and are not crowded or overlapping (Figure 1-57). In lesions with degenerative changes, the follicular cells may be somewhat oxyphilic. Reactive or reparative follicular cells may be present; they are elongated, and may demonstrate nuclear enlargement and prominent nucleoli. Occasionally, aspirates of cellular adenomatoid nodules which have little colloid are indistinguishable from those of follicular neoplasms based on cytologic examination alone. These are considered to be indeterminate or 'suggestive of neoplasm'; surgical removal of the nodule is usually required in such cases.

DIFFERENTIAL DIAGNOSIS

The chief differential diagnostic problems arise when adenomatoid nodules are cellular or when papillary hyperplasia is present, requiring separation from follicular neoplasms and papillary carcinoma. Cellular adenomatoid nodules may have a pseudocapsule associated with degenerative changes; prominent cystic degeneration is more often found in adenomatoid nodules than in follicular neoplasms, although FNA may induce such changes in neoplasms. Examination of the nodule's periphery for capsular or vascular invasion is necessary to exclude a minimally invasive follicular carcinoma. Once invasion is excluded, the distinction between an adenomatoid nodule and a follicular adenoma is of no clinical significance, and may, in fact, be impossible. Adenomatoid nodules with extensive papillae lack the nuclear features of papillary carcinoma and have an orderly, polarized arrangement of their cells.

PROGNOSIS AND THERAPY

Multinodular goiters are not life-threatening and treatment is usually sought for cosmetic or comfort issues. There is no increased incidence of thyroid carcinomas

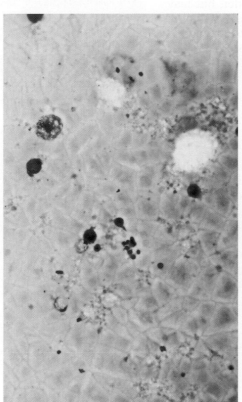
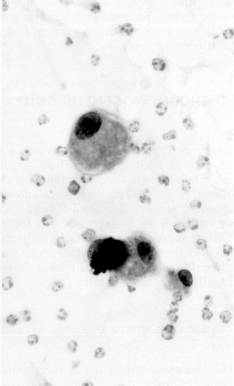

FIGURE 1-56

Left: Colloid is abundant in fine needle aspiration biopsies of typical adenomatoid nodules. The colloid often has a wavy or cracked appearance (Diff Quick stain). Right: Cystic degeneration or hemorrhage result in the presence of hemosiderin-laden macrophages in many cases (Papanicolaou stain).

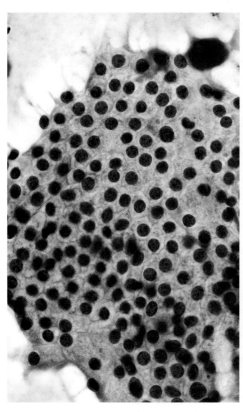
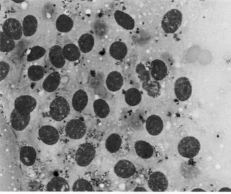
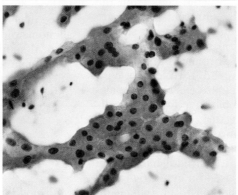

FIGURE 1-57

Left: The sheets of follicular epithelium usually have a 'honeycomb' appearance due to their polarity and distinct cell borders (Papanicolaou stain). Right upper: The follicular epithelium appears as flat sheets, in this case with hemosiderin present within the cytoplasm (Diff-Quick stain). Right lower: This cellular adenomatoid nodule has scant colloid, high cellularity, and oxyphilic change; separation from a neoplasm is often impossible on FNA (Papanicolaou stain).

in patients with multinodular goiters. The therapeutic approach to multinodular goiter includes medical therapy (thyroxin administration for suppression of the gland), radioactive iodine ablation, and thyroidectomy. Radioactive iodine ablation is not widely used in the US for treatment of multinodular goiter, but may be useful in patients who are not surgical candidates or for those with toxic multinodular goiter. Hypothyroidism is a risk in any patient treated surgically for multinodular goiter.

DYSHORMONOGENETIC GOITER

Dyshormonogenetic goiter represents a hyperplastic thyroid with hypothyroidism resulting from an inherited defect in the production of thyroid hormone. Several major enzyme defects are known, resulting in absent or severely decreased thyroid hormone synthesis, which leads to increased but futile secretion of TSH in response to functional hypothyroidism; the end result is thyroid hyperplasia with no improvement in thyroid function. The genetic mode of transmission is usually autosomal recessive.

CLINICAL FEATURES

Dyshormonogenetic goiter is rare, with a prevalence estimated to be 1 in 30 000–50 000 population. It is

---

**DYSHORMONOGENETIC GOITER
DISEASE FACT SHEET**

Definition
▸ Thyroid hyperplasia with hypothyroidism resulting from a number of inherited defects in thyroid hormone production

Incidence and Location
▸ Rare (estimated 1 in 30 000–50 000)
▸ Family history of hypothyroidism in 20%

Gender, Race and Age Distribution
▸ Female slightly > Male
▸ Mean, 16 years (wide age range)

Clinical Features
▸ Permanent congenital hypothyroidism
▸ Severe impairment presents in infancy; may be associated with cretinism; partial defects in hormone synthesis may present later in life
▸ Hypothyroidism recognized prior to goiter in two-thirds of patients
▸ Diffuse thyroid enlargement, often nodular with time
▸ Rarely Pendred's syndrome (familial deaf-mutism and dyshormonogenetic goiter)

Prognosis and Therapy
▸ No increased risk of thyroid carcinoma
▸ Lifelong treatment with thyroxin necessary
▸ Symptomatic goiter treated with total thyroidectomy

the second most frequent cause of permanent congenital hypothyroidism. However, only patients with the most severe impairment in thyroid hormone production present clinically in infancy with cretinism. Approximately two thirds of patients are known to have hypothyroidism prior to recognition of the goiter, which tends to develop later in life.

The average age at presentation is 16 years, but ranges from neonates to adults. There is a slight female predominance. A family history of hypothyroidism and/or goiter is elicited in 20% of patients. Pendred's syndrome is an association of dyshormonogenetic goiter with familial deaf-mutism due to sensorineural deafness; it is very rare.

PATHOLOGIC FEATURES

GROSS FINDINGS

The thyroid gland is enlarged, asymmetric, and nodular, with weights up to 600 g. The nodules resemble adenomatoid nodules, but colloid does not exude from the cut surfaces. The nodules tend to have a more opaque appearance in contrast to the somewhat translucent appearance of adenomatoid nodules.

**DYSHORMONOGENETIC GOITER
PATHOLOGIC FEATURES**

Gross Findings
▸ Thyroid enlarged, asymmetric, nodular
▸ Weights up to 600 g
▸ Nodules have more opaque appearance

Microscopic Findings
▸ Most often nodules are hypercellular, with microfollicular or solid patterns, and little, if any, colloid
▸ Some glands may have hyperplastic appearance similar to Graves' disease, with empty follicles
▸ Fibrosis often prominent and may distort the borders of the nodules
▸ Cytologic atypia may be striking, especially in parenchyma between nodules

Fine Needle Aspiration
▸ Highly cellular aspirate, with small sheets and clusters of follicular epithelial cells
▸ Little or no colloid
▸ Follicular cells often have cytoplasmic oxyphilia and marked nuclear atypia, with enlarged, hyperchromatic, and irregularly shaped nuclei
▸ Impossible to exclude a follicular neoplasm based on cytology alone

Pathologic Differential Diagnosis
▸ Follicular neoplasm, diffuse hyperplasia, radiation thyroiditis

---

MICROSCOPIC FINDINGS

All of the thyroid tissue has an abnormal histologic appearance (Figure 1-58), different from the relatively normal thyroid seen between adenomatoid nodules. The nodules of dyshormonogenetic goiter vary in their appearances, probably as a result of the different enzyme defects and the duration of the disease (age of patient) at the time of diagnosis (Figure 1-59). The most common finding is the presence of hypercellular nodules with solid or microfollicular patterns (Figure 1-60). Papillary and insular patterns may also be observed. Colloid is usually scant if it is present at all (Figure 1-60). Fibrosis is often a prominent finding and may be so extensive that it distorts the contours of the nodules, suggesting an invasive pattern as seen in follicular carcinoma. Cytologic atypia is present in many cases, and may be quite striking, similar to that seen in radiation thyroiditis (Figure 1-61), with an accentuation of this finding in the cells between the nodules, while usually not in the nodules.

ANCILLARY STUDIES

The aspirates are remarkably cellular, with little or no colloid, and often with prominent nuclear atypia. These findings make exclusion of a follicular neoplasm impossible, even if the history of dyshormonogenetic goiter is known. Aspiration cytology in these cases is useful primarily for ruling out papillary thyroid carcinoma.

DIFFERENTIAL DIAGNOSIS

The differential diagnosis includes follicular carcinoma, diffuse hyperplasia (Graves' disease) and radiation thyroiditis. A follicular carcinoma is cellular, often with an irregular contour and the presence of definitive invasion. However, the cellularity, fibrosis, and cellular atypia make a diagnosis of follicular carcinoma extremely challenging in the setting of dyshormonogenetic goiter. Only when there is *definitive* invasion should the diagnosis be made. Diffuse hyperplasia has clinical hyperthyroidism, often has lymphoid aggregates, and usually has colloid present. Radiation thyroiditis may demonstrate cellular nodules with cytologic atypia and increased fibrosis within the gland. An accurate clinical history should readily make the distinction between dyshormonogenetic goiter and these two entities.

PROGNOSIS AND THERAPY

Patients have a favorable outcome with thyroid hormone replacement therapy. There is no increased risk of thyroid carcinoma. Treatment of the

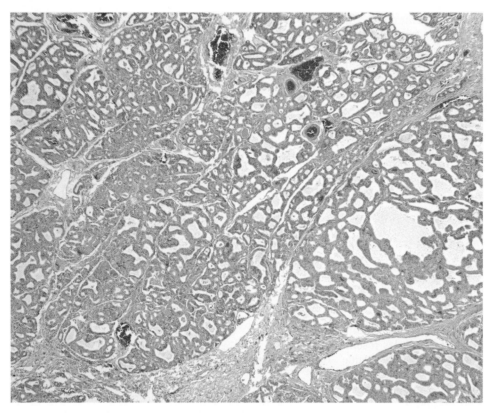

FIGURE 1-58

This example of dyshormonogenetic goiter bears a striking resemblance to Graves' disease, with diffuse hyperplastic changes throughout the gland. Note the abscence of well-formed colloid.

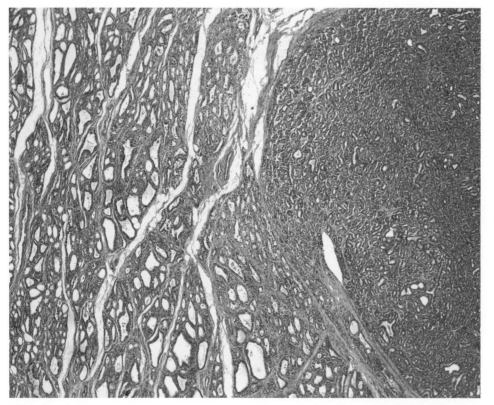

FIGURE 1-59

This gland contains numerous cellular nodules with abnormal thyroid parenchyma between the nodules.

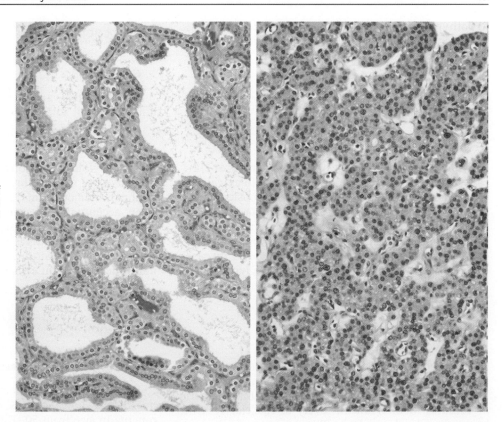

FIGURE 1-60

Left: There is a complete lack of normal colloid. Right: The nodules may be quite cellular, so as to suggest a follicular neoplasm.

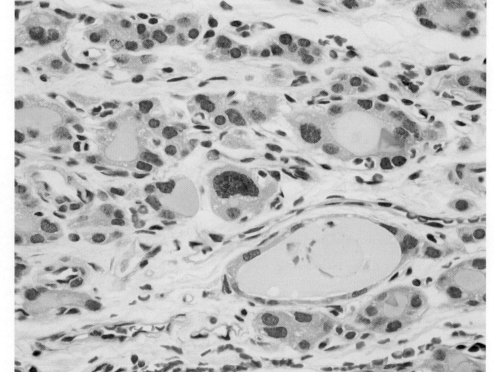

FIGURE 1-61

Cytologic atypia is common in dys-hormonogenetic goiter. It should not be over interpreted as suggesting malignancy. The atypical cells are usually noted in the parenchyma between the nodules.

hypothyroidism associated with dyshormonogenetic goiter is the primary goal. For symptomatic goiter, total thyroidectomy is the procedure of choice.

AMYLOID GOITER

Amyloid goiter represents a symptomatic mass or clinically detectable thyroid enlargement due to extracellular deposition of amyloid. The amyloid deposits may be related to primary systemic amyloidosis or to secondary amyloidosis associated with chronic inflammatory disease (such as rheumatoid arthritis, Crohn disease, familial Mediterranean fever) or neoplastic diseases (plasma cell dyscrasia/myeloma, Hodgkin lymphoma).

CLINICAL FEATURES

Amyloid goiter is very rare, without a known gender predilection. It occurs over a wide age range from adolescents (especially with juvenile rheumatoid arthritis or familial Mediterranean fever) to the elderly with hematolymphoid neoplasia. The majority of cases are associated with secondary amyloidosis. Patients usually identify a palpable mass which, if symptomatic, may cause dysphagia, dyspnea, and hoarseness. Patients are usually euthyroid.

**AMYLOID GOITER
DISEASE FACT SHEET**

Definition
▸ Amyloid goiter represents thyroid enlargement due to the intercellular deposition of amyloid

Incidence and Location
▸ Extremely rare

Gender, Race and Age Distribution
▸ Equal gender distribution
▸ Wide age range

Clinical Features
▸ Most cases associated with secondary amyloidosis
▸ Palpable mass
▸ May have dysphagia, dyspnea and hoarseness
▸ Patients are usually euthyroid
▸ Associated diseases: Juvenile rheumatoid arthritis, other rheumatologic diseases, Familial Mediterranean Fever, hematolymphoid neoplasms

Prognosis and Therapy
▸ Prognosis largely related to underlying disorder (especially hematolymphoid malignancy)
▸ Compressive symptoms may be relieved by thyroidectomy

PATHOLOGIC FEATURES

GROSS FINDINGS

The thyroid is variably enlarged and firm, with a pale tan, 'waxy' cut surface; nodules may be present.

MICROSCOPIC FINDINGS

The amyloid deposition is usually diffuse, but nodular deposits may occur. Amyloid appears as extracellular, acellular, homogeneous eosinophilic matrix material, often accentuated in and around vessels (Figure 1-62). Adipose tissue and squamous metaplasia are frequent coexisting findings (Figure 1-63). In some cases a chronic inflammatory cell infiltrate and, sometimes, multinucleated giant cells may be present.

ANCILLARY STUDIES

ULTRASTRUCTURAL FEATURES

Electron microscopy is rarely necessary for the diagnosis, but shows masses of nonbranching filaments ranging in size from 50–150 Å.

**AMYLOID GOITER
PATHOLOGIC FEATURES**

Gross Findings
▸ Thyroid diffusely enlarged with a firm, pale, tan, waxy cut surface
▸ Nodules may be present

Microscopic Findings
▸ Amyloid deposits usually diffuse, but occasionally nodular
▸ Extracellular accumulation of acellular, homogeneous, eosinophilic matrix material with 'smudgy' appearance
▸ Angiocentric deposits and amyloid in walls of blood vessels common
▸ Atrophy of follicular component with scattered follicles entrapped in amyloid deposits
▸ Groups of fat cells scattered throughout the gland
▸ Squamous metaplasia is common
▸ Chronic inflammatory infiltrate, sometimes with multinucleated giant cells

Ancillary Studies
▸ Most cases are positive for amyloid AA, while cases associated with plasma cells dyscrasia may be positive for amyloid AL
▸ Crystal violet: Amyloid is metachromatic
▸ Thioflavin T-positive
▸ Congo red: Deposits are rose-colored, with apple-green birefringence with polarization

Pathologic Differential Diagnosis
▸ Fibrous variant of Hashimoto thyroiditis, Riedel thyroiditis, adenomatoid nodules, lymphoplasmacytic neoplasm

---

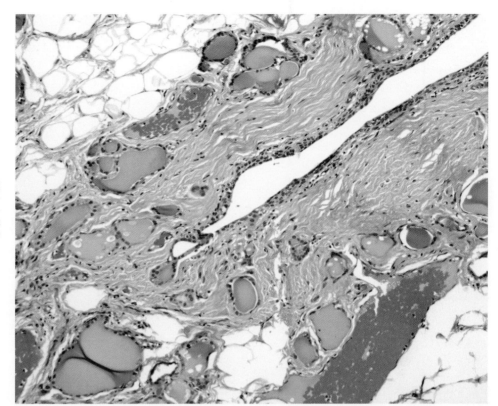

FIGURE 1-62

The thyroid is diffusely infiltrated by intercellular deposits of amorphous eosinophilic amyloid, crowding out the thyroid follicles. Fat cells and squamous metaplasia are frequently observed.

FIGURE 1-63

Left: Squamous metaplasia and adipose tissue with eosinophilic material in the background. Right: The eosinophilic amyloid pushes the thyroid follicular epithelium. Squamous metaplasia and fat are strongly associated with amyloid goiter.

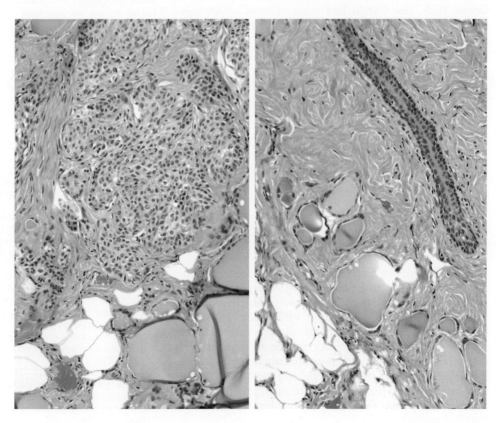

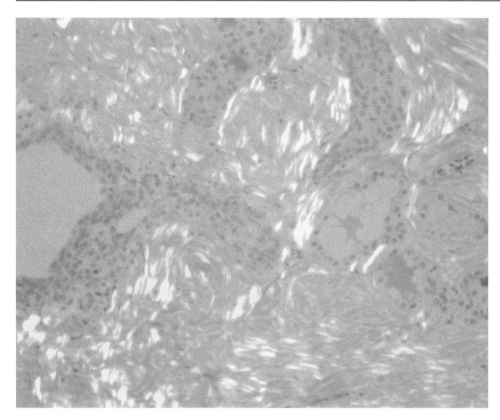

FIGURE 1-64
A Congo red stain highlights the amyloid deposits with 'apple-green' birefringence when polarized.

HISTOCHEMISTRY

Amyloid can be demonstrated with crystal violet (metachromatic amorphous material), thioflavin-T and Congo Red. The Congo Red stain is most commonly employed and exhibits apple-green birefringence when polarized (Figure 1-64).

IMMUNOHISTOCHEMICAL RESULTS

Most examples of amyloid goiter are positive for Amyloid AA immunohistochemistry, though cases associated with plasma cell dyscrasias may be positive for amyloid AL. Light chain restriction may be seen if the patient has a plasma cell dyscrasia or lymphoplasmacytic lymphoma.

DIFFERENTIAL DIAGNOSIS

Amyloid is usually distinctive, with the adipose tissue an initial clue to the diagnosis. Collagenous tissue seen in the fibrous variant of Hashimoto thyroiditis or Riedel thyroiditis will stain differently with histochemical stains. A neoplastic plasma cell or lymphoplasmacytic neoplasm may not be obvious in the setting of amyloid goiter; immunohistochemical stains for assessing immunophenotype and clonality (kappa and lambda) are useful in this regard. Adenomatoid nodules may have fatty infiltration, but do not have amyloid present.

PROGNOSIS AND THERAPY

Both prognosis and therapy are dependent on the underlying cause of amyloid goiter: chronic inflammatory disease, primary systemic amyloidosis, or associated with neoplasia. If there are compressive symptoms, thyroidectomy may be necessary. The more ominous findings are involvement of other organs such as the heart, kidneys, or liver.

SUGGESTED READING

Thyroglossal Duct Cyst

Brousseau VJ, Solares CA, Xu M, et al. Thyroglossal duct cysts: presentation and management in children versus adults. Int J Pediatric Otorhinolaryngol 2003;67:1285–1290.

Dedivitis RA, Camargo DL, Peixoto GL, et al. Thyroglossal duct: a review of 55 cases. J Am Coll Surg 2002;194:274–277.

Doshi SV, Cruz RM, Hilsinger RL. Thyroglossal duct carcinoma: a large case series. Ann Otol Rhinol Laryngol 2001;110:734–738.

Lloyd RV, Douglas BR, Young WF Jr. Thyroid gland. Endocrine Diseases. Atlas of Nontumor Pathology, First Series, Fascicle 1. Washington, DC: Armed Forces Institute of Pathology, 2002:91–170.

Luna-Ortiz K, Hurtado-Lopez LM, Valdarrama-Landaeta JL, Ruiz-Vega A. Thyroglossal duct cyst with papillary carcinoma: what must be done? Thyroid 2004;14:363–366.

Miccoli P, Minuto MN, Galleri D, et al. Extent of surgery in thyroglossal duct carcinoma: reflections on a series of eighteen cases. Thyroid 2004; 14:121–123.

Motamed M, McGlashan JA. Thyroglossal duct carcinoma. Curr Opin Otolaryngol Head Neck Surg 2004;12:106–109.

Patel SG, Escrig M, Shaha AR, et al. Management of well-differentiated thyroid carcinoma presenting within a thyroglossal duct cyst. J Surg Oncol 2002;79:134–139.

Shaffer MM, Oertel YC, Oertel JE. Thyroglossal duct cysts: diagnostic criteria by fine-needle aspiration. Arch Pathol Lab Med 1996;120:1039–1043.

Ultimobranchial Body Remnants

Abscher KJ, Truong LD, Khurana KK, Ramzy I. Parathyroid cytology: avoiding diagnostic pitfalls. Head Neck 2002;24:157–164.

Beckner ME, Shultz JJ, Richardson T. Solid and cystic ultimobranchial body remnants in the thyroid. Arch Pathol Lab Med 1992;116:461.

Buyukyavuz I, Otcu S, Karnak I, et al. Ectopic thymic tissue as a rare and confusing entity. Eur J Pediatri Surg 2002;12:327–329.

Cameselle-Teijeiro J, Varela-Duran J, Sambade C, et al. Solid cell nests of the thyroid: light microscopy and immunohistochemical profile. Hum Pathol 1994;25:684–693.

Cameselle-Teijeiro J, Varela-Duran J. Intrathyroidal salivary gland-type tissue in multinodular goiter. Virchow's Arch 1994;425:331–334.

de la Cruz Vigo F, Ortega J, Gonzalez S, Martinez JI, et al. Pathologic intrathyroidal parathyroid glands. Int Surg 1997;82:87–90.

Harach HR. Solid cell nests of the thyroid. J Pathol 1988;155:191–200.

McIntyre RC, Eisenach JH, Pearlman NW, et al. Intrathyroidal parathyroid glands can be a cause of failed cervical exploration for hyperparathyroidism. Am J Surg 1997;174:750–753.

Sawady J, Mendelsohn G, Sirota TL, Taxy JB. The intrathyroidal hyperfunctioning parathyroid gland. Mod Pathol 1989;2:652–657.

Black Thyroid

Bell CD, Kovacs K, Horvath E, Rotondo F. Histologic, immunohistochemical, and ultrastructural findings in a case of minocycline-associated 'black thyroid'. Endocr Pathol 2001;12:443–451.

Enochs WS, Nilges MJ, Swartz HM. The minocycline-induced thyroid pigment and several synthetic models: identification and characterization by electron paramagnetic resonance spectroscopy. J Pharmacol Exp Ther 1993;266:1164–1176.

Hecht DA, Wenig BM, Sessions RB. Black thyroid: a collaborative series. Otolaryngol Head Neck Surg 1999;12:293–296.

Keyhani-Rofagha S, Koober DS, Landas SK, Keyhani M. Black thyroid: a pitfall for aspiration cytology. Diagn Cytopathol 1991;7:640–643.

Lloyd RV, Douglas BR, Young WF Jr. Thyroid gland. Endocrine Diseases. Atlas of Nontumor Pathology, First Series, Fascicle 1. Washington, DC: Armed Forces Institute of Pathology, 2002:91–170.

Tarjan G, Nayar R. Black thyroid syndrome. Thyroid 2002;12:343–344.

Taurog A, Dorris ML, Doerge DR. Minocycline and the thyroid: antithyroid effects of the drug, and the role of thyroid peroxidase in minocycline-induced black pigmentation of the gland. Thyroid 1996;6:211–219.

Thompson AD, Pasieka JL, Kneafsky P, DiFrancesco LM. Hypopigmentation of a papillary carcinoma arising in a black thyroid. Mod Pathol 1999;12:1181–1185.

Acute Thyroiditis

Berger SA, Zonszein J, Villamena P, Mittman N. Infectious diseases of the thyroid gland. Rev Infect Dis 1983;5:108–122.

Singer PA. Thyroiditis. Acute, subacute, and chronic. Med Clin North Am 1991;75:61–77.

Granulomatous Thyroiditis

deBruin TW, Riekhoff FP, deBoer JJ. An outbreak of thyrotoxicosis due to atypical subacute thyroiditis. J Clin Endocrinol Metab 1990;70:396–402.

Fatourechi V, Aniszewski JP, Fatourechi GZE, et al. Clinical features and outcome of subacute thyroiditis in an incidence cohort: Olmstead County, Minnesota study. J Clin Endocrinol Metab 2003;88:2100–2105.

Lloyd RV, Douglas BR, Young WF Jr. Thyroid gland. Endocrine Diseases. Atlas of Nontumor Pathology, First Series, Fascicle 1. Washington, DC: Armed Forces Institute of Pathology, 2002:91–170.

Manson CM, Cross P, DeSousa B. Postoperative necrotizing granulomas of the thyroid. Histopathology 1992;21:392–393.

Mizukami V, Nomomura A, Michigishi T, et al. Sarcoidosis of the thyroid gland manifested initially as thyroid tumor. Pathol Res Pract 1994;190:1201–1205.

Oksa H, Jarvenpaa, Metsahonkala L, et al. No seasonal distribution in subacute deQuervain's thyroiditis in Finland. J Endocrinol Invest 1989;12:495.

Singer PA. Thyroiditis. Acute, subacute and chronic. Med Clin North Am 1991;75:61–77.

Volpe R. The management of subacute (deQuervain's) thyroiditis. Thyroid 1993;3:253–255.

Walfish PG. Syndromes of thyrotoxicosis with low radioactive iodine uptake. Endocrinol Metab Clin North Am 1998;27:169–185.

Palpation Thyroiditis

Buergi U, Gebel E, Maier E, et al. Serum thyroglobulin before and after palpation of the thyroid. N Engl J Med 1983;308:777.

Carney JA, Moore SB, Northcutt RC, et al. Palpation thyroiditis (multifocal granulomatous thyroiditis). Am J Surg Pathol 1975;64:639–647.

Riedel's Disease

Blumenfeld W. Correlation of cytologic and histologic findings in fibrosing thyroiditis. Acta Cytol 1997;41:1337–1340.

Caraway NP, Sneige N, Samaan NA. Diagnostic pitfalls in thyroid fine-needle aspiration: a review of 394 cases. Diagn Cytopathol 1993;9:345–350.

Dehner LP, Coffin CM. Idiopathic fibrosclerotic disorders and other inflammatory pseudotumors. Semin Diagn Pathol 1998;15:161–173.

Heufelder AE, Hay ID. Evidence of autoimmune mechanisms in the evolution of invasive fibrous thyroiditis (Riedel's struma). Clin Invest 1994;72:788–793.

Lloyd RV, Douglas BR, Young WF Jr. Thyroid gland. Endocrine Diseases. Atlas of Nontumor Pathology, First Series, Fascicle 1. Washington, DC: Armed Forces Institute of Pathology, 2002:91–170.

Papi G, Corrado S, Carapezzi C, et al. Riedel's thyroiditis and fibrous variant of Hashimoto's thyroiditis: a clinicopathologic and immunohistochemical study. J Endocrinol Inest 2003;26:444–449.

Papi G, Corrado S, Cesinaro AM, et al. Riedel thyroiditis: clinical, pathological, and imaging features. Int J Clin Pract 2002;56:65–67.

Papi G, LiVolsi VA. Current concepts on Riedel thyroiditis. Am J Clin Pathol 2004;121(Suppl 1):S50-S63.

Tutuncu NB, Erbas T, Bayraktar M, et al. Multifocal idiopathic fibrosclerosis manifesting with Reidel's thyroiditis. Endocr Pract 2000;6:447–449.

Vaidya B, Harris PE, Barrett P, et al. Corticosteroid therapy in Riedel's thyroiditis. Postgrad Med J 1997;73:817–819.

Wan S, Chan KHC, Tang S. Paucicellular variant of anaplastic thyroid carcinoma: a mimic of Riedel's thyroiditis. Am J Clin Pathol 1996;105:388–393.

Chronic Lymphocytic Thyroiditis (Hashimoto's thyroiditis)

Dayan CM, Daniels GH. Chronic autoimmune thyroiditis. N Engl J Med 1996;335:99–107.

LiVolsi VA. The pathology of autoimmune thyroid disease: a review. Thyroid 1994;4:333–339.

Lloyd RV, Douglas BR, Young WF Jr. Thyroid gland. Endocrine Diseases. Atlas of Nontumor Pathology, First Series, Fascicle 1. Washington, DC: Armed Forces Institute of Pathology, 2002:91–170.

Louis DN, Vickery AL, Rosai J, Wang CA. Multiple branchial cleft-like cysts in Hashimoto's thyroiditis. Am J Surg Pathol 1989;13:45–49.

Roman SH, Greensberg D, Rubinstein P, et al. Genetics of autoimmune thyroid disease: lack of evidence for linkage to HLA within families. J Clin Endocrinol Metab 1992;74:496–503.

Tamai H, Kimura A, Dong R-P, et al. Resistance to autoimmune thyroid disease is associated with HLA-DQ. J Clin Endocrinol Metab 1994;78:94–97.

Vanderpump MP, Tunbridge WM, French JM, et al. The incidence of thyroid disorders in the community: a twenty-year follow-up of the Wickham survey. Clin Endocrinol 1995;43:55–68.

Volpe R. A perspective on human autoimmune thyroid disease: is there an abnormality of the target cell which predisposes to the disorder? Autoimmunity 1992;13:3–9.

Weetman AP, McGregor AM. Autoimmune thyroiditis: further developments in our understanding. Endocr Rev 1994;15:788–830.

Diffuse Hyperplasia (Graves' Disease)

Alsanea O, Clark OH. Treatment of Graves' disease: the advantage of surgery. Endocrinol Metab Clin North Am 2000;29:321–337.

Bahn RS. Understanding the immunology of Graves' opthalmopathy. Is it an autoimmune disease? Endocrinol Metab Clin North Am 2000;29:287–296.

Brown RS. Immunoglobulins affecting thyroid growth: a continuing controversy. J Clin Endocrinol Metab 1995;80:1506–1508.

Carnell NE, Valente WA. Thyroid nodules in Graves' disease: classification, characterization, and response to treatment. Thyroid 1998;8:647–652.

Cooper DS. Antithyroid drugs for the treatment of hyperthyroidism caused by Graves' disease. Endocrinol Clin North Am 1998;27:225–246.

Dabon-Almirante CLM, Surks MI. Clinical and laboratory diagnosis of thyrotoxicosis. Endocrinol Metab Clin North Am 1998;27:25–35.

Gough SCL. The genetics of Graves' disease. Endocrinol Metab Clin North Am 2000;29:255–266.

Graves PN, Davies TF. New insights into the thyroid-stimulating hormone receptor. Endocrinol Clin North Am 2000;29:267–286.

Kaplan MM, Meier DA, Dworkin HJ. Treatment of hyperthyroidism with radioactive iodine. Endocrinol Metab Clin North Am 1998;27:205–223.

Lloyd RV, Douglas BR, Young WF Jr. Thyroid gland. Endocrine Diseases. Atlas of Nontumor Pathology, First Series, Fascicle 1. Washington, DC: Armed Forces Institute of Pathology, 2002:91–170.

McIver B, Morris JC. The pathogenesis of Graves' disease. Endocrinol Metab Clin North Am 1998;27:73–89.

Motomura K, Brent GA. Mechanisms of thyroid hormone action. Endocrinol Clin North Am 1998;27:1–23.

Adenomatoid Nodule (Nodular Goiter)

Aeschimann S, Kopp PA, Kimura ET, et al. Morphological and functional polymorphism within cloncal thyroid nodules. J Clin Endocrinol Metab 1993;77:846–851.

Apel RL, Ezzat S, Bapat BV, et al. Clonality of thyroid nodules in sporadic goiter. Diagn Mol Pathol 1995;4:113–121.

Berghout A, Wiersinga WM, Smits NJ, Touber JL. Interrelationships beween age, thyroid volume, thyroid nodularity, and thyroid function in patients with sporadic non-toxic goiter. Am J Med 1990;89:602–608.

Day TA, Chu A, Hoang KG. Multinodular goiter. Otolaryngol Clin North Am 2003;26:35–54.

Derwahl M, Studer H. Nodular goiter and goiter nodules: where iodine deficiency falls short of explaining the facts. Exp Clin Endocrinol Diabetes 2001;109:250–260.

Glinoer D, Leone M. Goiter and pregnancy: a new insight into an old problem. Thyroid 1992;2:65–70.

Glinoer D. Radioiodine therapy of non-toxic multinodular goiter. Clin Endocrinol 1994;41:713–714.

Lloyd RV, Douglas BR, Young WF Jr. Thyroid gland. Endocrine Diseases. Atlas of Nontumor Pathology, First Series, Fascicle 1. Washington, DC: Armed Forces Institute of Pathology, 2002:91–170.

Siegel RD, Lee SL. Toxic nodular goiter. Endocrinol Metab Clin North Am 1998;27:151–168.

Studer H, Peter HJ, Gerber H. Natural heterogeneity of thyroid cells: the basis for understanding thyroid function and nodular goiter growth. Endocr Rev 1989;10:125–135.

Tollin SR, Mery GM, Jelveh N, et al. The use of fine-needle aspiration biopsy under untrasound guidance to assess the risk of malignancy in patients with a multinodular goiter. Thyroid 2000;10:235–241.

Dyshormonogenetic Goiter

Ghossein RA, Rosai J, Heffess C. Dyshormonogenetic goiter: a clinicopathologic study of 56 cases. Endocr Pathol 1997;8:283–292.

Matos PS, Bisi H, Medeiros-Neto G. Dyshormonogenetic goiter. A morphological and immunohistochemical study. Endocr Pathol 1994;5:49–58.

Medeiros-Neto GA, Billerbeck AE, Wajchenberg BL, Targovnik HM. Defective organification of iodide causing hereditary goitrous hypothyroidism. Thyroid 1993;3:143–159.

Amyloid Goiter

Alvarez-Sala R, Prados C, Sastre Marcos J, et al. Amyloid goiter and hypothyroidism secondary to cystic fibrosis. Postgrad Med J 1995;7:307–308.

Hamed G, Heffess CS, Schmookler BM, Wenig BM. Amyloid goiter. A clinicopathologic study of 14 cases and review of the literature. Am J Clin Pathol 1995;104:306–312.

2

Benign Neoplasms of the Thyroid Gland

Lester DR Thompson

Most thyroid neoplasms are benign, with the vast majority accounted for by follicular adenoma. While follicular adenoma may be difficult to separate from adenomatoid nodule, many do not make this distinction in a multinodular gland. Even though there are variants of follicular adenoma, they are of no clinical consequence, but are diagnosed to exclude the lesions raised in the differential diagnosis. Fine needle aspiration (FNA) is an excellent screening tool to diagnose follicular lesions and separate them from other thyroid disease and neoplasms, but FNA will not reproducibly or accurately separate a follicular adenoma from follicular carcinoma. Furthermore, intraoperative consultation cannot reliably separate a follicular adenoma from follicular carcinoma, and therefore is not helpful. Finally, how much of the periphery should be sampled in order to adequately assess the capsule for invasion? It is my practice to submit at least one section per centimeter of tumor diameter, but furthermore, I try to submit the whole periphery if possible. If the tumor looks macroscopically homogeneous, then the center of the tumor is not of interest. The tumor is halved, with 2–3 mm thick sections created. Then only the very periphery of the tumor to capsule to parenchymal interface is embedded. As many as five sections, 3 mm thick and up to 3 cm long can be placed side by side in the 2.5 cm wide cassette. With this technique, most tumors can be placed in 4–8 blocks, allowing for complete evaluation of the capsule (Figure 2-1).

FOLLICULAR ADENOMA

Follicular adenoma is a benign encapsulated tumor with evidence of follicular differentiation and is the most common neoplasm of the thyroid gland. Nearly 70% of solitary nodules are follicular adenomas, although about 5% of palpable masses are carcinoma.

CLINICAL FEATURES

The most common tumor of the thyroid gland, the solitary, painless mass is often discovered incidentally during routine physical exam, during radiographic studies for other reasons, or as a slow growing nodule present for months to years. Women are affected more frequently than men. Patients present over a wide age range, but there is a peak in the fifth to sixth decades. Patients are typically euthyroid and only rarely develop hyper- or hypofunction. Neck pain or pressure may be reported if bleeding into the tumor has occurred. Initial management includes a fine needle aspiration with or without an ultrasound examination.

**FOLLICULAR ADENOMA
DISEASE FACT SHEET**

Definition
▸ Benign encapsulated tumor with evidence of follicular cell differentiation

Incidence and Location
▸ About 5 % of population has palpable thyroid nodule (up to 20 % if ultrasound is used)

Morbidity and Mortality
▸ None (although hypoparathyroidism or recurrent laryngeal nerve damage may occur during surgery)

Gender, Race and Age Distribution
▸ Female > Male
▸ Wide age range, but usually fifth to sixth decade

Clinical Features
▸ Painless neck mass, often present for years
▸ Solitary nodule involving only one lobe

Radiologic Features
▸ Ultrasound shows size, character, and location
▸ Usually 'cold' nodule on nuclear imaging

Prognosis and Therapy
▸ Excellent
▸ Surgery (lobectomy)

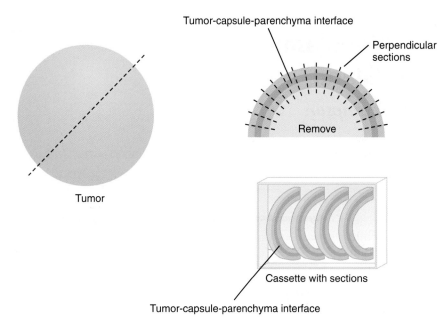

FIGURE 2-1
The tumor is cross sectioned. The central portion is removed. Serial sections are cut perpendicular to the tumor-capsule-parenchymal interface. Sections are submitted to ensure the interface is examined.

RADIOLOGIC FEATURES

Ultrasound will identify the size, location and character of the nodule and may aid in guiding a fine needle aspiration if the mass is not clinically palpable or if deeply seated. Since adenomas are encapsulated, they are easily identified radiographically. Nuclear imaging studies are invariably 'cold', although a functional or 'hot' nodule can be seen (Figure 2-2). In current medical practice these studies are not used nearly as frequently as in the past. CT and MRI techniques are generally not employed.

PATHOLOGIC FEATURES

GROSS FINDINGS

Follicular adenomas are solitary, well demarcated and encapsulated masses identified in a single lobe (Figure 2-3). The capsule is usually thin, but distinct; a thick capsule should raise suspicion for a follicular carcinoma (Figure 2-4). Adenomas are usually spherical, measuring about 3 cm on average, although quite variable depending upon clinical presentation (palpable versus incidental radiographic finding). The cut surface is rubbery to firm with a homogeneous appearance. Grey-white lesions are usually more cellular, while brown-tan lesions tend to have more colloid. Cystic change, degeneration, calcification, and infarction are common and may alter the physical appearance.

**FOLLICULAR ADENOMA
PATHOLOGIC FEATURES**

Gross Findings
▸ Solitary, encapsulated mass
▸ Mean size: 3 cm
▸ Well demarcated with interior of tumor distinct from remaining thyroid parenchyma

Microscopic Findings
▸ Surrounded by intact capsule (no invasion)
▸ Smooth muscle-walled vessels present in fibrous connective tissue capsule
▸ Histology 'inside' mass is distinct and separate from parenchyma
▸ Colloid is usually present
▸ Variants include trabecular, oncocytic, fetal, clear cell, signet-ring cell

Immunohistochemical Results
▸ TTF-1, thyroglobulin, keratin

Fine Needle Aspiration
▸ Cellular smears
▸ Colloid present
▸ Follicular groups without nuclear features of papillary carcinoma
▸ Cannot separate between adenomatoid nodule, follicular adenoma and follicular carcinoma

Pathologic Differential Diagnosis
▸ Cellular/dominant adenomatoid nodule, follicular carcinoma, papillary carcinoma, trabecular neoplasm, metastatic carcinoma

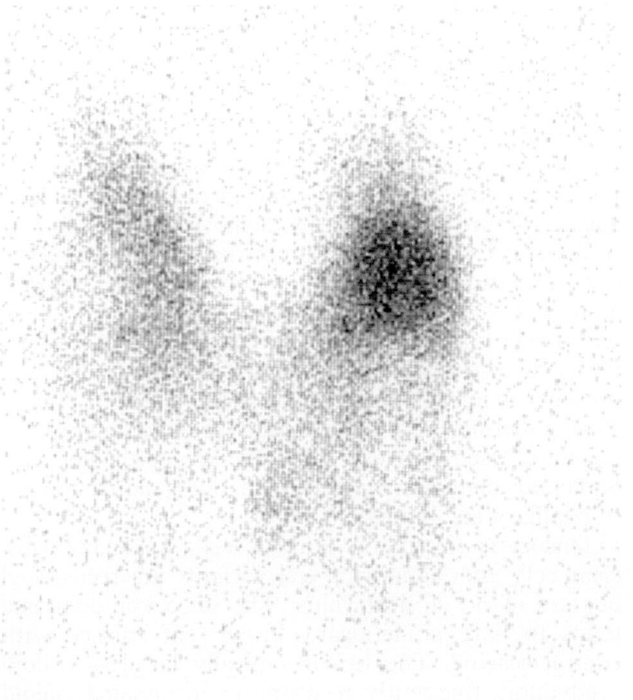

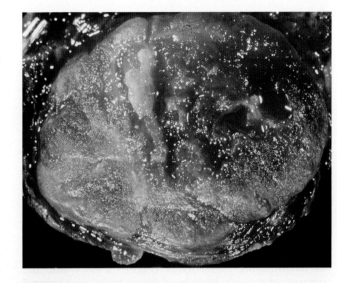

FIGURE 2-3

The thinly encapsulated follicular adenoma has a different appearance than the surrounding thyroid parenchyma. The tumor has focal cystic change.

FIGURE 2-2

A 'hot' nodule on in the left lobe of the thyroid gland demonstrates increased uptake of the radiolabelled iodine (Courtesy of Dr W Chen).

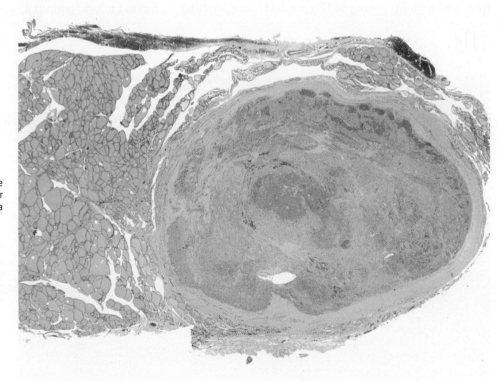

FIGURE 2-4

A variably thick fibrous connective tissue capsule surrounds a follicular adenoma. Central degeneration is a result of previous FNA.

MICROSCOPIC FINDINGS

A well-defined, albeit thin fibrous connective tissue capsule encloses the neoplastic cells, separating them from the compressed or atrophic thyroid parenchyma (Figure 2-5). Small to medium sized, smooth muscle-walled vessels can usually be seen within the fibrous connective tissue (Figure 2-6). No invasion is present by definition. FNA may result in iatrogenic defects in the capsule, but these are usually associated with a linear tract, extravasated erythrocytes, hemosiderin laden macrophages, 'reactive' fibrosis and endothelial hyperplasia (Figure 2-7). The site of puncture often has a 'sharp edge' of transgression, suggesting a mechanical device rather than biologic aggression (Figure 2-8).

The cells are arranged in a variety of patterns with a variable amount of colloid, usually distinctive from the surrounding parenchyma (Figure 2-9). While the patterns of growth have been given 'type' or 'variant' designations (normofollicular, macrofollicular [Figure 2-9], microfollicular, fetal, embryonal, solid, trabecular [Figure 2-10], insular, organoid), these terms are of no clinical consequence. The follicles are usually uniform with a single architectural pattern predominating. Colloid may be highlighted by a PAS stain if it is limited. While the cells are slightly enlarged, there is a low nuclear-to-cytoplasmic ratio with well-defined cell borders in the cuboidal to columnar cells. The nuclei are usually aligned in an orderly arrangement along the basal aspect of the cell (Figure 2-10). Ample cytoplasm, ranging from eosinophilic, oncocytic (Figure 2-11), amphophilic

(Figure 2-12), granular (Figure 2-13) to clear, surrounds round and regular nuclei with coarse to heavy nuclear chromatin distribution. Nucleoli are inconspicuous, although they may be prominent and centrally placed in an oncocytic follicular adenoma. Nuclear pleomorphism can be seen, but is usually focal. Mitotic figures are inconspicuous. Degenerative and cystic changes include edema (Figure 2-14), fibrosis, hemorrhage, cyst formation and calcification, but tumor necrosis is not identified. Infarction, especially in oncocytic tumors, may be associated with FNA or decreased blood supply. Viable tumor cells may be limited to the periphery. Fat is rarely noted (lipid-rich adenoma) within the tumor cells and presents as intracytoplasmic, oil red O positive vesicles. This is distinct from lipoadenoma in which mature fat is interspersed between the follicular epithelial cells. Squamous metaplasia may be seen, but is more common in papillary carcinoma.

Oncocytic (oxyphilic, Hürthle cell, Askanazy cell), clear cell, and signet-ring cell variants are recognized but are of no clinical value. The oncocytic adenoma tends to have a mahogany brown cut surface with central scaring. The tumor typically has less colloid production, frequently resulting in inspissated colloid that can mimic psammoma bodies (Figure 2-10, left). Tumor cells tend to have a greater degree of nuclear pleomorphism, with vesicular nuclear chromatin and prominent nucleoli. The cytoplasm often has a 'glassy' opaque appearance (Figure 2-11). However, oncocytic adenoma is a description only and *does not* imply a different biologic potential.

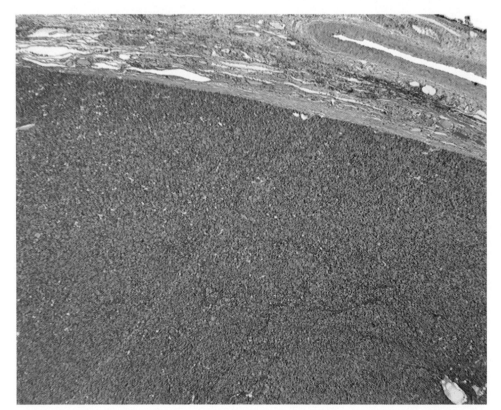

FIGURE 2-5

A cellular follicular adenoma is surrounded by a thin, but well formed capsule. Compressed parenchyma is noted at the periphery.

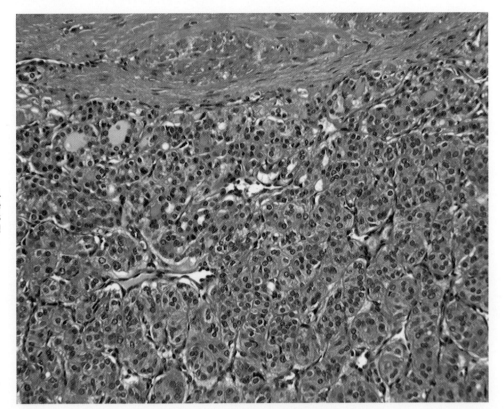

FIGURE 2-6

A smooth muscle-walled vessel is identified within the capsule of a follicular adenoma. The cells are arranged in follicles and trabeculae.

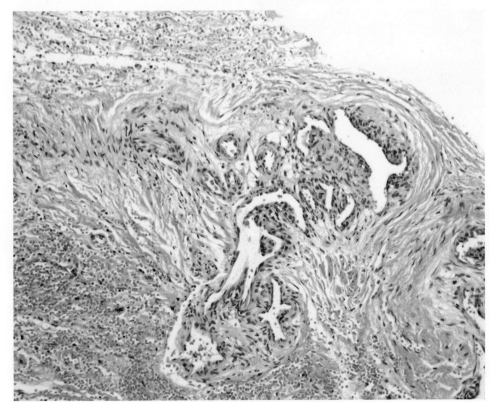

FIGURE 2-7

This FNA site shows distortion of the fibrosis and extravasated erythrocytes and an associated vascular proliferation similar to vegetant endothelial hyperplasia or organizing thrombus.

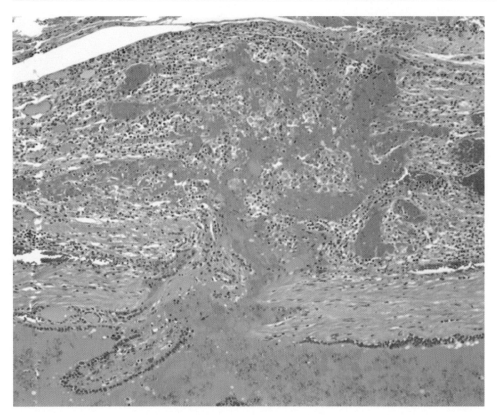

FIGURE 2-8
Extravasated erythrocytes, disruption of the capsule, hemosiderin laden macrophages and endothelial hyperplasia are seen in a site of previous FNA.

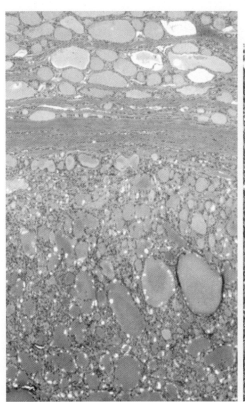
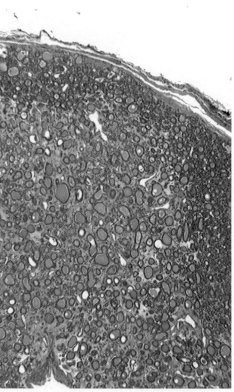

FIGURE 2-9
Left: A capsule separates the tumor from the thyroid parenchyma. Abundant colloid is present within this 'macrofollicular variant' follicular adenoma. Right: Most of the follicles are similar size and shape (normofollicular), but there is a thin capsule at the periphery.

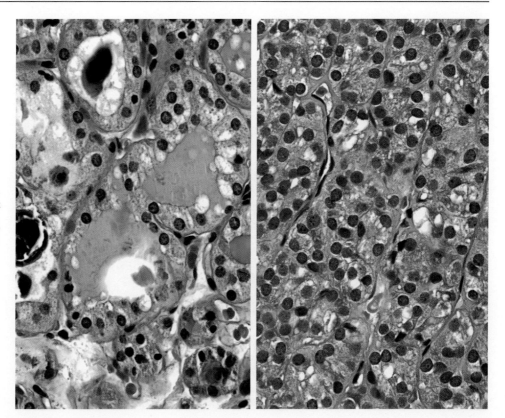

FIGURE 2-10

Left: Colloid has become inspissated and calcified (far left), but the nuclei are round and regular. Right: A trabecular architecture with cuboidal cells and round nuclei with coarse nuclear chromatin.

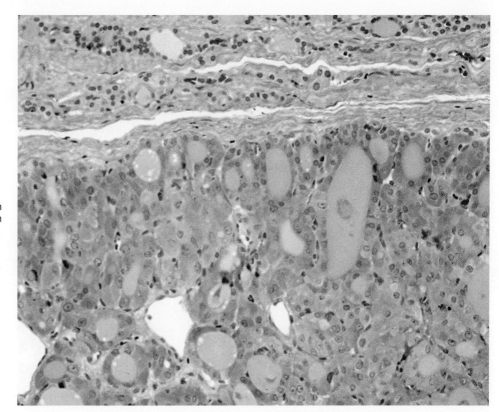

FIGURE 2-11

Oncocytic cytoplasm is seen in this adenoma surrounded by a thin capsule.

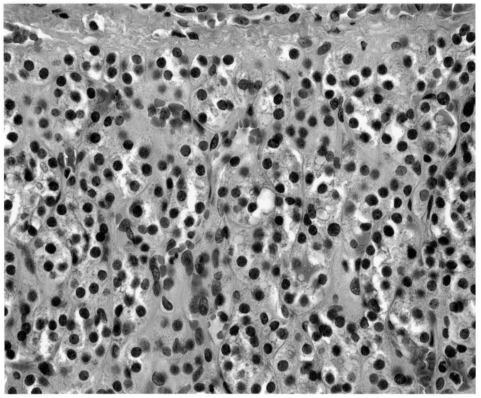

FIGURE 2-12
Amphophilic cytoplasm surrounds small, round, hyperchromatic nuclei.

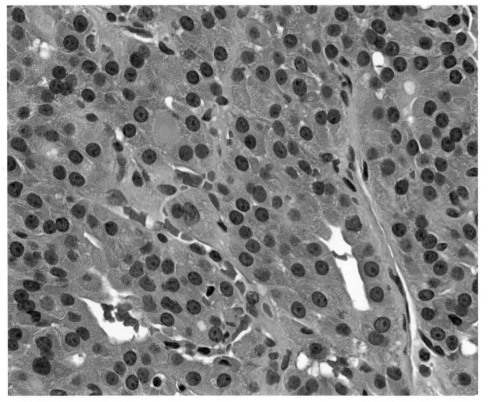

FIGURE 2-13
Granular, slightly basophilic cytoplasm surrounds nuclei with small nucleoli. Colloid is scant in this adenoma.

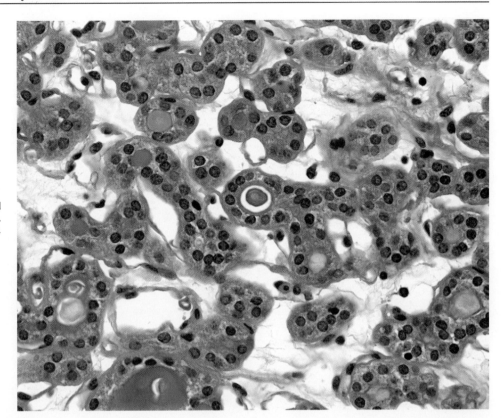

FIGURE 2-14

Edematous change is noted around the follicles in this adenoma. The colloid is focally inspissated, forming a pseudo-psammona body.

Clear cell tumors, such as medullary carcinoma, parathyroid neoplasms, or metastatic renal cell carcinoma (CD10, RCC), can usually be separated on immunohistochemical grounds. To be qualified as a clear cell variant, the tumor should be predominantly or exclusively composed of cells with clear cytoplasm (Figure 2-15). The nuclei are usually centrally situated and are hyperchromatic.

Signet-ring cell adenoma is extremely rare, but has cells with large intracytoplasmic vacuoles which compress the nucleus to the side (Figure 2-16). This vacuole contains diastase-resistant, PAS positive material which is strongly thyroglobulin immunoreactive, suggesting an abnormal thyroglobulin accumulation. Metastatic adenocarcinoma may rarely give a similar histologic appearance.

adenoma or a follicular carcinoma with any degree of reliability or reproducibility. As discussed in Chapter 3 (Malignant Neoplasms), after adequacy is assessed, a follicular neoplasm may be favored over adenomatoid nodule (colloid goiter). Features that favor a neoplasm are syncytial groups with a microfollicular arrangement in a cellular smear in which there is increased cellularity compared to the amount of colloid, and uniform, monotonous cells that vary little from one another (Figures 2-17 and 2-18). Oncocytic adenomas have large, polygonal cells with granular cytoplasm (Figures 2-19 and 2-20). The nucleoli tend to be more prominent. Adenomatoid nodules tend to have cellular variability and often have extensive degenerative changes present. The diagnosis of *'thyroid follicular epithelial proliferation, favor neoplasm'* will result in appropriate surgery for a solitary thyroid mass.

ANCILLARY STUDIES

IMMUNOHISTOCHEMICAL RESULTS

Immunohistochemistry is seldom necessary for the diagnosis, but in cases where the diagnosis is in question, the neoplastic cells will be thyroglobulin, TTF-1 and keratin immunoreactive.

FINE NEEDLE ASPIRATION

Fine needle aspiration is the first line evaluation technique. Unfortunately, FNA does not separate between a cellular or dominant adenomatoid nodule, follicular

DIFFERENTIAL DIAGNOSIS

The differential diagnosis includes cellular or dominant adenomatoid nodules, follicular carcinoma, papillary carcinoma, medullary carcinoma, trabecular tumor, and metastatic carcinomas. Definitive separation between a follicular adenoma and adenomatoid nodule is arbitrary and sometimes semantic, as both are benign lesions requiring no difference in management. With that said, adenomatoid nodules are usually multiple, lack a capsule with smooth-muscle walled vessels, and usually have much more abundant colloid and degenerative changes than an adenoma (Figure 2-21).

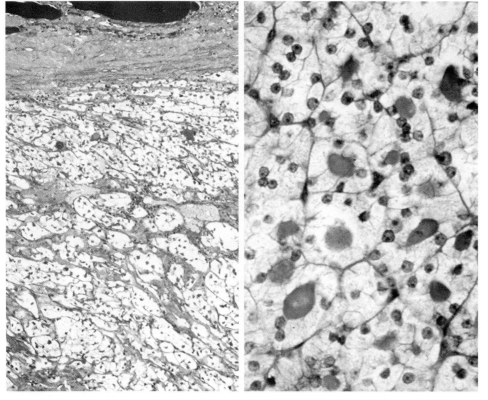

FIGURE 2-15

A follicular adenoma is composed exclusively of clear cells (left), although colloid production can still be identified (right).

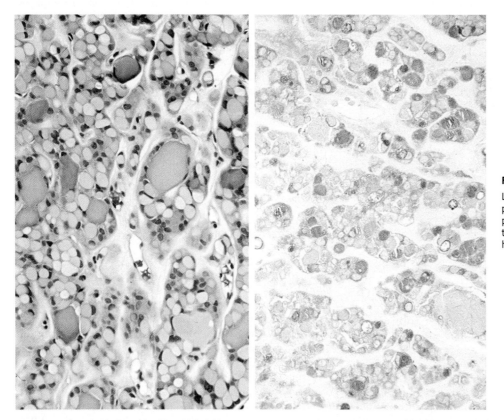

FIGURE 2-16

Left: Signet ring adenoma is composed of cells with a large cytoplasmic vacuole which compresses the nucleus. Right: Thyroglobulin highlights the vacuoles.

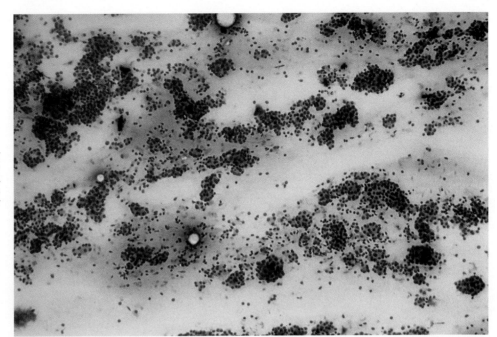

FIGURE 2-17

FNA smear of 'thyroid follicular epithelial proliferation, favor neoplasm.' Cellular, with syncytial groups of uniform and monotonous cells. Scant colloid present (air dried, Diff-Quick).

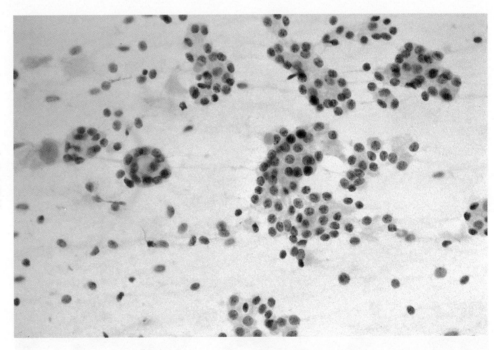

FIGURE 2-18

FNA smear of 'thyroid follicular epithelial proliferation, favor neoplasm.' Cellular smear with monotonous cells arranged in follicles and sheets. Small nuclei and a low N:C ratio (alcohol fixed, Papanicolau).

Oncocytic cells can be seen. Without capsular or vascular invasion a diagnosis of carcinoma cannot be rendered in follicular neoplasms. However, features which raise the suspicion of carcinoma include a remarkably thickened fibrous capsule, increased cellularity (especially at the periphery of the tumor), increased mitotic activity, atypical mitotic figures, and tumor necrosis (Figure 2-22). Still, invasion must be present to call the

tumor a follicular carcinoma. Atypical adenoma may be employed in these circumstances where a definitive separation is impossible (Figure 2-23). To date, cytogenetic and molecular studies cannot reliably separate follicular tumors. Oxyphilia often results in nuclear contour irregularities and intranuclear cytoplasmic inclusions (any cell with abundant cytoplasm is prone to intranuclear cytoplasmic invaginations), both

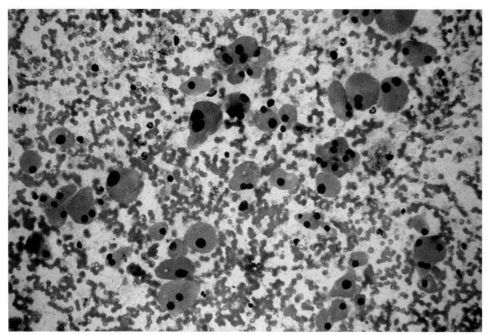

FIGURE 2-19

FNA smear of 'thyroid follicular epithelial proliferation, favor neoplasm with oncocytic cells.' Oncocytic cells are polygonal with abundant, opaque cytoplasm with slight granularity (alcohol fixed, Papanicolau).

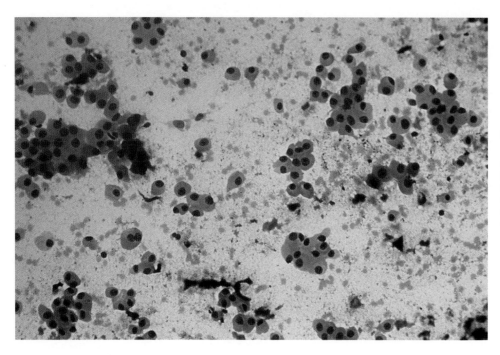

FIGURE 2-20

FNA smear of 'thyroid follicular epithelial proliferation, favor neoplasm with oncocytic cells.' Sheets and small groups of oncocytic cells with abundant, heavy, opaque, cytoplasm surrounding small nuclei (air dried, Diff-Quick).

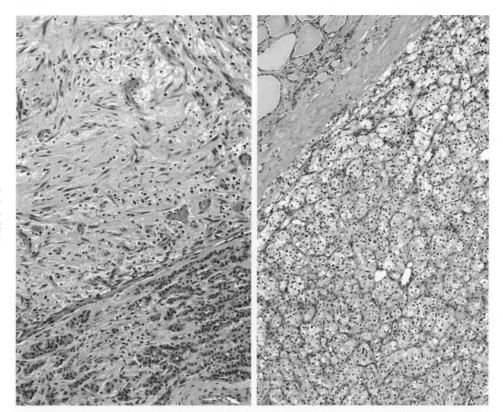

FIGURE 2-21

Left: Degenerative changes with myxoid areas and fibroblastic proliferation are more common in adenomatoid nodules. Right: A metastatic renal cell carcinoma can mimic a clear cell adenoma.

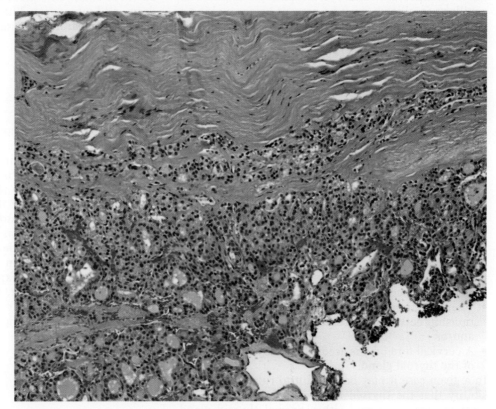

FIGURE 2-22

New collagen deposition has created a thick capsule, entrapping lesional cells. However, these changes alone are not sufficient to warrant a diagnosis of atypical adenoma.

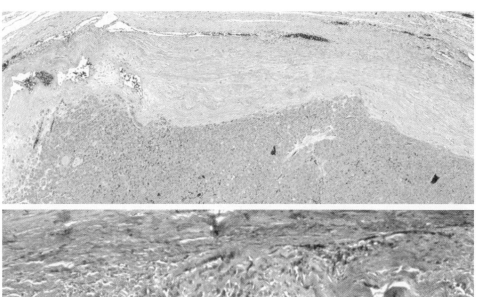

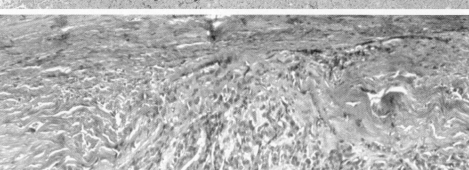

FIGURE 2-23
A very thick fibrous connective tissue capsule with irregularities in the contour, focal areas of 'pushing' and an increased cellularity at the periphery are worrisome for a follicular carcinoma, but not quite definitive for invasion. 'Atypical adenoma' may be employed as the diagnosis.

features seen in papillary carcinoma. However, additional architectural and cytomorphologic features of papillary carcinoma must be present before making a diagnosis of papillary carcinoma.

PROGNOSIS AND THERAPY

Excellent long term clinical prognosis without recurrences or metastasis when removed by conservative surgery (lobectomy alone).

TERATOMA

Tumors of the cervical region are regarded as thyroid teratomas if:
• The tumor occupies a portion of the thyroid gland;
• There is direct continuity or close anatomic relationship between the tumor and the thyroid gland; and/or
• A cervical teratoma is accompanied by total absence of the thyroid gland.
In a given case it may be difficult to rule out the possibility that the thyroid tissue found adjacent to the teratoma may represent either normal thyroid gland secondarily replaced by a primary teratoma or just another component of the teratoma. The tumors his-

tologically display mature or immature tissues from all three embryonic germ cell layers: ectoderm, endoderm, and mesoderm. The percentage of each element is used to separate the tumors into mature, immature, and malignant types.

CLINICAL FEATURES

Teratoma is a rare tumor comprising <0.1% of all primary thyroid neoplasms. Patients range from newborn to 85 years at initial presentation, although the peak and median is 'newborn'. The average age is skewed by older patients who usually have malignant teratomas. Over 90% of the tumors in the neonatal group will be benign teratomas, whereas 50% or more of the children/adult group will have malignant teratomas. There is no gender predilection. All patients present with a mass lesion, often reaching a significant size. Patients may also experience dyspnea, difficulty breathing, and/or stridor. Benign teratomas, whether mature or immature, may result in the patient's death due to tracheal compression or maldevelopment of the neck organs.

RADIOLOGIC FEATURES

Radiographic images can be obtained *in utero*, at the time of birth or in the adult patient. Plain films and

TERATOMA
DISEASE FACT SHEET

Definition

▸ Neoplasm within the thyroid displaying mature or immature tissues from ectoderm, endoderm, and mesoderm

Incidence and Location

▸ <0.1 % of all thyroid primary neoplasms

Morbidity and Mortality

▸ Significant respiratory distress and associated malformations of neck vital structures due to mass effect
▸ Malignant teratomas have a high mortality rate

Gender, Race and Age Distribution

▸ Equal gender distribution
▸ Biphasic age distribution: benign in neonates and infants; malignant in older children and adults

Clinical Features

▸ Mass lesion of significant size
▸ Dyspnea, difficulty breathing and stridor
▸ Maldevelopment of neck organs and/or tracheal compression

Radiologic Features

▸ *In utero* ultrasound may define extent of disease
▸ Multicystic mass lesions
▸ Inhomogeneous mass arising within the thyroid/anterior neck

Prognosis and Therapy

▸ Size, age at presentation and proportion of immaturity determines prognosis
▸ Death may occur due to tracheal compression or lack of development of neck organs
▸ 30 % of malignant teratomas have recurrence and dissemination

TERATOMA
PATHOLOGIC FEATURES

Gross Findings

▸ Mean size 6 cm
▸ Lobulated, smooth with variable consistency
▸ Multiloculated cysts with white-tan creamy material, mucoid glairy material or dark hemorrhagic fluid with necrotic debris
▸ 'Brain' tissue is usually present
▸ Gritty material represents bone or cartilage

Microscopic Findings

▸ Thyroid parenchyma should be identified
▸ Mature or immature tissues from all germ cell layers
▸ Squamous, respiratory, glandular and cuboidal epithelium
▸ Organ differentiation may be seen
▸ Neural tissues, including glial elements, choroid plexus, immature neuroblastema and pigmented retinal anlage
▸ Bone, cartilage, muscle and fat
▸ Separated into benign, immature and malignant based on degree and extent of immature neuroectodermal elements

Immunohistochemical Results

▸ Variable for each specific element within teratoma
▸ Immature glial elements can be highlighted with S-100 protein, GFAP, NSE and NFP

Fine Needle Aspiration

▸ Cellular smears with various elements often misdiagnosed as 'contamination' or 'missed lesion'
▸ Immature/malignant neural elements are called 'malignant' but not specific for teratoma

Pathologic Differential Diagnosis

▸ Benign: Choristoma, hamartoma, heterotopia, dermoid
▸ Malignant: Ewing sarcoma, lymphoma, rhabdomyosarcoma, small cell carcinoma

---

ultrasonographic techniques provide the best information and are easiest to perform. A multicystic mass lesion of the thyroid gland is most frequently identified. Computed tomography images show an inhomogeneous mass arising in the thyroid gland and compressing the upper airway in either the benign or malignant teratomas (Figure 2-24). The presence of enlarged, peripherally enhancing lymph nodes in the neck suggest a malignant teratoma.

PATHOLOGIC FEATURES

GROSS FINDINGS

The tumors average 6 cm, but can be quite large. The outer tumor surface is lobulated and smooth with a variable consistency from firm to soft and cystic (Figure 2-25). A gray-tan to translucent cut surface is common. Small, multiloculated cysts may contain white-tan creamy material, mucoid glairy material or dark brown hemorrhagic fluid with necrotic debris. 'Brain' tissue is frequent. Bone and cartilage can be recognized macroscopically.

MICROSCOPIC FINDINGS

Teratoma, choristoma, hamartoma, heterotopia, epignathus, and dermoid are all unique lesions, and while semantic, these separations are well accepted. Teratoma should only be applied to a tumor with tri-lineage differentiation. Thyroid parenchyma should be identified somewhere within the mass to qualify as a thyroid teratoma (Figure 2-26), although in malignant teratomas residual thyroid follicles are frequently scarce or absent. Tumors display a wide array of tissue types and growth patterns within a single lesion (Figure 2-27). A host of small cystic spaces are lined by a variety of different epithelia (Figure 2-28): squamous, pseudostratified ciliated columnar (respiratory), cuboidal (with and without goblet cells), glandular, and transitional epithelia (Figure 2-29). Pilosebaceous and other adnexal structures are seen in association with squamous

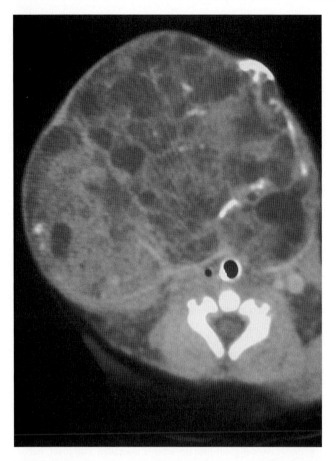

epithelium. True 'organ' differentiation (pancreas, liver, lung) is uncommonly noted. Nearly all cases contain neural tissue, which consists of mature glial elements, choroid plexus, pigmented retinal anlage (Figure 2-30), or immature neuroblastemal elements. Neuroblastic elements often arranged in sheets or rosette-like structures are characterized by small to medium-sized cells with dense hyperchromatic nuclei and mitoses (Figure 2-31). Cartilage, bone, striated skeletal muscle (Figure 2-32), smooth muscle, adipose tissue, and loose myxoid to fibrous embryonic mesenchymal connective tissue is seen intermixed with the neural and epithelial elements.

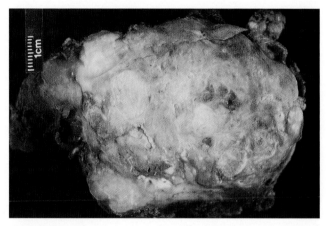

FIGURE 2-24

This CT scan demonstrates a large multicystic thyroid teratoma in the anterior neck that completely replaces the thyroid gland.

FIGURE 2-25

The teratoma has a multinodular appearance and has completely replaced the thyroid gland. Cystic and calcified areas are noted.

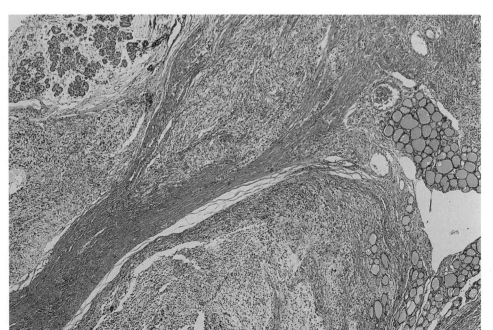

FIGURE 2-26

Benign mature teratoma. Mature thyroid follicular epithelium is compressed to the periphery by mature glial tissue and salivary gland tissue.

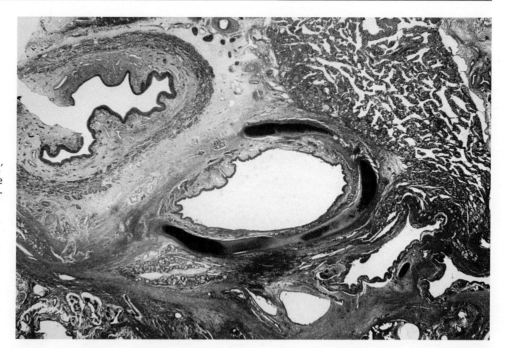

FIGURE 2-27

A mature 'esophagus,' 'trachea,' and 'lung' are seen in this mature thyroid teratoma, forming an 'epignathus' type lesion.

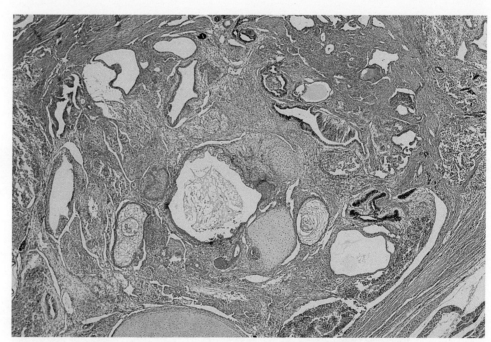

FIGURE 2-28

Multiple cystic spaces are lined by squamous, cuboidal and respiratory type epithelium in this benign mature teratoma. Neural tissue and pigmented retinal anlage is also noted.

The maturation of the neural-type tissue determines the grade. Benign mature teratomas contain only mature elements (grade 0). The term 'Benign, immature teratoma' encompasses tumors with a limited degree of immaturity (embryonal-type tissue in only 1 low power field [grade 1]) and tumors with >1 but <4 low power fields of immature foci (grade 2). Malignant teratomas contain >4 low power fields of immature tissue (Figure 2-33), along with mitoses and cellular atypia (grade 3). The presence of embryonal carcinoma or yolk sac tumor would place a teratoma into the malignant category by definition.

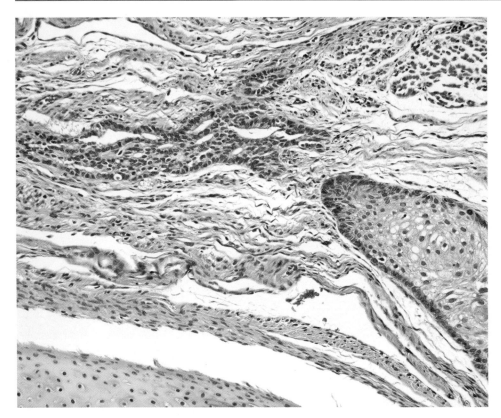

FIGURE 2-29
Benign mature teratoma. Mature squamous epithelium, cuboidal epithelium, cartilage and mature skeletal muscle are haphazardly arranged.

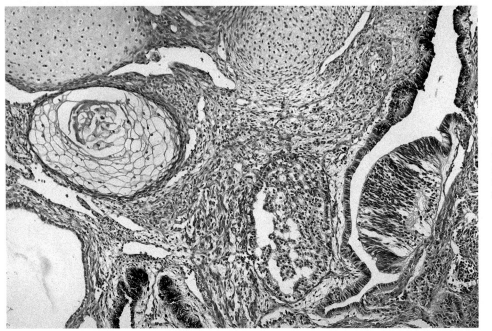

FIGURE 2-30
Benign mature teratoma. Mature squamous epithelium, cartilage, mesenchyme and pigmented retinal anlage comprise this teratoma.

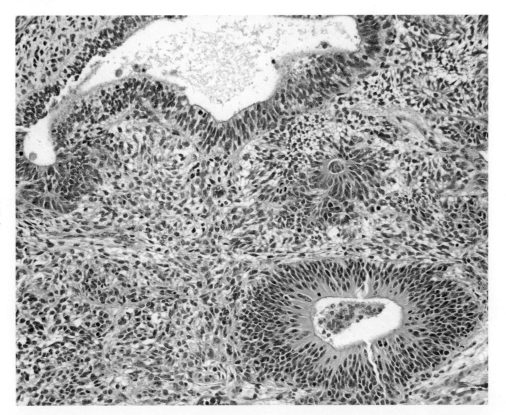

FIGURE 2-31

Benign immature teratoma. Immature neuroectodermal tissue arranged in Flexner-Wintersteiner rosettes.

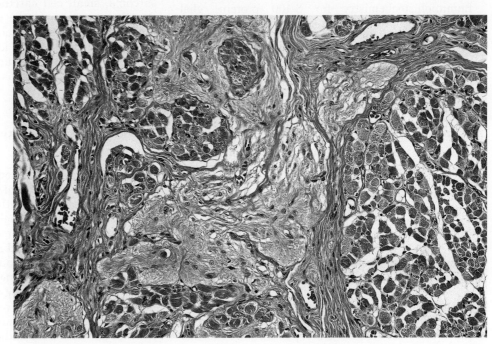

FIGURE 2-32

This benign mature teratoma has a haphazard arrangement of skeletal muscle with mature glial tissue.

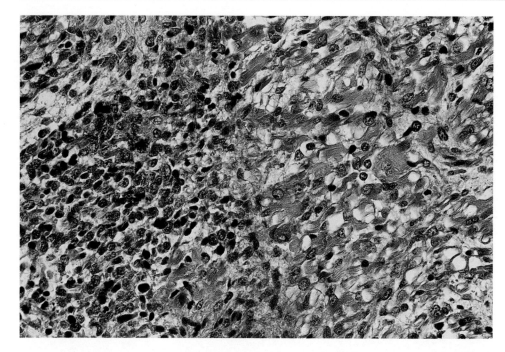

FIGURE 2-33
Malignant teratoma. This tumor has immature neuroectodermal and rhabdomyosarcomatous differentiation.

ANCILLARY STUDIES

IMMUNOHISTOCHEMICAL RESULTS

Immunohistochemistry for S-100 protein, glial fibrillary acidic protein, neuron specific enolase, neurofilament and myo-D1 may be of value for the characterization of the various immature elements.

FINE NEEDLE ASPIRATION

Smears will demonstrate various cellular components, often misinterpreted to represent a contamination or a 'missed' lesion. In malignant teratomas, the FNA smears will show a 'neuroepithelial' small-blue-round cell appearance when taken from the immature/malignant neural elements. These cells are frequently interpreted as 'malignant cells' rather than giving a specific diagnosis of malignant teratoma.

DIFFERENTIAL DIAGNOSIS

Choristoma is used for histologically normal tissues for a location other than the site at which it is detected. Hamartoma refers to a disorganized collection of normal mature tissues for the anatomic area. Heterotopias are normal tissue in an abnormal location (misplaced or displaced). Epignathus is used for tumors of the palate, sometimes considered to be a parasitic fetus in which the tumor contains nearly all of the tissues seen in a complete fetus. Dermoid ('resembling skin') generally contains only ectodermal and mesodermal elements,

specifically skin and hair. The majority of thyroid teratomas are easily recognizable as such on clinical, radiographic, and pathologic grounds. However, when immature elements predominate, extraskeletal Ewing sarcoma, small cell carcinoma, lymphoma and rhabdomyosarcoma enter the differential diagnosis. The diagnosis of teratoma under these circumstances is largely dependent on the identification of other tissue elements, the immature/malignant neural tissues, and a confirmatory immunohistochemical panel.

PROGNOSIS AND THERAPY

The outcome for thyroid teratomas is dependent largely on the age of the patient, the size of the tumor at initial presentation, and the presence and proportion of immaturity. Even though histologically benign teratomas (whether mature or immature) do not invade or metastasize, they can still result in the patient's death due to tracheal compression or a lack of development of vital neck structures during fetal growth. Prompt surgical intervention, including *in utero* procedures, may be necessary to yield a good patient outcome. Recurrence and dissemination are known to occur in about one third of patients with malignant teratomas, nearly all of whom are adults. Lymph node metastasis is usually followed by lung disease. These patients are managed with radiation and chemotherapy, although it is generally considered palliative with an almost uniformly fatal outcome. Staging is not usually applied since the local effect is more prognostically significant than other features.

HYALINIZING TRABECULAR TUMOR

Also known as a paraganglioma-like adenoma, this is a very uncommon follicular neoplasm with trabecular growth and intratrabecular hyalinization which seems to have a molecular link to papillary thyroid carcinoma.

CLINICAL FEATURES

Women are affected much more commonly than men with a wide age range at initial presentation, although most patients are in the middle to later decades of life. Patients usually have an asymptomatic neck mass. Association with radiation has been documented.

PATHOLOGIC FEATURES

GROSS FINDINGS

A solitary, encapsulated thyroid tumor that is usually small, with a mean size of 2.5 cm. The cut surface is usually solid with a slight yellow tinge and occasionally patulous vessels.

HYALINIZING TRABECULAR TUMOR
DISEASE FACT SHEET

Definition
▸ Hyalinizing trabecular adenoma is a follicular cell tumor with a trabecular growth pattern and heavy intratrabecular hyalinization

Incidence and Location
▸ Rare

Morbidity and Mortality
▸ None (although trabecular pattern can be seen in follicular carcinoma)

Gender, Race and Age Distribution
▸ Female ≫ Male
▸ Usually presents in fifth to sixth decades

Clinical Features
▸ Palpable, solitary mass
▸ Usually asymptomatic and incidentally found
▸ Rare association with radiation

Prognosis and Therapy
▸ By definition, excellent
▸ Reports of lymph node metastases may suggest a relationship with papillary carcinoma

---

HYALINIZING TRABECULAR TUMOR
PATHOLOGIC FEATURES

Gross Findings
▸ Solitary, solid, encapsulated neoplasm
▸ Usually small, 2.5 cm mean size

Microscopic Findings
▸ Thin fibrous connective tissue capsule
▸ Trabecular to insular growth pattern
▸ Scant to absent colloid
▸ Calcific bodies
▸ Medium to large polygonal to fusiform cells
▸ Variable cytoplasm, sometimes containing yellow paranuclear bodies
▸ Prominent nuclear grooves and perinucleolar halos
▸ Prominent intranuclear cytoplasmic inclusions
▸ Hyalinized stroma separating neoplastic cells into trabeculae
▸ Associated lymphocytic thyroiditis

Immunohistochemical Results
▸ Thyroglobulin and TTF-1 immunoreactive
▸ Membrane MIB-1 immunoreactivity

Fine Needle Aspiration
▸ Cellular aspirates
▸ Elongated nuclei may be misinterpreted as papillary carcinoma
▸ Lumpy basement membrane material

Pathologic Differential Diagnosis
▸ Papillary carcinoma, follicular adenoma, follicular carcinoma, medullary thyroid carcinoma, paraganglioma

---

MICROSCOPIC FINDINGS

The cellular and solid tumors are surrounded by a well formed, but thin fibrous connective tissue capsule (Figure 2-34). The cells are arranged in trabecular and insular patterns (Figure 2-35), the nests formed by a dense, heavily hyalinized fibrovascular stroma. Colloid is limited to absent. The nuclei are arranged perpendicular to the fibrovascular stroma (Figure 2-36). The cells are medium to large, polygonal to fusiform, with variable cytoplasm surrounding the oval to elongated nuclei. Intranuclear cytoplasmic inclusions are common, while nuclear grooves are easy to identify. Perinucleolar halos are common. Small, slightly yellow intracytoplasmic vacuoles/bodies are seen in a paranuclear distribution (Figure 2-37). Lymphocytic thyroiditis may be present in the background thyroid parenchyma as may an occasional calcospherite (psammoma body) (Figure 2-38).

ANCILLARY STUDIES

IMMUNOHISTOCHEMICAL RESULTS

The neoplastic cells are thyroglobulin (Figure 2-39), TTF-1, keratin and vimentin reactive, while nonreactive with chromogranin and calcitonin. Membrane MIB-1 staining is distinctive.

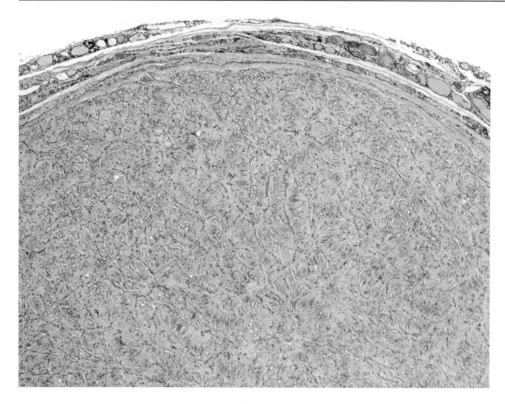

FIGURE 2-34
A well circumscribed hyalinizing trabecular tumor with cells arranged in trabeculae separated by fibrous connective tissue.

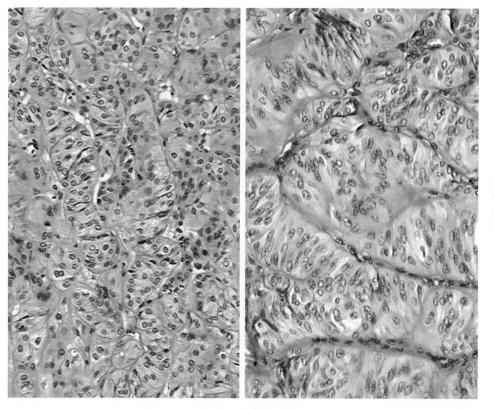

FIGURE 2-35
Trabecular and insular patterns are formed by fibrous bands in these hyalinizing trabecular tumors.

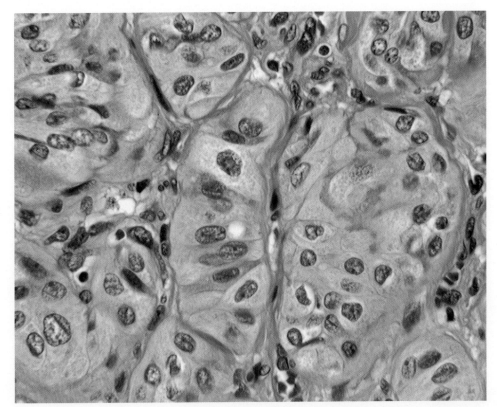

FIGURE 2-36
The fusiform cells are arranged perpendicular to the fibrovascular stroma in this hyalinizing trabecular adenoma.

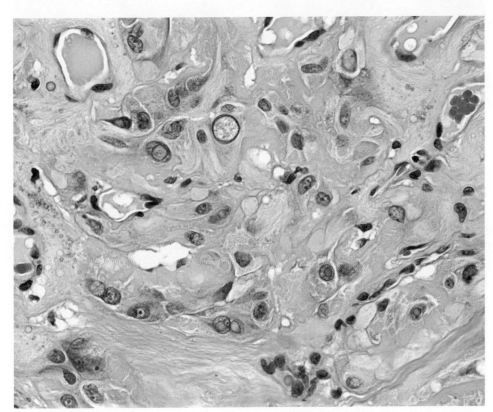

FIGURE 2-37
Multiple intranuclear cytoplasmic inclusions and perinucleolar halos are seen. Slightly yellow, paranuclear cytoplasmic bodies are noted.

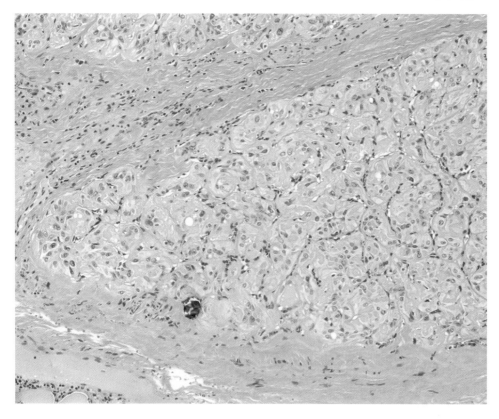

FIGURE 2-38

Dense fibrosis separates the tumor nests and nodules. Small psammoma-like bodies are noted in this hyalinizing trabecular adenoma.

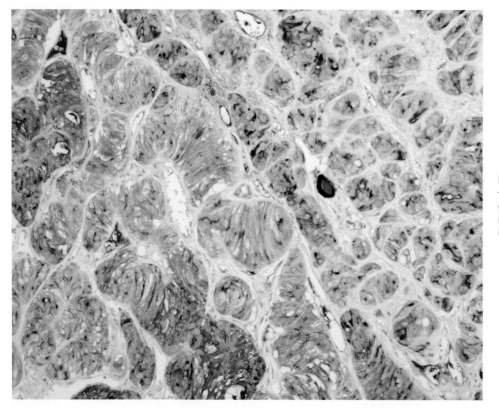

FIGURE 2-39

There is a cytoplasmic immunoreactivity with thyroglobulin, although membrane accentuation is also noted.

FINE NEEDLE ASPIRATION

Cellular aspirates are often misinterpreted as papillary carcinoma due to the similar nuclear features. The dense, lumpy basement membrane material may help with the diagnosis, but it is often difficult.

DIFFERENTIAL DIAGNOSIS

The differential diagnosis includes papillary carcinoma, medullary carcinoma, paraganglioma, follicular adenoma and follicular carcinoma. Paragangliomas are rare and have a characteristic immunophenotype. Trabecular pattern of growth can be seen in papillary, medullary and follicular neoplasms. Follicular carcinoma with trabecular architecture by definition will have invasion. Recent molecular studies have shown a possible link with papillary carcinoma, and so the separation may sometimes be challenging. A trabecular growth, lack of colloid, and the yellowish bodies/vacuoles are not usually present in papillary carcinoma.

PROGNOSIS AND THERAPY

Complete, but conservative surgery yields an excellent prognosis. Isolated case reports of lymph node metastases may suggest that the relationship with papillary carcinoma needs further exploration.

SUGGESTED READING

Follicular Adenoma

Bocker W, Dralle H, Koch G, et al. Immunohistochemical and electron microscope analysis of adenomas of the thyroid gland. II. Adenomas with specific cytological differentiation. Virchows Arch A Pathol Anat Histol 1978;380:205–220.

Carcangiu ML, Bianchi S, Savino D, et al. Follicular Hurthle cell tumors of the thyroid gland. Cancer 1991;68:1944–1953.

Carcangiu ML, Sibley RK, Rosai J. Clear cell change in primary thyroid tumors: a study of 38 cases. Am J Surg Pathol 1985;9;705–722.

Chan JKC, Hirokawa M, Evans H, et al. Follicular adenoma. *In*: DeLellis RA, Lloyd RV, Heitz PU, Eng C (eds). Pathology and Genetics of Tumours of Endocrine Organs. Kleihues P, Sobin LH, series eds. World Health Organization Classification of Tumours. Lyon, France: IARC Press, 2004:98–103.

Thyroid Carcinoma Task Force. AACE/AAES medical/surgical guidelines for clinical practice: management of thyroid carcinoma. American Association of Clinical Endocrinologists. American College of Endocrinology. Endocr Pract 2001;7:202–220.

Flint A, Lloyd RV. Hürthle-cell neoplasms of the thyroid gland. Pathol Annu 1990;25:37–52.

Gherardi G. Signet ring cell 'mucinous' thyroid adenoma: a follicle cell tumour with abnormal accumulation of thyroglobulin and a peculiar histochemical profile. Histopathology 1987;11:317–326.

Gnepp DR, Ogorzalek JM, Heffess CS. Fat-containing lesions of the thyroid gland. Am J Surg Pathol 1989;13;605–612.

Ko HM, Jhu IK, Yang SH, et al. Clinicopathologic analysis of fine needle aspiration cytology of the thyroid. A review of 1,613 cases and correlation with histopathologic diagnoses. Acta Cytol 2003;47:727–732.

Rigaud C, Peltier F, Bogomoletz WV. Mucin producing microfollicular adenoma of the thyroid. J Clin Pathol 1985;38:277–280.

Schröder S, Böcker W. Signet-ring-cell thyroid tumors: Follicle cell tumors with arrest of folliculogenesis. Am J Surg Pathol 1985;9:619–629.

Yamashina M. Follicular neoplasms of the thyroid. Total circumferential evaluation of the fibrous capsule. Am J Surg Pathol 1992;16:392–400.

Teratoma

Craver RD, Lipscomb JT, Suskind D, Velez MC. Malignant teratoma of the thyroid with primitive neuroepithelial and mesenchymal sarcomatous components. Ann Diagn Pathol 2001;5:285–292.

Jayaram G, Cheah PL, Yip CH. Malignant teratoma of the thyroid with predominantly neuroepithelial differentiation. Fine needle aspiration cytologic, histologic and immunocytochemical features of a case. Acta Cytol 2000;44:375–379.

Jordan RB, Gauderer MWL. Cervical teratomas: an analysis, literature review and proposed classification. J Pediatr Surg 1988;23:583–591.

Lack EE. Extragonadal germ cell tumors of the head and neck region: review of 16 cases. Hum Pathol 1985;16:56–64.

Thompson LDR, Craver RD. Teratoma. *In*: DeLellis RA, Lloyd RV, Heitz PU, Eng C (eds). Pathology and Genetics of Tumours of Endocrine Organs. Kleihues P, Sobin LH, series eds. World Health Organization Classification of Tumours. Lyon, France: IARC Press, 2004:106–108.

Thompson LDR, Rosai J, Heffess CS. Primary thyroid teratomas: a clinicopathological study of 30 cases. Cancer 2000;88:1149–1158.

Hyalinizing Trabecular Adenoma

Bronner MP, LiVolsi VA, Jennings TA. PLAT: paraganglioma-like adenomas of the thyroid. Surg Pathol 1988;1:383–389.

Carney JA, Ryan J, Goellner JR: Hyalinizing trabecular adenoma of the thyroid gland. Am J Surg Pathol 1987;11:583–591.

Carney JA, Volante M, Papotti M, Asa S. Hyalinizing trabecular tumour. *In*: DeLellis RA, Lloyd RV, Heitz PU, Eng C (eds). Pathology and Genetics of Tumours of Endocrine Organs. Kleihues P, Sobin LH, series eds. World Health Organization Classification of Tumours. Lyon, France: IARC Press, 2004:104–105.

Cheung CC, Boerner SL, MacMillan CM, et al. Hyalinizing trabecular tumor of the thyroid: a variant of papillary carcinoma proved by molecular genetics. Am J Surg Pathol 2000;24:1622–1626.

Hirokawa M, Carney JA. Cell membrane and cytoplasmic staining for MIB-1 in hyalinizing trabecular adenoma of the thyroid gland. Am J Surg Pathol 2000;24:575–578.

3 Malignant Neoplasms of the Thyroid Gland

Lester DR Thompson

Thyroid neoplasms account for about 1% of all cancers, but they represent the most common malignancy of the endocrine system, posing a substantial diagnostic challenge to pathologists. In general, thyroid cancer afflicts young to middle aged adults with environmental, genetic and hormonal factors often playing an etiologic role. Iodine is essential for normal thyroid function and consequently radioactive iodine can be used in treatment. Women are affected by thyroid lesions nearly four times as frequently as men. Fine needle aspiration (FNA) has contributed significantly to the assessment of thyroid nodules, especially ultrasound detected masses, with a corresponding decline in use of nuclear scintigraphy. FNA is satisfactory or unsatisfactory, and then divided into benign, malignant and indeterminate or suspicious, with a sensitivity for cancer of 65–98%, specificity of 72–100%, and a positive predictive value of 50–96%. Most of the tumors are of thyroid follicular cell derivation and for the most part carry an excellent long term prognosis.

PAPILLARY CARCINOMA

'A malignant epithelial tumour showing evidence of follicular cell differentiation and characterized by distinctive nuclear features' is the somewhat vague World Health Organization definition of this tumor. However, with a constellation of architectural and cytomorphologic features, accurate diagnosis of papillary carcinoma is achievable.

CLINICAL FEATURES

Papillary carcinoma represents about 80% of all malignant thyroid neoplasms and occurs largely in young to middle aged adults with a 4:1 female to male ratio. Even though rare, papillary carcinoma is still the most common pediatric thyroid malignancy. Curiously, there is about a 20% prevalence of papillary thyroid carcinoma (autopsy studies), supporting the overall excellent long term prognosis and highlighting the difficulty in deciding appropriate patient management. There is

---

PAPILLARY CARCINOMA
DISEASE FACT SHEET

Definition
- A malignant epithelial tumor showing evidence of follicular cell differentiation and characterized by distinctive nuclear features

Incidence and Location
- Thyroid malignancies represent about 1% of all carcinomas
- About 80% of thyroid malignancies are papillary carcinoma

Morbidity and Mortality
- Recurrent laryngeal nerve damage and hypoparathyroidism
- Excellent long term outcome (>98% 20-year survival)

Gender, Race and Age Distribution
- Female >> Male (4:1)
- 20–50 years

Clinical Features
- Associated with radiation
- Usually a palpable mass lesion, often with neck lymph nodes
- Rarely dysphagia or hoarseness

Radiologic Features
- Ultrasound shows a solid or cystic mass
- CT is useful to determine extent of the mass and lymph node disease
- Nuclear scintigraphy no longer necessary or used

Prognosis and Therapy
- Excellent long term prognosis (>98% 20-year survival)
- Surgery (lobectomy or thyroidectomy) with radioactive iodine

---

a close link with radiation exposure, an association much more highly developed in young patients. Patients present with a solitary thyroid mass or with cervical lymph adenopathy (metastatic disease). Dysphagia, stridor and cough are usually seen in patients with large tumors. There are many 'incidental' papillary carcinomas (discussed below), which are frequently discovered during routine radiographic studies for unrelated reasons or in patients with other thyroid diseases. Fine needle aspiration (FNA) is the initial study of choice for a thyroid nodule, with excellent positive predictive value. Thyroid function studies are

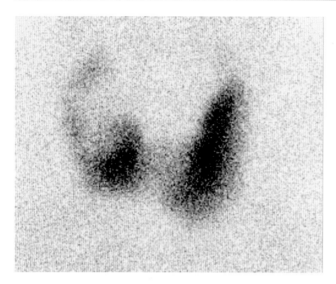

FIGURE 3-1

[131]I scan showing a cold nodule in the right upper lobe of the thyroid gland. No separation can be made between benign and malignant (Courtesy of Dr W Chen).

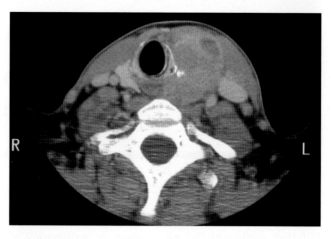

FIGURE 3-2

A CT scan of a large thyroid tumor with extensive infiltration of the soft tissue of the neck and cystic change in lymph nodes.

not useful in the initial evaluation of patients as there is rarely functional compromise.

RADIOLOGIC FEATURES

Ultrasound will usually establish the size and whether the lesion is solid or cystic, while also being a valuable adjunct for guiding FNA. While nuclear scintigraphy was widely used to demonstrate functionality ('cold' without uptake [Figure 3-1]; 'hot' increased uptake) in comparison to the uninvolved thyroid parenchyma, it has been almost completely replaced by ultrasound and FNA as the techniques of choice in initial evaluation of a thyroid nodule. CT or MRI scans are valuable in highlighting enlarged, cystic lymph nodes, which may suggest metastatic disease (Figure 3-2), showing increased signal intensity on T1 weighted images and may reveal punctate calcifications.

PATHOLOGIC FEATURES

GROSS FINDINGS

Most clinical tumors are circumscribed often with an irregular and infiltrative border. A gritty, dystrophic calcification is common. Extension beyond the thyroid gland capsule can be identified along with infiltrating into the surrounding thyroid parenchyma. Cystic change with hemorrhage is common. Multifocality is occasional identified macroscopically (Figure 3-3).

PAPILLARY CARCINOMA PATHOLOGIC FEATURES

Gross Findings
▸ Grey-white, firm mass with irregular borders, although often circumscribed
▸ Calcifications give a 'gritty' cut surface
▸ Extrathyroidal capsular extension can be seen

Microscopic Findings
▸ *Architecture*: Variable growth patterns, complex papillae, elongated and twisted follicles, invasive growth, psammoma bodies, 'bright eosinophilic' colloid, intratumoral sclerosis, crystals and giant cells in colloid
▸ *Cytology*: Enlarged cells, increased nuclear to cytoplasmic ratio, nuclear enlargement, nuclear overlapping and crowding, loss of polarity, nuclear contour irregularities and grooves, folds or 'crescent moons', pale nuclear chromatin, nuclear chromatin clearing, intranuclear cytoplasmic inclusions

Immunohistochemical Results
▸ TTF-1, thyroglobulin, S-100 protein, CK19, HBME-1, *RET* positive

Fine Needle Aspiration
▸ Cellular aspirate with papillary and monolayered sheets, cuboidal cells with enlarged and overlapped nuclei, powdery nuclear chromatin with nuclear grooves and intranuclear cytoplasmic inclusions, and ropy, 'bubble-gum' colloid

Pathologic Differential Diagnosis
▸ Adenomatoid nodules, diffuse hyperplasia (Graves' disease), dyshormonogenetic goiter, follicular adenoma, follicular carcinoma, medullary carcinoma, metastatic carcinoma

---

MICROSCOPIC FINDINGS

The diagnosis of papillary carcinoma is made by using an assemblage of architectural and cytologic features, with no one single feature being diagnostic. The exact

number of features necessary for the diagnosis is undefined. Multinodular and multifocal tumors are common
(Figure 3-4). The architectural features include variable
growth patterns (papillary, solid, trabecular, micro- or
macrofollicular, cystic), elongated and/or twisted follicles, complex, arborizing, delicate, narrow papillae, intra-

tumoral dense fibrosis, 'bright', eosinophilic colloid
(distinct from surrounding thyroid parenchyma), and
psammoma bodies (concentrically laminated calcific
bodies)(Figures 3-5 to 3-11). If a single tumor has many
different growth patterns, suspicion for papillary carcinoma should be raised. The cytomorphologic and nuclear
features are vital in the diagnosis of papillary carcinoma
and are usually constant even between the variants. The
features include enlarged cells with a high nuclear to
cytoplasmic ratio. There is nuclear enlargement of oval
to elongated nuclei, variability in size and shape, with
nuclear overlapping and crowding, loss of polarity and
disorganized nuclear arrangement within the cell. The
nuclear chromatin is pale ('ground glass') with chromatin margination or condensation and clearing ('Orphan
Annie' nuclei). Nuclear grooves and folds, creating 'crescent moon' or convoluted shapes are characteristic
(Figure 3-7). Intranuclear cytoplasmic inclusions are recognized by the contents of the inclusion having an
appearance similar to the cytoplasm – not artifactual
'vacuole' formation, a fixation artifact (Figure 3-11).
Nucleoli, if present are usually small and inconspicuous
and seem to touch the nuclear membrane rather than
being centrally located (Figure 3-10). The cytoplasm is
variable and usually not helpful in the diagnosis, although
variants are named according to the cytoplasm (clear,
oncocytic). Giant cells in the colloid and crystals are
'soft' criteria, not seen as frequently (Figure 3-10). Squamous metaplasia, cyst formation, and degeneration are
not uncommon, with infarction seen after FNA (Figure
3-8). Psammoma bodies are **not** the same as dystrophic
calcification of colloid in the center of a follicle.
Psammoma bodies (Greek for 'salt-like') represent

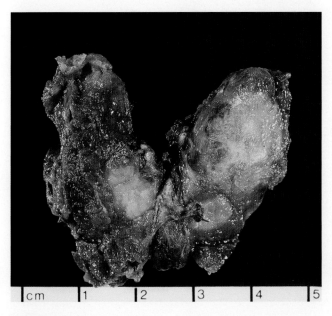

FIGURE 3-3

Three separate primaries are noted, with the largest lesion in the left
upper lobe. There is an infiltrative border of these sclerotic tumors
(Courtesy of Dr JA Ohara).

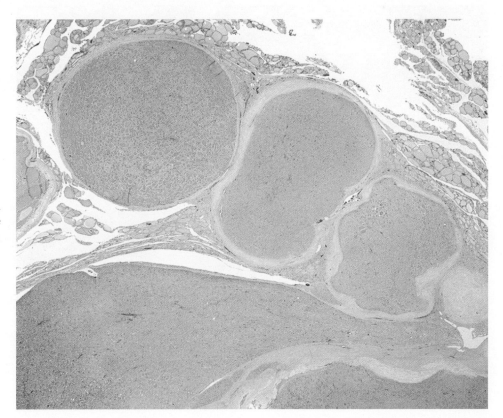

FIGURE 3-4

Multiple nodules of papillary carcinoma are surrounded by dense
fibrosis.

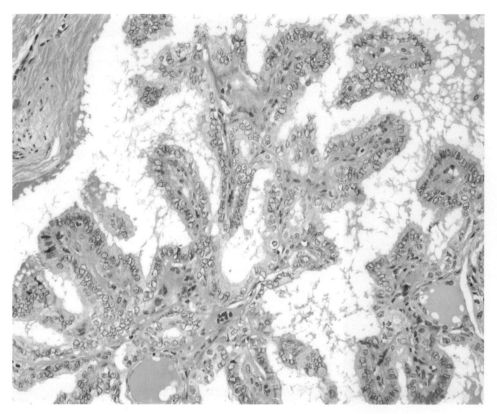

FIGURE 3-5
Delicate and complex papillary fronds lined by cells with an increased nuclear to cytoplasmic ratio, disorganized placement of the nuclei within the cell and nuclear crowding and overlap.

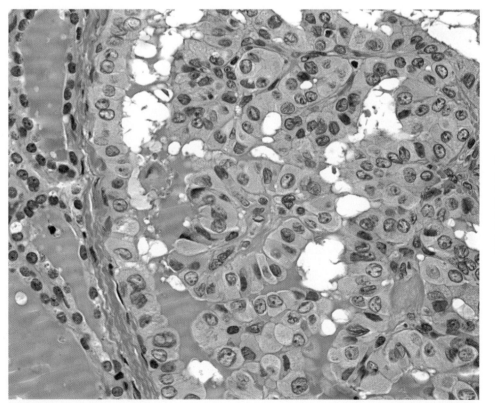

FIGURE 3-6
Normal thyroid follicles (left) contain much smaller cells than the papillary carcinoma, where the cells are enlarged with an increased nuclear to cytoplasmic ratio, nuclear grooves and intranuclear inclusions. Colloid scalloping is present.

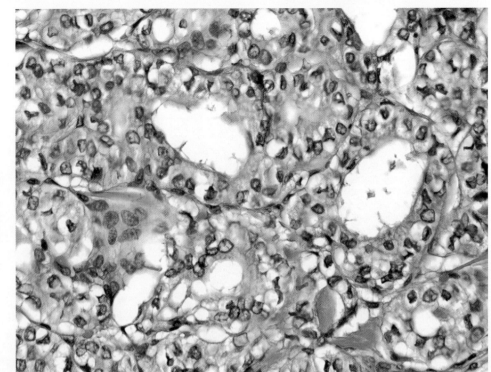

FIGURE 3-7

Irregular placement of the nuclei around the follicle, nuclear crowding, nuclear contour irregularities, nuclear 'crescent-moon' formation, nuclear grooves, nuclear folds and nuclear chromatin clearing seen in papillary carcinoma.

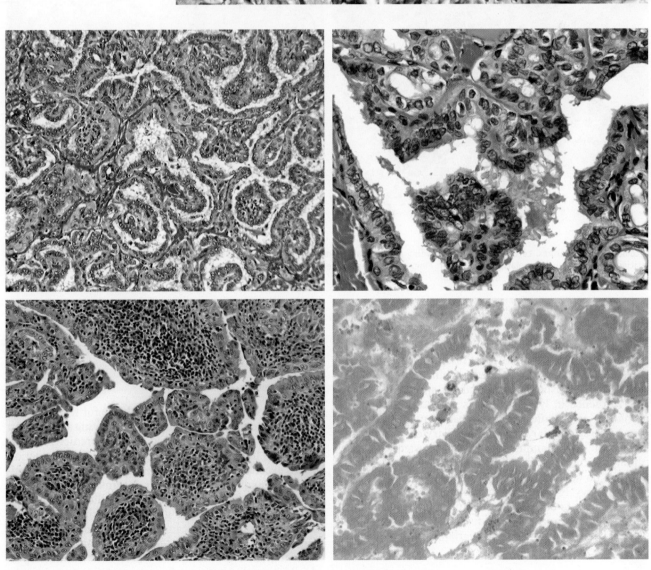

FIGURE 3-8

Patterns of papillary growth. Left upper: Complex, arborizing, delicate papillary structures. Left lower: Oncocytic granular cells with associated lymphoid stroma (so called 'Warthin's variant'). Right upper: Papillary structure with crowded nuclei. Right lower: Infarcted tumor with only ghost cell outlines remaining.

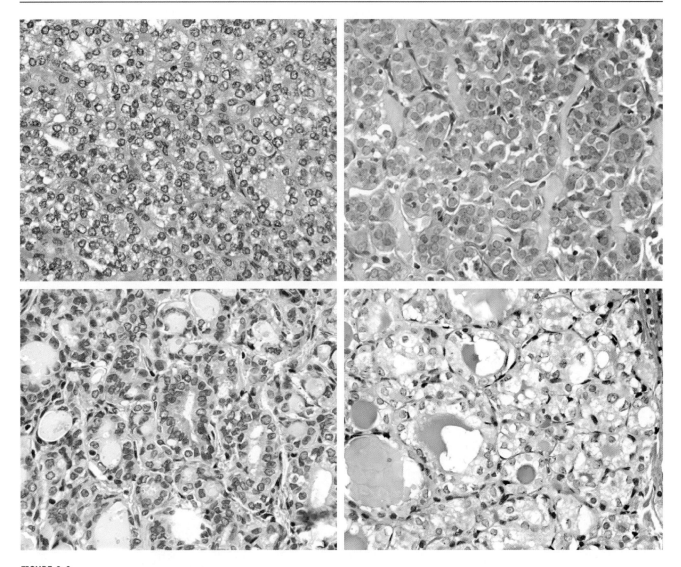

FIGURE 3-9
Cytomorphologic features. Left upper: Nuclear crowding and nuclear chromatin clearing. Left lower: Nuclear overlapping, nuclear chromatin irregularities and loss of nuclear polarity. Right upper: Fine, ground glass nuclear chromatin. Right lower: Pale nuclear chromatin in irregular nuclei surrounding follicles with scalloped, dense colloid.

apoptotic cells that form the nidus for concentric lamellation of calcium (Figure 3-11). Present in up to 50% of cases, they are often identified within lymph-vascular channels, diagnostic of intraglandular spread. Likewise, their presence in lymph nodes is practically pathognomonic for metastatic disease. Separation of multifocal versus intraglandular spread of papillary carcinoma can be difficult. Intraglandular spread is suggested when the tumor is within a septae, within a lymphvascular channel and has no stellate fibrosis at the periphery (Figure 3-12). A heavy lymphocytic response is frequently seen both adjacent to and within the tumor (see Figure 3-8). Papillary carcinoma is not graded, as nearly all are considered well differentiated. The variants are described in the next section.

ANCILLARY STUDIES

FINE NEEDLE ASPIRATION

FNA is considered the test of choice for the diagnosis and management of thyroid nodules, having an excellent sensitivity and specificity and positive predictive value. An initial pass using a 25 gauge needle without suction yields excellent material uncontaminated by blood. Aspirates are qualified as satisfactory or unsatisfactory based on adequacy (at least six groups of follicular cells with 15–20 follicular cells per group). The smears are then separated into benign, indeterminate/suspicious, and malignant categories. Indeterminate lesions include cellular follicular proliferations where FNA cannot reproducibly or reliably separate between follicular adenoma and follicular carcinoma. In general practice, about 70%

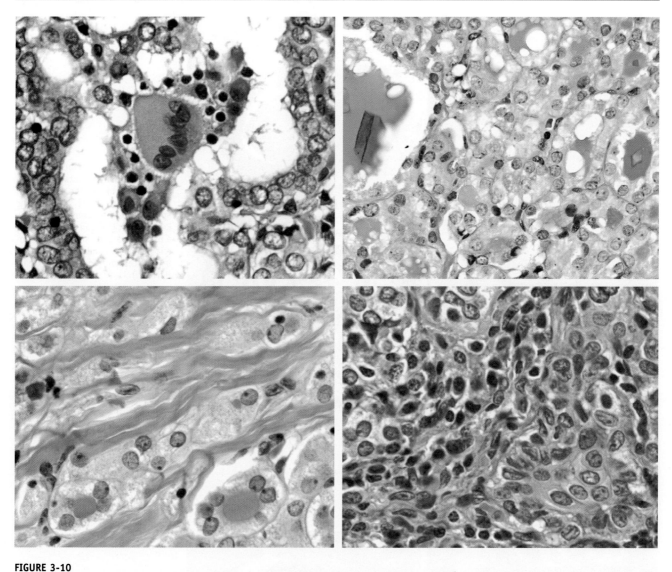

FIGURE 3-10
Associated findings in papillary carcinoma. Left upper: Giant cells within the colloid. Left lower: Dense fibrosis separating the tumor cells. Nucleoli are noted along the nuclear membrane. Right upper: Crystals within the colloid. Right lower: Squamous metaplasia within a papillary carcinoma.

of thyroid FNAs are benign, 10% are indeterminate, 15% are unsatisfactory, and 5% are malignant.

Aspirates from papillary carcinomas are usually diagnostic and are characteristically cellular, with monolayered sheets (syncytium) and three dimensional clusters of enlarged cells (Figures 3-13 and 3-14). The nuclei are enlarged and overlapped with irregular borders, but with a powdery/dusty, delicate nuclear chromatin on alcohol fixed preparations. Nuclear folds or grooves and intranuclear cytoplasmic inclusions are also common. The cytoplasm is often pale or foamy, but not distinctive on FNA. Colloid is often scant and thickened ('chewing gum' or ropey), with occasional multinucleate giant cells and rarely psammoma bodies. The features of papillary carcinoma are best appreciated with alcohol pre-

served Papanicolau preparations rather than with air-dried material.

IMMUNOHISTOCHEMICAL RESULTS

Immunohistochemistry is seldom of value in diagnosing papillary carcinoma, although it may play a role in metastatic disease. The neoplastic cells are strongly and diffusely immunoreactive with keratin, CK7, thyroglobulin, and TTF-1 (Figure 3-15), while other markers (S-100 protein, CK19, HBME-1, galectin-3, RET) yield variable results. p27 (lost) and cyclin D1 (up regulation) shows differential staining in tumors which are more likely to metastasize.

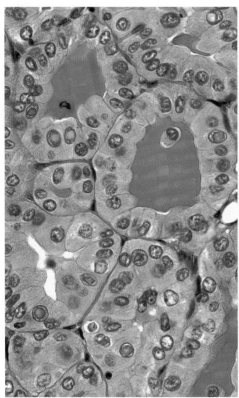

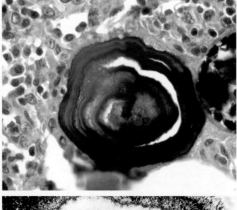

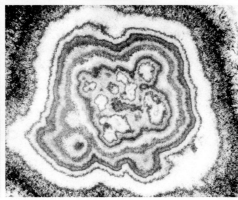

FIGURE 3-11

Left: Multiple intranuclear cytoplasmic inclusions contain material the same color as the cytoplasm. Right upper: Light microscopic appearance of a psammoma body. Right lower: Electron micrograph of a psammoma body showing concentric lamination and crenated nuclei in the center. (Courtesy of Dr CS Heffess.)

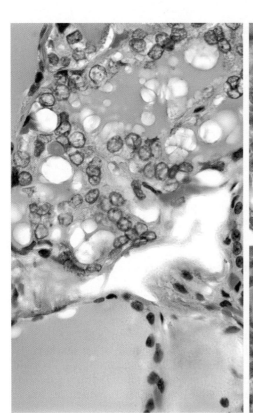

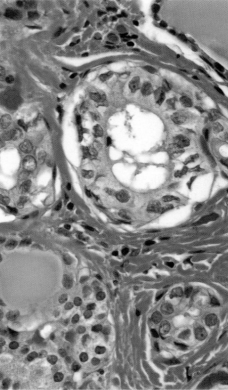

FIGURE 3-12

Intraglandular spread with foci of papillary carcinoma confined to the septae (left) and within lymphvascular channels surrounded by fibrosis (right). Benign thyroid parenchyma is noted in the lower portions of each figure as a point of comparison.

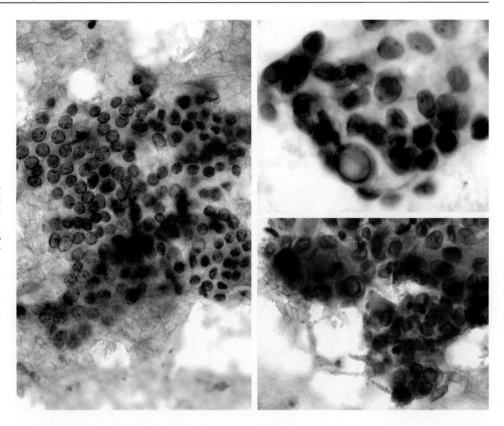

FIGURE 3-13

Papanicolau preparation. Left: Syncytium of cells with enlarged nuclei and nuclear grooves. Right upper: Intranuclear cytoplasmic inclusion. Right lower: Three-dimensional papillae with intranuclear cytoplasmic inclusions.

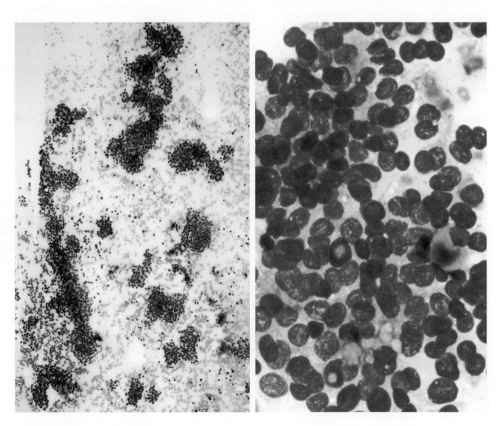

FIGURE 3-14

Air dried, MGG preparation. Left: cellular smear with monolayered sheets and three dimensional clusters without colloid. Right: Nuclear crowding, overlapping, grooves and intranuclear cytoplasmic inclusions. Heavy, 'chewing gum' colloid.

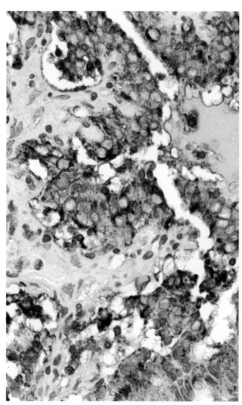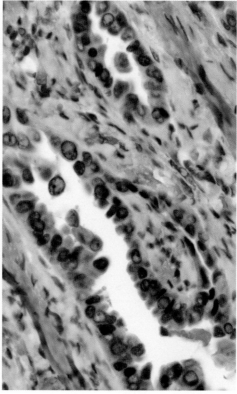

FIGURE 3-15

Papillary carcinoma immunohisto-chemistry. Left: Thyroglobulin stains the cytoplasm and the colloid. However, there is significant diffusion and background staining. Right: Strong, diffuse, nuclear immunoreactivity with TTF-1. Note the lack of diffusion artifact. Cytoplasmic staining alone is *not* interpreted to be positive.

MOLECULAR ANALYSIS

Rearrangements or mutations involving *BRAF* (part of the RAF family of protein kinases), *RET* gene, and *RAS* are structural genetic alterations identified to a variable degree in papillary thyroid carcinoma. Point mutations in the *BRAF* gene are identified in up to 60 % of papillary carcinomas, while *RET*/PTC1 or *RET*/PTC3 is detected in a highly variable frequency from 0–80 % of cases. RAS mutations are seen in up to 15 % of tumors. Each of these results are extremely dependent upon the technique used, whether by immunohistochemistry or in situ hybridization, in adults or children, if there is a history of radiation, and the variant histology present. Therefore, until greater standardization, molecular studies at present do not add to the diagnosis. One caveat may be in inherited papillary carcinoma syndromes, such as familial adenomatous polyposis coli or Cowden syndrome, where genetic studies may help in patient management.

DIFFERENTIAL DIAGNOSIS

The differential diagnosis includes a number disorders with papillae, including adenomatoid nodules (Figures 3-16 and 3-17), diffuse hyperplasia (Graves' disease), and dyshormonogenetic goiter, while follicular adenoma, follicular carcinoma, medullary carcinoma, and metastatic tumors are also considered. In general, the papillae of all of these other lesions are short, simple, non-branching and often 'thick'. The nuclei are round, regular, basally located and hyperchromatic. Intracytoplasmic

hemosiderin pigment is lacking in papillary carcinoma. Although a nuclear feature or two may be present in these other lesions, there is both a qualitative and quantitative difference in their appearance. Many lesions that have oncocytic cytoplasm may induce nuclear enlargement, but other features of papillary carcinoma are lacking. Alcohol fixatives will often cause nuclear enlargement and 'optical clearing', and so caution must be used when making a diagnosis of papillary carcinoma when non-formalin based fixatives have been used.

PROGNOSIS AND THERAPY

Papillary carcinoma spreads preferentially by lymphatic channels, with the regional lymph nodes affected most commonly, and in a significant proportion of cases (Figure 3-18). Intraglandular spread, including the contralateral lobe, is common. However, the prognosis is excellent, with >98 % 20-year survival rate and a <0.2 % mortality rate. The age (<45 years) and gender (female) are the most important prognostic factors, although tumor size, extrathyroidal extension and metastasis are significant for patients >45 years. Surgery is the treatment of choice, although the extent of surgery (lobectomy, subtotal or total thyroidectomy) remains controversial. Recurrent laryngeal nerve damage and hypoparathyroidism are known surgical complications. Radioablative iodine therapy is incorporated after a total thyroidectomy. Lymph node sampling is advocated only if there is clinical or radiographic enlargement.

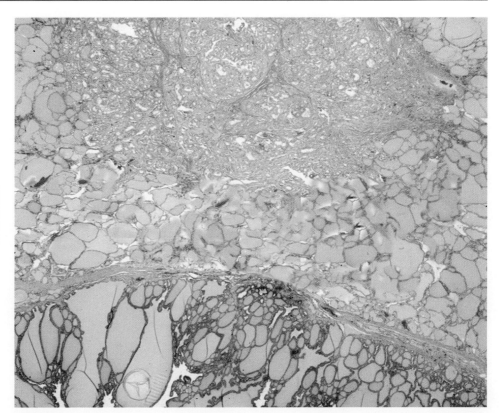

FIGURE 3-16

Adenomatoid nodule (lower half) and papillary carcinoma (upper half) frequently co-exist. There are differences in architecture and cytology, even at this low magnification.

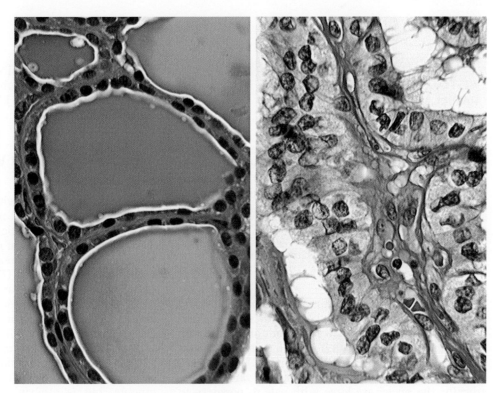

FIGURE 3-17

Left: An adenomatoid nodule has small cells in an orderly arrangement around the follicles with coarse/heavy nuclear chromatin distribution. Right: Papillary carcinoma has large cells with an increased nuclear to cytoplasmic ratio, irregular placement of the nuclei, nuclear contour irregularities, nuclear grooves and folds and delicate to fine nuclear chromatin distribution (identical magnification).

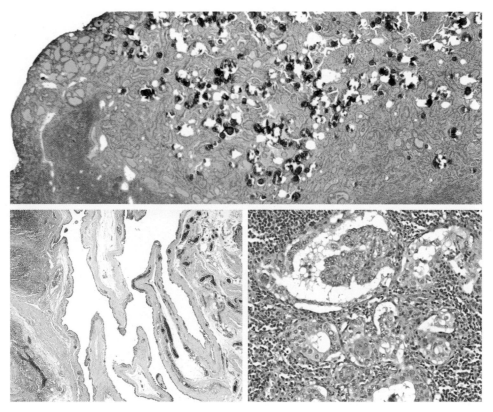

FIGURE 3-18

Upper half: Numerous psammoma bodies and papillary carcinoma have nearly completely replaced this lymph node. Left lower: A predominantly cystic metastasis can sometimes simulate a lymphangioma or branchial cyst. Right lower: Papillary projections and follicles of metastatic papillary carcinoma in a lymph node.

HISTOLOGICAL VARIANTS OF PAPILLARY CARCINOMA

Variants of papillary carcinomas have specific features which may be associated with a different patient outcome or cause difficulty with differential diagnosis. In general, the changes should be the dominant finding to qualify as a histologic variant.

FOLLICULAR VARIANT

Usually encapsulated, the tumor must be exclusively comprised of small, tight follicles with scant, hypereosinophilic colloid. Papillae are absent or vanishingly rare (Figure 3-19), although if enough sections are submitted papillary structures can be found. The nuclear features determine the diagnosis in this variant. Specifically, the nuclei are large with pale to powdery to cleared nuclear chromatin and an increased number of nuclear grooves. Internal sclerosis or fibrosis is seen (Figure 3-20). This variant has no impact on patient management and has an identical outcome to conventional papillary carcinoma.

MACROFOLLICULAR VARIANT

An uncommon variant which is difficult to recognize as it has an architectural resemblance to adenomatoid nodules or hyperplastic nodules (Figure 3-21). The tumor is composed of predominantly large/macrofollicles with a subtle increased cellularity, often accentuated at the periphery (Figure 3-22). The colloid is often scalloped or vacuolated. The nuclei are often flattened and hyperchromatic, although classic papillary nuclei are scattered throughout the tumor (Figure 3-23). Abortive, 'rigid' or straight papillary structures will extend into the center of the colloid filled follicle, usually lined by the atypical cells. This variant seems to metastasize less frequently than classic papillary carcinoma, but is otherwise similar in treatment and outcome.

VARIANTS OF PAPILLARY CARCINOMA

Follicular Variant

▸ Almost exclusively small follicles with scant colloid
▸ Classic nuclear features of papillary carcinoma

Macrofollicular Variant

▸ Enlarged follicles with remaining features similar to follicular variant although nuclei are often flattened
▸ Abortive, rigid papillae may be seen
▸ Separation from adenomatoid nodule is imperative

Oncocytic Variant

▸ >70 % papillary architecture
▸ Enlarged cells with abundant oncocytic cytoplasm, apically oriented enlarged nuclei, increased number of intranuclear cytoplasmic inclusions
▸ Degenerative change common

Clear Cell Variant

▸ Clear cytoplasm, although occasionally oncocytic and clear cells are combined
▸ Must be separated from medullary and metastatic renal cell carcinoma

Diffuse Sclerosing Variant

▸ Diffuse, bilateral involvement, extensive fibrosis, innumerable psammoma bodies, extensive intravascular growth and extrathyroidal extension, florid squamous metaplasia, dense lymphocytic thyroiditis, solid or papillary growth of papillary carcinoma cells

Tall Cell Variant

▸ >70 % of tumor area composed of cells which are at least three times as tall as they are wide, usually oncocytic cytoplasm, sharply defined cellular borders, increased intranuclear cytoplasmic inclusions, centrally placed nuclei within the cell

Columnar Cell Variant

▸ Prominent papillary growth, parallel follicles ('railroad tracks'), scant colloid, syncytial architecture with prominent nuclear stratification, coarse nuclear chromatin, subnuclear cytoplasmic vacuolization, squamous metaplasia as 'morules', and increased mitotic figures

Solid/Insular Variant

▸ Solid or insular pattern with nuclear features of papillary carcinoma

Size variation

▸ Incidentally found, <1 cm papillary carcinoma with a proclivity for thyroid subcapsular location – designated 'microcarcinoma'

ONCOCYTIC VARIANT

The macroscopic appearance is of a deep brown ('mahogany') encapsulated neoplasm, which tends to be large and have cystic change. Lymphocytic infiltrate is common. More than 70 % of the tumor should have complex, arborizing papillary structures (Figure 3-24) with fibrovascular stromal cores lined by enlarged cells with abundant oncocytic (oxyphilic, Askanazy, Hürthle) cytoplasm. The oncocytic cytoplasm is compact and 'glassy' with a fine granularity, representing an increased number of mitochondria. The enlarged nuclei tend to be apically oriented and slightly more hyperchromatic than classic papillary carcinoma (Figures 3-25 and 3-26), with numerous intranuclear cytoplasmic inclusions (the latter a common finding in any tumor with abundant cytoplasm). Psammoma bodies are occasionally present. Degenerative changes are common. The cells are frequently immunoreactive with K19, but this finding is non-specific (Figure 3-26). The diagnosis by FNA is very difficult, but clear nuclei with grooves and inclusions may help to separate it from a follicular neoplasm. Oncocytic cells can be seen in the tall cell variant of papillary carcinoma, from which it should be separated. The patient outcome and management for the oncocytic variant is identical to classical papillary carcinoma.

CLEAR CELL VARIANT

This is a very uncommon variant which predominantly is comprised of cells with clear cytoplasm (Figure 3-27). Papillary or follicular patterns may predominate. Occasionally, a mixture of oncocytic and clear cells may be seen, as clearing results from degeneration of the oncocytic cells. Separation from metastatic renal cell carcinoma or medullary carcinoma can be made by the presence of colloid, but may require the use of TTF-1, thyroglobulin, and calcitonin. The treatment and prognosis are identical to classic papillary carcinoma.

DIFFUSE SCLEROSING VARIANT

Usually developing in young patients (mean, 18 years), the tumor is characterized by diffuse involvement of one or both lobes with nearly 100 % of patients demonstrating cervical lymph node metastasis at the time of presentation. The gland is firm, with white streaks and a gritty cut consistency, with ill defined tumor border if a dominant mass is noted. The histology shows an exaggeration of features of papillary carcinoma, with extensive fibrosis, innumerable psammoma bodies, extensive intravascular and extrathyroidal extension, florid squamous metaplasia and a background of dense lymphocytic thyroiditis (Figures 3-28 and 3-29). Nuclear features of papillary carcinoma are present, often identified in papillary or solid groups of cells within vascular spaces (Figure 3-30). Total thyroidectomy, lymph node dissection and radioablative therapy will yield an excellent long term prognosis despite the 'biologically' aggressive clinical presentation. Lung metastases occurs in up to 25 % of patients, necessitating close and careful patient follow-up.

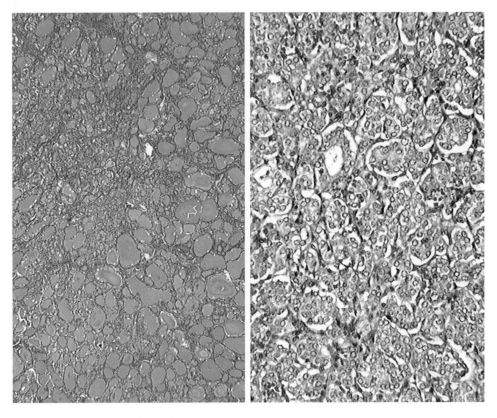

FIGURE 3-19

Left: Small, tight follicles with hypereosinophilic colloid in this follicular variant of papillary carcinoma. Right: Nuclear chromatin clearing and overlap with small tight follicles and no colloid production.

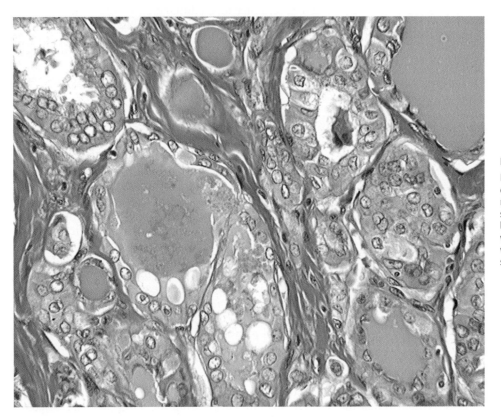

FIGURE 3-20

Follicle formation lined by irregular cells with optically clear nuclei. The nuclear are irregular in shape and size and misplaced around the follicle. Giant cell formation is seen within the hypereosinophilic colloid with scalloping. Tumoral fibrosis separates the follicles.

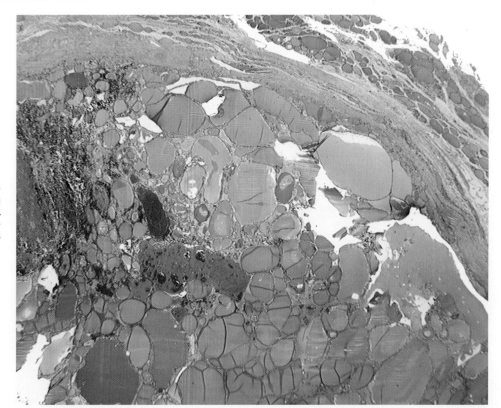

FIGURE 3-21

This macrofollicular variant of papillary carcinoma is surrounded by a capsule, compressing the peripheral parenchyma. The low power resemblance to adenomatoid nodule is deceiving.

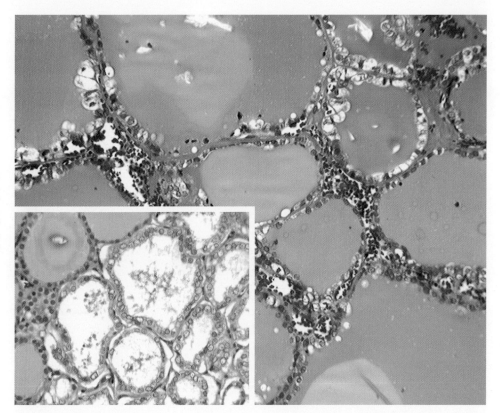

FIGURE 3-22

Large follicles are lined by flattened to atypical follicular cells with scalloped colloid in this macrofollicular variant of papillary carcinoma. Inset demonstrates an area of increased cellularity and the cytologic features of papillary carcinoma.

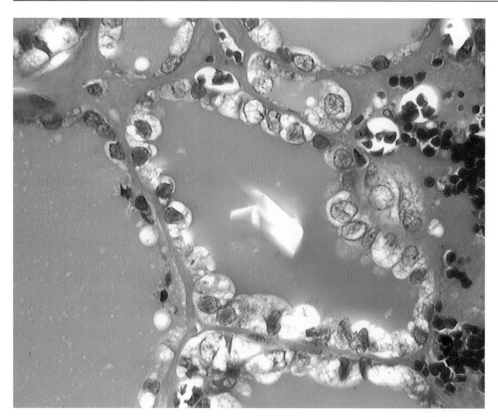

FIGURE 3-23
The nuclear features are well demonstrated in this macrofollicular variant of papillary carcinoma. A crystalloid is seen in the center. Nuclear grooves, nuclear contour irregularities and nuclear chromatin clearing is accentuated.

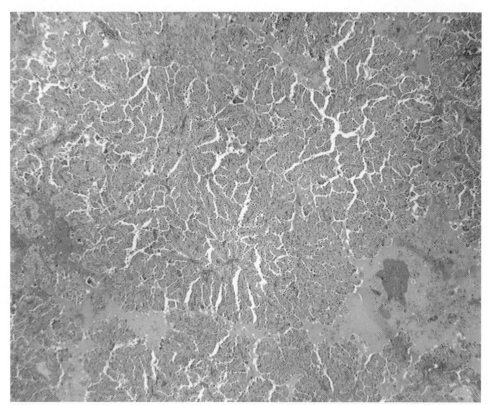

FIGURE 3-24
Complex, arborizing papillary structures are composed of oncocytic cells in this papillary carcinoma variant. Hemorrhage and degeneration is noted.

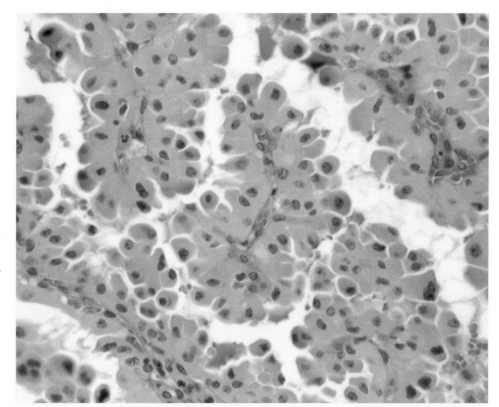

FIGURE 3-25

Tumor nuclei show apical polarization on the papillary fronds with deeply eosinophilic cytoplasm in this oncocytic variant of papillary carcinoma.

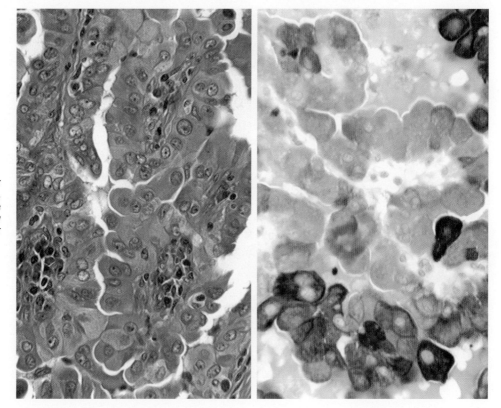

FIGURE 3-26

Left: Oncocytic cells with nuclear features of papillary carcinoma. Right: K19 is known to be positive in the oncocytic variant of papillary carcinoma, but is not specific or sensitive.

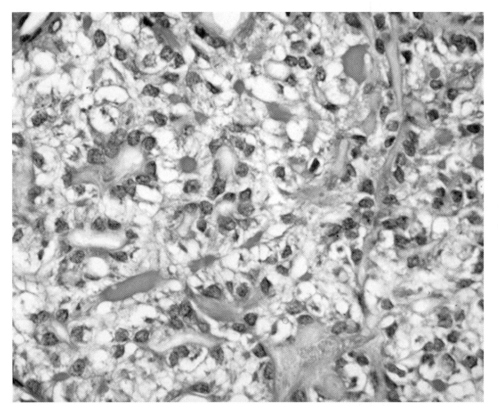

FIGURE 3-27

A cleared cytoplasm dominates this papillary thyroid carcinoma. Colloid is focally noted.

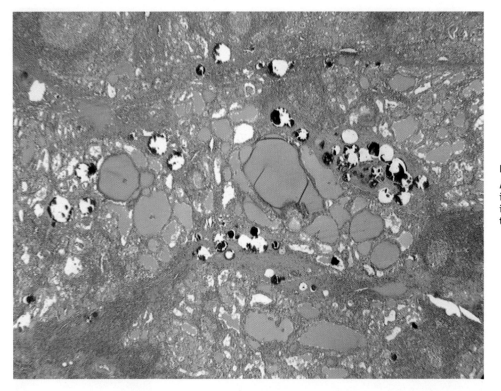

FIGURE 3-28

A low magnification demonstrating innumerable psammoma bodies in clusters with lymphocytic thyroiditis.

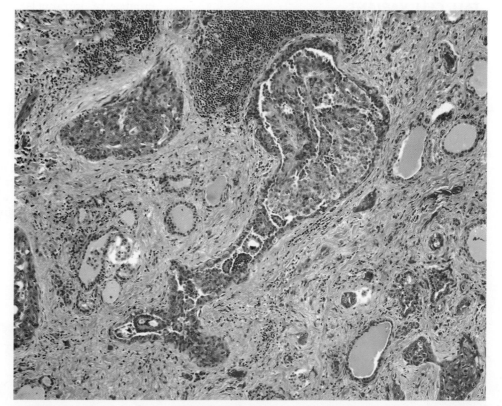

FIGURE 3-29

Dense fibrosis separates the tumor into nodules. Lymph-vascular invasion is noted, along with lymphocytic thyroiditis and squamous metaplasia.

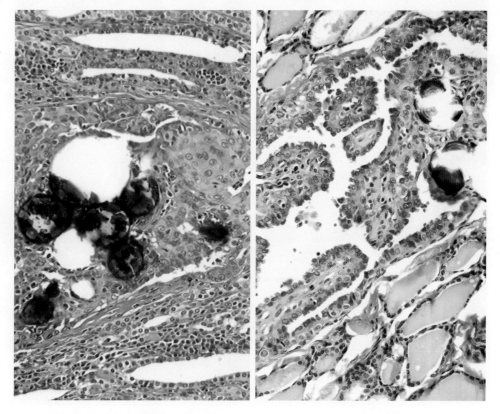

FIGURE 3-30

Left: Papillary carcinoma with squamous metaplasia associated with numerous psammoma bodies. Right: Psammoma bodies and papillary carcinoma are noted within a lymph-vascular channel.

TALL CELL VARIANT

There is controversy as to whether the 'tall cell' is a variant or just a pattern of growth within papillary carcinoma. When this cell type is the dominant finding in the neoplasm (>70% of the tumor area), the patients tend to be older (>60 years) with an increased proportion of men, the tumor tends to be large (>5 cm) and exhibits extrathyroidal extension. Microscopic tumors can occur. Papillary structures and elongated parallel follicles with scant or no colloid are common, along with intratumoral fibrosis. By definition, a tall cell is at least three times as high as it is wide (plane of section must be taken into consideration). There is usually abundant, granular cytoplasm, resulting in an increased number of intranuclear cytoplasmic inclusions and nuclear grooves (Figure 3-31). Intercellular borders are sharply demarcated (Figure 3-32). Necrosis and mitotic activity is present. The nuclei are enlarged with a central position of the nucleus rather than at the lumenal aspect as seen in the oncocytic variant. Since most of these tumors occur in older patients who have large tumors with extrathyroidal extension, perhaps the histologic variant has only a minor influence on the patient's outcome. There does tend to be an increased incidence of lymph node metastasis and hematogenous spread to bone and lung, with a tendency for local recurrence and invasion into adjacent structures. Surgery and adjuvant therapy are necessary, with a worse prognosis than classic papillary carcinoma.

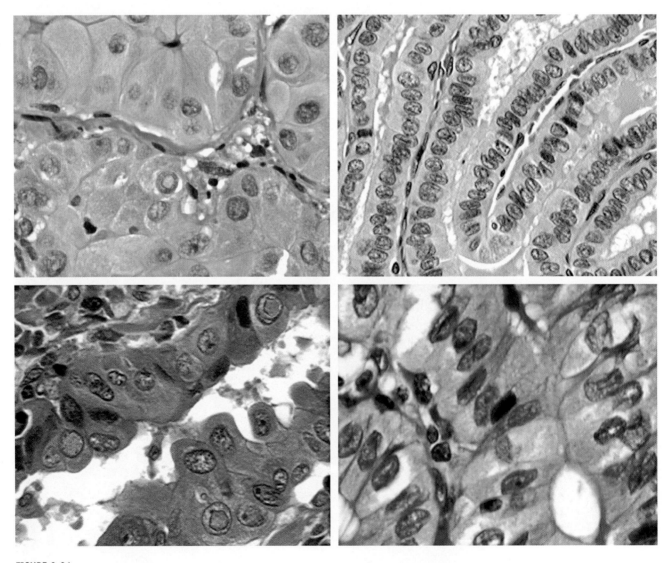

FIGURE 3-31

Various patterns seen in tall cell variant of papillary carcinoma. The cells are each at least three times taller than they are wide with prominent cellular borders. The cytoplasm ranges from oncocytic, amphophilic, basophilic and clear. Intranuclear cytoplasmic inclusions are common.

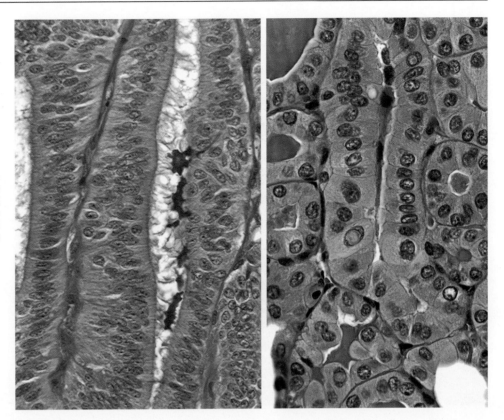

FIGURE 3-32

Left: Columnar variant with pseudostratification of nuclei with no colloid present. Right: Tall cell variant with oncocytic cells, intranuclear cytoplasmic inclusions and cells three times as tall as they are wide.

COLUMNAR CELL VARIANT

Men and women are equally affected by this rare variant. Tumors are usually large (>5 cm) and are encapsulated, but have intra- and extrathyroidal spread. There is prominent papillary growth with markedly elongated, parallel follicles ('railroad tracks') which are separated by scant colloid (Figure 3-33). The cells are tall with a syncytial arrangement. There is prominent nuclear stratification of elongated nuclei with coarse and heavy chromatin deposition, distinctly different from classic papillary carcinoma. Sub-nuclear or supranuclear vacuolization of the cytoplasm is common (Figure 3-34). Squamous metaplasia in the form of 'morules' is common ('endometrioid pattern'; Figure 3-33). Mitotic figures may be present, along with necrosis in a few cases (Figure 3-35). If the patient is older with a large tumor that has extrathyroidal extension, more aggressive surgery and radioablative therapy may be necessary. The prognosis is worse than classic papillary carcinoma.

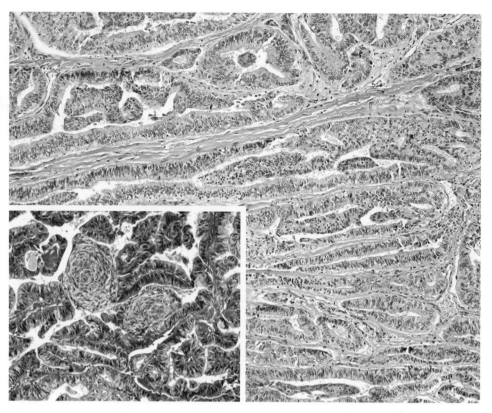

FIGURE 3-33

The cells are arranged in elongated follicles with papillary structures. Fibrosis is seen. The inset demonstrates squamous morules.

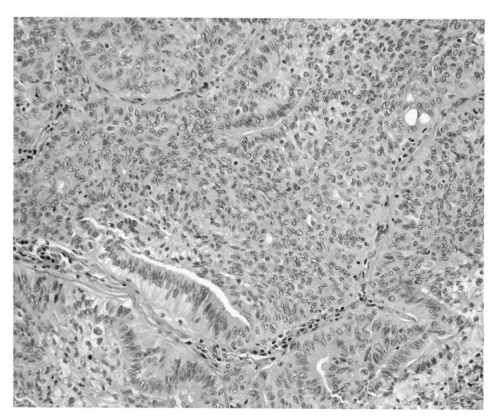

FIGURE 3-34

A syncytial architecture predominates in this tumor. Nuclear stratification with subnuclear vacuoles are noted.

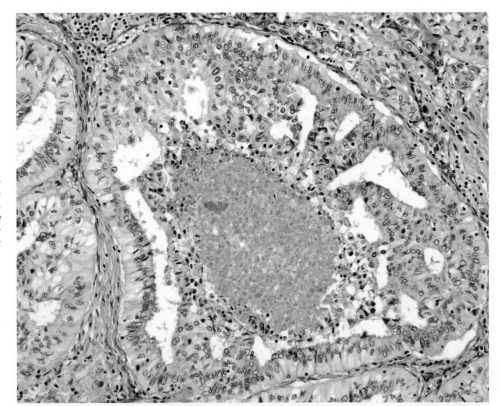

FIGURE 3-35

The tumor cell nuclei have an elongate shape and demonstrate pronounced pseudostratification. Prominent subnuclear vacuoles are seen in cells arranged in a cribriform architecture. Central comedonecrosis is present.

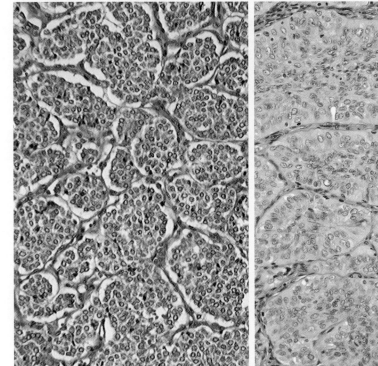

FIGURE 3-36

An insular architecture can be the predominant pattern in any thyroid tumor. Left: Classic papillary carcinoma with an insular architecture. Right: Columnar variant with an insular pattern.

INSULAR/SOLID

Papillary carcinoma may have a solid or insular pattern, with oval nests or islands with scant colloid, and cells with a high nuclear to cytoplasmic ratio (Figure 3-36). Sometimes the pattern is classified as poorly differentiated, but if the nuclear features of papillary carcinoma are present, then this pattern does not influence the management or the outcome.

PAPILLARY CARCINOMA-SIZE VARIATION

Any of the papillary carcinoma variants may be <1 cm in size, which is referred to as microscopic papillary carcinoma, occult or microcarcinoma (Figure 3-37). This qualification should only be applied when the tumor is found incidentally in a thyroid gland removed for other reasons. The tumor has a proclivity to develop in the subcapsular region and is frequently sclerotic with a radiating 'scar-like' infiltration into the surrounding parenchyma (Figure 3-38). The term 'microcarcinoma' should be used for adult patients, since children with small tumors may still have biologically aggressive neoplasms. Separation from intraglandular metastasis may be difficult, although the intravascular location, lack of capsule and sclerosis and lack of 'stellate' growth supports intraglandular metastasis. Most of these tumors are <2 mm in size and are of limited clinical consequence, with an outcome indistinguishable from the general population. Therefore, no additional therapy is necessary for tumors of this size.

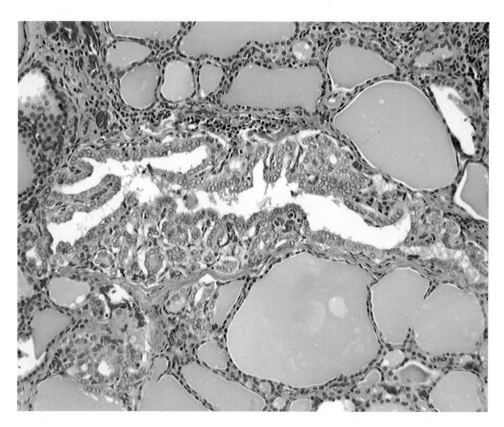

FIGURE 3-37

Microscopic papillary carcinoma is distinct from the surrounding tissue and has both papillary architecture and shows typical nuclear features. Fibrosis is present.

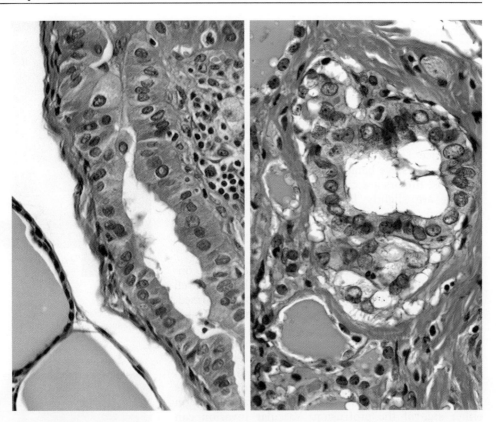

FIGURE 3-38
Left: A tall cell pattern is noted in this microscopic papillary carcinoma. Normal parenchyma is at the left. Right: Sclerosis surrounds this small focus of papillary carcinoma. Normal parenchyma is present at the bottom.

FOLLICULAR CARCINOMA

Follicular carcinoma is the second most common malignant neoplasm of the thyroid gland, defined by invasive growth of a follicular epithelial derived cell that lacks the nuclear features of papillary carcinoma.

CLINICAL FEATURES

About 10–15% of thyroid carcinomas are follicular carcinomas. They are more common in women than men (about 2:1), with a peak incidence in the fifth and sixth decades, although recently the gender difference is not as distinct. The oncocytic type tends to occur in patients about a decade older. Iodine-deficient areas have a higher incidence of follicular carcinoma. Radiation exposure is significantly less important as an epidemiologic factor than in papillary carcinoma. Patients usually present with an asymptomatic solitary, painless thyroid mass, which is usually solid on radiographic imaging. Lymph node metastasis is uncommon, although slightly more common in the oncocytic variant, as hematogenous spread is more common than lymphatic spread.

FOLLICULAR CARCINOMA DISEASE FACT SHEET

Definition
▶ A malignant epithelial neoplasm with follicular cell differentiation and lacking the nuclear features of papillary carcinoma

Incidence and Location
▶ About 10 % of thyroid malignancies
▶ Increased in iodine-deficient areas

Morbidity and Mortality
▶ Recurrent laryngeal nerve damage and hypoparathyroidism
▶ Excellent long term outcome (>90 % 20-year survival)

Gender, Race and Age Distribution
▶ Female > Male
▶ Usually in the fifth decade

Clinical Features
▶ Usually an asymptomatic, palpable mass
▶ Rarely dysphagia or hoarseness

Radiologic Features
▶ Ultrasound shows a solid or cystic mass
▶ CT is useful to determine extent of the mass and lymph node disease
▶ Nuclear scintigraphy no longer necessary or used

Prognosis and Therapy
▶ Excellent long term prognosis (>90 % 20-year survival)
▶ Surgery (lobectomy or thyroidectomy) with radioactive iodine

PATHOLOGIC FEATURES

GROSS FINDINGS

The tumors are usually solitary masses, well circumscribed and surrounded by a variably thick capsule separating them from the uninvolved parenchyma. The cut surface is often bulging and has a light tan to brown appearance (Figure 3-39), although widely invasive tumors often have hemorrhage and necrosis (Figure 3-40). Most tumors are <5 cm in size, although oncocytic tumors are slightly larger. The tumors are rarely multifocal.

MICROSCOPIC FINDINGS

The tumors are surrounded by a variable fibrous connective tissue capsule, which ranges from thick and well formed to thin, irregular, uneven and poorly formed. The diagnostic feature of follicular carcinoma is invasion: capsular and/or vascular penetration. Single or multiple foci of tumor cells identified penetrating into (partial capsule) and through the capsule (entire thickness) are classified as capsular invasion (Figure 3-41). Parenchymal extension is defined by neoplastic cells surrounded by uninvolved thyroid parenchyma on either side of the protrusion. Vascular invasion can

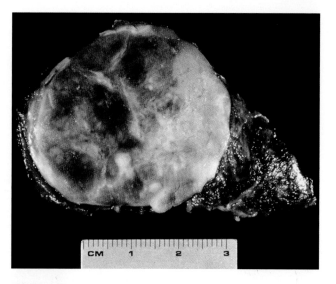

FIGURE 3-39
A solitary mass surrounded by a capsule has a distinctly different appearance from the surrounding uninvolved thyroid parenchyma.

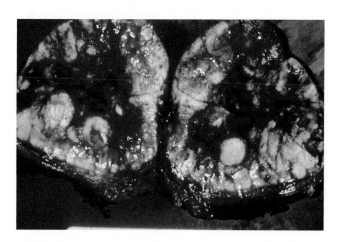

FIGURE 3-40
A widely invasive tumor with central hemorrhage, necrosis and degeneration.

FOLLICULAR CARCINOMA
PATHOLOGIC FEATURES

Gross Findings
▸ Solitary, encapsulated mass
▸ Invasive growth difficult to see on macroscopic examination (in low grade carcinomas)

Microscopic Findings
▸ Capsular and/or vascular invasion (separates into minimally invasive versus widely invasive depending on degree of invasion)
▸ Cellular tumors with follicular, solid and trabecular growth
▸ Slightly enlarged cells with round to oval nuclei and coarse nuclear chromatin
▸ Oncocytic cells often have large, centrally placed macronucleoli within the nuclei

Immunohistochemical Results
▸ Thyroglobulin and TTF-1 positive

Fine Needle Aspiration
▸ Cellular aspirates with dispersed microfollicular arrangements of cells forming small 'ring-like' structures; colloid is scant
▸ Cannot be reliably separated from follicular adenoma and adenomatoid nodules

Pathologic Differential Diagnosis
▸ Follicular adenoma, papillary carcinoma, medullary carcinoma and adenomatoid nodules

---

involve single or multiple foci within small, medium, or large vessels (Figure 3-42). Small vessels, usually within the capsule, have a limited caliber, while medium sized vessels with or without smooth muscle walls, are noted within or immediately adjacent to the capsule. Vascular invasion is defined by direct extension of tumor cells into the vessel lumen, tumor thrombi adherent to the vessel wall (often associated with blood clot), and/or tumor nests covered by endothelium. Tumor plugs in vascular spaces *within* the tumor mass do not qualify as vascular invasion; nor do detached or artifactually dislodged tumor fragments free floating in vascular spaces. An intravascular organizing thrombus (Masson's disease) does not qualify as invasion.

Many different patterns of growth can be seen in follicular carcinoma (follicular, trabecular, insular, solid; Figure 3-43). The tumors are usually cellular with

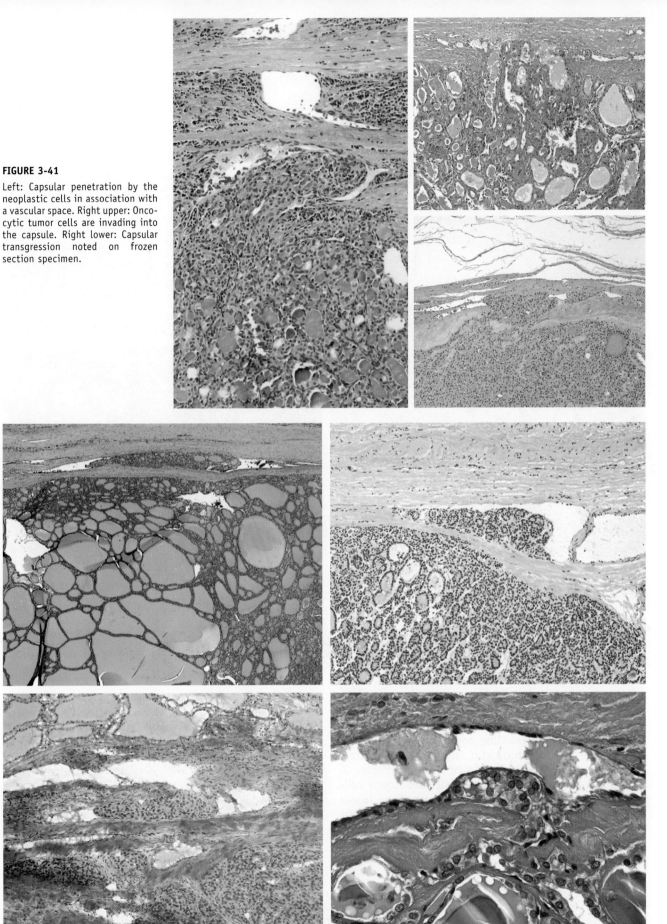

FIGURE 3-41

Left: Capsular penetration by the neoplastic cells in association with a vascular space. Right upper: Onco-cytic tumor cells are invading into the capsule. Right lower: Capsular transgression noted on frozen section specimen.

FIGURE 3-42

Vascular invasion in follicular carcinoma. Left upper: Tumor thrombus filling a vascular space. Left lower: A frozen section showing tumor attached to the wall of an intermediate vessel. Right upper: A tumor fragment attached to a vessel wall within the tumor capsule. Right lower: The point of vascular invasion is noted, with an endothelial lining covering the tumor nest.

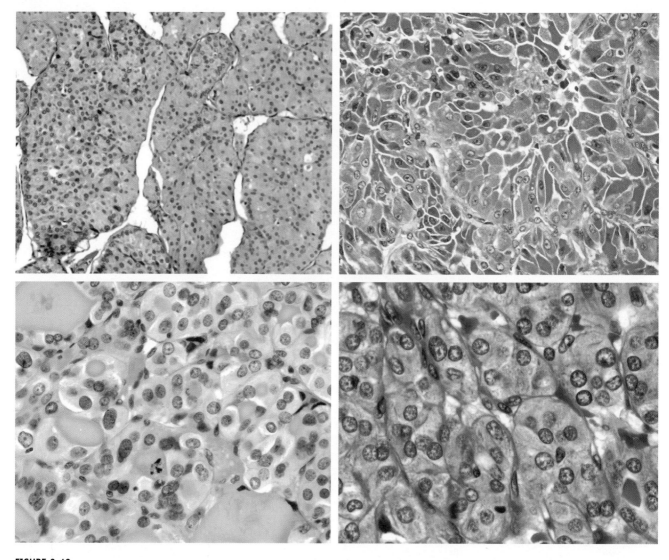

FIGURE 3-43

Patterns of growth and cytoplasmic appearance of follicular carcinoma. Left upper: Trabecular pattern with granular cytoplasm. Left lower: Slight nuclear variability in a follicular pattern. Right upper: Solid pattern with oncocytic cytoplasm. Right lower: Insular growth with focal colloid.

colloid easily identified (Figure 3-44). Oncocytic cells (cytoplasmic oxyphilia, 'Askanazy-cell' or Hürthle cell) have fine to slightly coarse, granular, abundant eosinophilic cytoplasm surrounding round to regular nuclei with coarse nuclear chromatin and frequently prominent, eosinophilic, centrally placed nucleoli (Figure 3-43). While the majority of cases will have tumor cells which are round and regular, occasionally, focal tumor cell spindling may be present (Figure 3-45). Mitotic figures and necrosis can be seen (Figure 3-46), but degenerative changes are more common, especially in the central regions of the tumor or post fine needle aspiration.

A number of variants or qualifiers are used in describing follicular carcinomas, identified as follows:

- *Minimally invasive:* limited capsular and/or vascular invasion, although exact number of foci is undefined. Invasion is limited to small or medium capsular or pericapsular vascular spaces.

- *Widely invasive:* uncommon type with extensive infiltration beyond the tumor capsule ('mushroom' invasion), into large vessels, and shows nodules of tumor within the parenchyma. As the degree of invasion increases, the biologic behavior becomes more aggressive (Figures 3-40, 3-47 and 3-48).

- *Oncocytic variant:* greater than 75% of the tumor is composed of oncocytic cells (Figure 3-43), the cytoplasm of which are filled with abnormal mitochondria (abnormal dense bodies).The tumors have scant or absent colloid, occasionally containing calcifications which can resemble psammoma bodies. The nuclei often contain large, centrally placed, eosinophilic nucleoli. There is no difference in outcome or management, although follicular carcinomas with oncocytic cells tend to occur in older patients, have larger tumors, and more commonly have lymph node metastasis (up to 30%). FNA will frequently result in infarction with associated hemorrhage, cyst formation and eventual fibrosis.

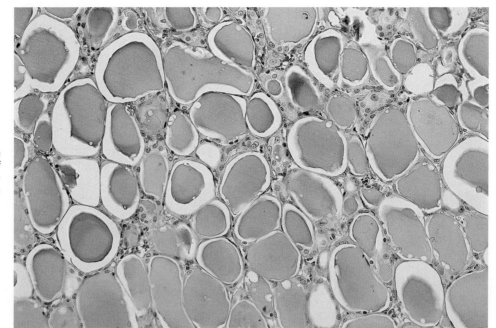

FIGURE 3-44

Abundant colloid is noted with the nuclei compressed to the edges of the follicles in this minimally invasive follicular carcinoma (invasion is not shown in this field).

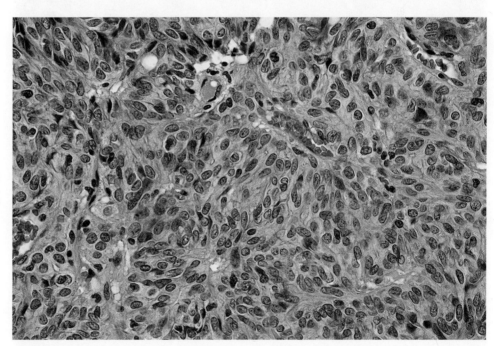

FIGURE 3-45

Focal tumor cell spindling is noted within this follicular carcinoma. Colloid is not appreciated in this focus.

• *Clear cell variant:* any tumor may have clear cell change, especially prominent in oncocytic neoplasms. It should be the dominant finding for this variant to be diagnosed.

ANCILLARY STUDIES

IMMUNOHISTOCHEMICAL RESULTS

Immunohistochemistry may be of value in confirming that the neoplasm is of follicular derivation, but it is seldom necessary for diagnostic purposes. The cells would be thyroglobulin, TTF-1, and CK7 immunoreactive, while chromogranin and calcitonin are negative. Stains for endothelial markers (CD34, CD31, factor VIII-RAg) to accentuate vessels is of only limited value, as the endothelial cells are frequently discontinuous or lost in deeper sections, making interpretation difficult.

FINE NEEDLE ASPIRATION

Separation between adenomatoid nodule, follicular adenoma and follicular carcinoma relies on the

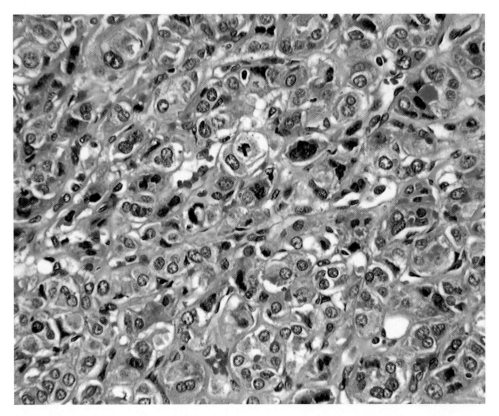

FIGURE 3-46

Nuclear pleomorphism and mitotic figures, including atypical forms can be seen in a number of different follicular neoplasms. Invasion would be required to confirm the diagnosis of follicular carcinoma.

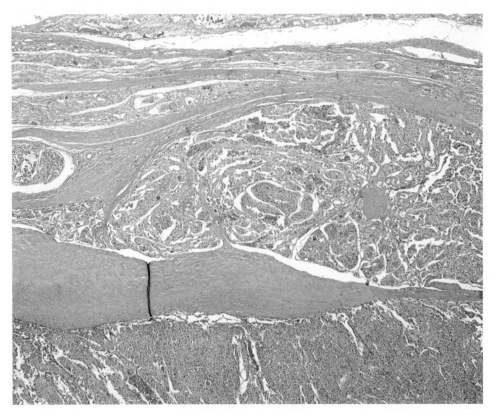

FIGURE 3-47

Large projections of tumor beyond the contour of the lesion with vascular invasion is diagnostic of a widely invasive follicular carcinoma.

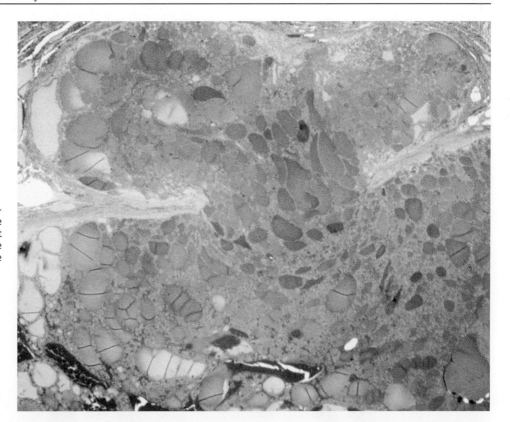

FIGURE 3-48

A large, 'mushroom-shaped' projection of neoplastic cells out into the surrounding parenchyma. Note that the capsule has 'traveled' with the tumor and is still present at the advancing edge.

demonstration of capsular or vascular invasion, making FNA of no value in making such a distinction. However, FNA is an excellent screening tool. The aspirates are hypercellular with a dispersed microfollicular architecture or small three-dimensional clusters. The cells are enlarged with uniform, round nuclei with coarse nuclear chromatin. Nuclear size and shape variability may be present (Figure 3-49). Oncocytic cells may be the dominant finding (Figure 3-50). There is usually scant or absent colloid. These findings are reported as 'thyroid follicular epithelial proliferation, favor neoplasm', which translates into a tumor requiring surgical excision.

MOLECULAR ANALYSIS

Many follicular carcinomas (up to 40 %) will demonstrate rearrangements of the peroxisome proliferator-activated receptor gamma ($PPAR\gamma$) gene, which produces a number of fusion proteins of which $PAX8$-$PPAR\gamma$ is the most common. Additionally, RAS mutations are identified in about 45 % of follicular carcinomas and $p53$ alterations in about 10 %. However, the detection techniques are not universally detected, and there is some overlap with follicular adenomas, papillary carcinoma, and anaplastic carcinoma. This suggests additional studies are necessary before these molecular techniques are incorporated into daily use.

DIFFERENTIAL DIAGNOSIS

Follicular adenoma and cellular adenomatoid nodules, especially those with degenerative fibrosis, are some-

times difficult to separate from minimally invasive or low grade follicular carcinoma. Neoplasms usually have muscle-walled vessels in the fibrous capsule, while an adenomatoid nodule usually does not. Tangential sectioning, irregular tumor contour, fine needle aspiration, and frozen section artifacts all hamper interpretation (Figure 3-51). Adequate sampling of the *tumor-to-capsule-to-parenchymal* interface (at least one section per cm of tumor) is imperative before resorting to 'atypical follicular adenoma' or 'follicular neoplasm of uncertain malignant potential'.

Follicular variant of papillary carcinoma may occasionally be a problem, although the nuclear features should assist in the distinction. Medullary carcinoma can occasionally be oncocytic, but the nuclei tend to be finely stippled (neuroendocrine) and the cells are chromogranin, calcitonin and CEA immunoreactive. In the clear cell neoplasms, parathyroid tumors and metastatic renal cell carcinoma may need to be separated from follicular carcinoma by using immunohistochemical studies along with the clinical history.

PROGNOSIS AND THERAPY

There has been a change in patient outcome over the past decades, especially with more neoplasms being found earlier in their development and with correct classification as minimally invasive. Overall, minimally invasive follicular carcinoma have a >95 % 20-year survival, with survival curves approaching those of normal age and gender matched controls. Widely invasive tumors, on the other hand, portend a more aggressive biologic behavior with an approximately 30% 10-year survival. In any tumor type or grade, if metastasis develops, it occurs most commonly in lungs and bone, although the oncocytic type may have a higher frequency of lymph node metastases. When follicular carcinomas are stratified by gender, age, size and extent of invasion, there is no difference in recurrence or patient outcome when controlling for variant type, specifically oncocytic variant. Therefore, 'oncocytic' follicular car-

cinomas should be managed in a fashion identical to follicular carcinoma.

Conservative resection (lobectomy) versus radical surgery (total thyroidectomy) does not seem to yield statistically significant differences in patient outcome. Therefore, the most conservative treatment to completely remove the tumor is advocated. Staging of follicular carcinomas is discussed in the TNM classification appendix.

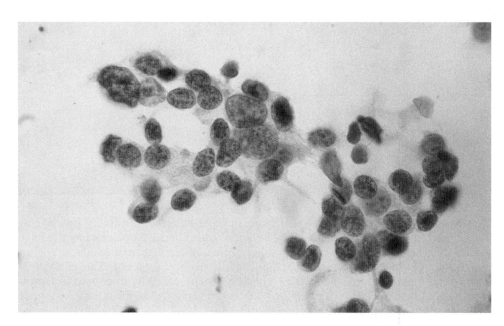

FIGURE 3-49

A FNA smear showing a microfollicular pattern with nuclear size and shape variability. (Papanicolau preparation).

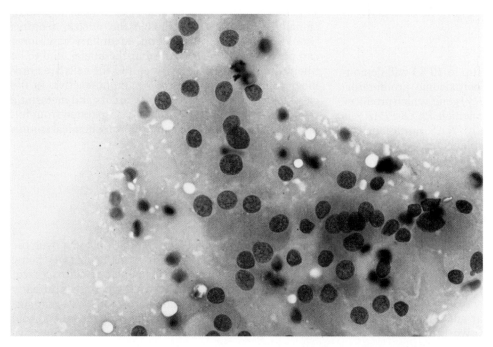

FIGURE 3-50

Small follicles and sheets of oncocytic cells in a 'thyroid follicular epithelial proliferation, favor neoplasm' FNA. (air dried preparation).

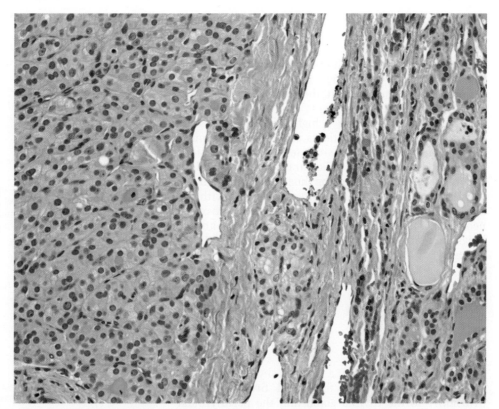

FIGURE 3-51
Entrapment of tumor cells between two vessels must not be over interpreted as capsular or vascular invasion. This represents entrapment in a follicular adenoma.

UNDIFFERENTIATED CARCINOMA

Accounting for <5% of all thyroid gland neoplasms, undifferentiated carcinoma (also known as *anaplastic carcinoma* and *pleomorphic carcinoma*), is a highly malignant neoplasm composed of undifferentiated cells which require immunohistochemical or ultrastructural support for their epithelial origin. All are T4 tumors by definition.

UNDIFFERENTIATED CARCINOMA DISEASE FACT SHEET

Definition
▶ Highly malignant neoplasm composed of undifferentiated cells that exhibit immunohistochemical or ultrastructural epithelial differentiation

Incidence and Location
▶ <5 % of all thyroid malignancies
▶ Higher in endemic goiter regions and in Europe

Morbidity and Mortality
▶ >90 % die of disease usually within 6 months

Gender, Race and Age Distribution
▶ Female > Male (1.5 : 1)
▶ Most patients >60 years

Clinical Features
▶ Rapidly expanding neck mass
▶ Usually have underlying long history of thyroid disease
▶ Hoarseness, dysphagia, and pain are common

Prognosis and Therapy
▶ Poor prognosis, >90 % die of disease usually in <6 months
▶ Surgery

CLINICAL FEATURES

The vast majority of patients are over 60 years, but the sharp female predilection for other thyroid gland neoplasms is not sustained in this neoplasm: the female to male ratio is 1.5:1. Patients who live in endemic goiter areas tend to have a higher incidence of this tumor. Nearly all of the patients present with a rapidly enlarging neck mass, often associated with a long history of thyroid disease (goiter, follicular carcinoma, papillary carcinoma). Furthermore, the hoarseness, dysphagia, vocal cord paralysis and pain often associated with the mass are indications of the widely invasive nature of the neoplasm. Metastases to cervical lymph nodes and/or lungs are noted at clinical presentation in about 50% of patients.

PATHOLOGIC FEATURES

GROSS FINDINGS

The tumors are usually a large, fleshy, pale-tan solitary mass (60%), often fixed and firm. Extensive invasion into the thyroid gland and the perithyroidal tissues is common: muscle, adipose tissue, trachea and esophagus. Necrosis and hemorrhage are almost ubiquitous.

MICROSCOPIC FINDINGS

The remarkably infiltrative tumor is comprised of a combination of pleomorphic, spindle and epithelioid cells arranged in solid sheets to fascicular bundles which nearly completely efface the thyroid parenchyma (Figures 3-52 to 3-54). One of the cell types may predominate; the spindle cell type often resembles various different sarcomas (Figure 3-53). Tumor giant cells filled with bizarre nuclei are common; non-tumor osteoclast-like giant cells are described infrequently (Figure 3-54). Squamous differentiation is also occasionally noted. Mitotic figures, including atypical forms, and necrosis are prominent features (Figure 3-54). A rich acute inflammatory infiltrate and a vascular component may also be present, the later a mimic of angiosarcoma (anastomosing) or hemangiopericytoma (staghorn). Colloid is absent within the tumor. Thoroughly sampled tumors will often demonstrate foci of papillary (Figure 3-52) or follicular carcinoma, suggesting dedifferentiation of a pre-existing neoplasm in the development of undifferentiated carcinoma.

ANCILLARY STUDIES

IMMUNOHISTOCHEMICAL RESULTS

Cytokeratin and epithelial membrane antigen are the most commonly identified 'epithelial' markers, present

---

UNDIFFERENTIATED CARCINOMA PATHOLOGIC FEATURES

Gross Findings

▶ Large, fleshy masses with necrosis and hemorrhage
▶ Infiltrating, often into adjacent soft tissues and organs

Microscopic Findings

▶ Poorly differentiated cells
▶ Polygonal, spindle and epithelioid
▶ Profound pleomorphism
▶ Tumor giant cells and osteoclast-like giant cells are common
▶ Increased mitotic figures, including atypical forms
▶ Necrosis, hemorrhage and degeneration

Immunohistochemical Results

▶ Keratin and EMA, in up to 80% of cases
▶ Vimentin in nearly all cases
▶ Thyroglobulin and TTF-1 are rarely positive

Ultrastructural Features

▶ Tight cell junctions and tonofilaments (although EM is usually not performed)

Fine Needle Aspiration

▶ Highly cellular with single cells and focal clusters composed of remarkable atypical cells; mitotic figures are prominent; background necrosis can be seen

Pathologic Differential Diagnosis

▶ Exclude metastatic disease to thyroid; primary thyroid sarcomas and anaplastic lymphoma

---

in up to 80% of cases, but often limited to focal areas and/or isolated cells (pleomorphic, spindle, and/or epithelioid cells). Vimentin is strongly positive. Thyroglobulin and TTF-1 are usually not identified. *TP53* mutations are common, with strong reactivity for this marker. When confronted with the differential diagnostic considerations, other specific sarcoma markers may help to separate these neoplasm. These markers may include desmin, myo-D1, smooth muscle actin, CD31, CD34, S-100 protein, HMB-45, CD30 and CD45RB.

FINE NEEDLE ASPIRATION

Aspirates are highly cellular, composed of single cells, small clusters or sheets of large, highly pleomorphic cells (Figure 3-55). Cytoplasm is often abundant, with prominent nucleoli. Mitotic figures, necrosis and acute inflammatory cells are present. While a diagnosis of 'poorly differentiated malignant neoplasm' can be rendered, separation between primary and metastatic tumor, and whether it is a carcinoma, sarcoma, lymphoma or melanoma would require ancillary techniques.

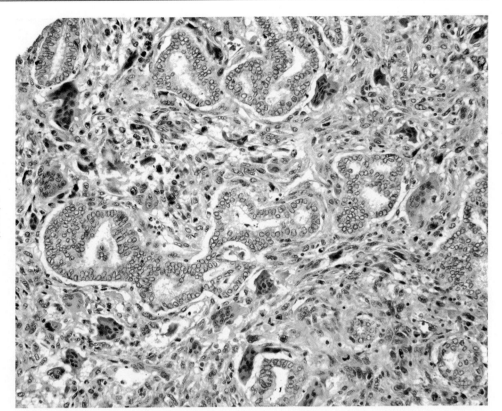

FIGURE 3-52

An undifferentiated carcinoma arising in association with papillary carcinoma. The undifferentiated component has spindle and giant cell features.

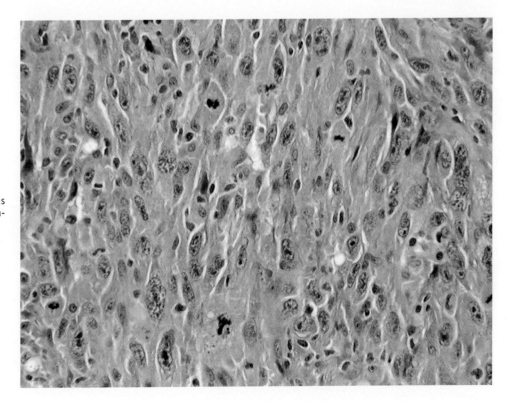

FIGURE 3-53

The spindle cells with numerous atypical mitoses comprise this anaplastic carcinoma.

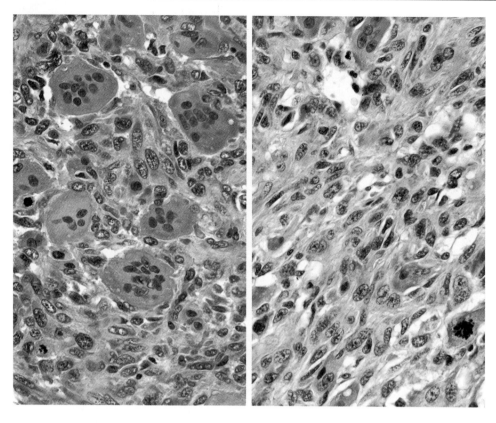

FIGURE 3-54
Left: Numerous osteoclast-like giant cells compose this tumor. Mitotic figures are noted. Right: Atypical mitotic figures and undifferentiated spindle cells are common findings in undifferentiated carcinoma.

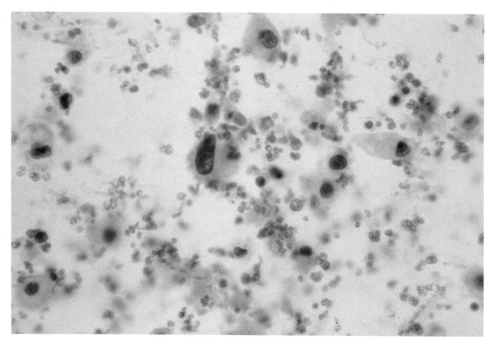

FIGURE 3-55
A fine needle demonstrates single cells with remarkable atypia in this undifferentiated carcinoma.

DIFFERENTIAL DIAGNOSIS

Metastatic tumors to the thyroid gland present the most common differential diagnostic difficulty, although primary sarcomas and lymphomas of the thyroid may also occur. A selection of various immunohistochemical markers will usually help make the separation.

PROGNOSIS AND THERAPY

The extremely grave clinical outcome of >90% of patients dying from disease in <6 months accounts for over 50% of *all* thyroid cancer deaths. In spite of surgery and combination multimodality therapy, the adverse prognosis seems unaltered. Only rarely will patients have a better prognosis when the undifferentiated carcinoma is a minor component of a thyroid neoplasm which has been completely excised and aggressively managed with adjuvant chemotherapy and radiation.

MEDULLARY CARCINOMA

The ultimobranchial body is thought to give rise to C-cells (parafollicular cells) which tend to be aggregated in the upper and middle lobes of the thyroid gland. Calcitonin is the main peptide secreted by these cells, a hormone involved in calcium homeostasis, usually causing the kidneys to secrete calcium and inhibiting osteoclastic bone resorption. Calcitonin gene-related peptide (CGRP) is also present, but tends to occur in extrathyroidal sites. The malignant neuroendocrine neoplasm of the thyroid gland with C-cell differentiation is referred to as medullary carcinoma. This tumor has a strong familial or inherited association with the multiple endocrine neoplasia (MEN) syndromes as well as other inherited forms of medullary carcinoma when there is a germ-line mutation in the *RET* proto-oncogene.

CLINICAL FEATURES

About 5–10% of all thyroid neoplasms are medullary carcinoma. The sporadic (non-familial) and inherited (familial) forms of the tumor determine the clinical presentation, although nearly 80% of medullary carcinoma are sporadic. In spite of this frequency, exclusion of an inherited form of the disease is mandatory.

Sporadic medullary carcinoma is slightly more common in women than men and tends to occur in the middle decades of life (fifth and sixth decades). Patients usually present with a unilateral palpable thyroid mass,

---

MEDULLARY CARCINOMA DISEASE FACT SHEET

Definition
▶ A malignant tumor of the thyroid gland showing C-cell differentiation

Incidence and Location
▶ About 5–10% of thyroid malignancies
▶ 80% sporadic; 20% inherited (familial)
▶ Usually develops in upper to middle thyroid lobes (never isthmus)

Morbidity and Mortality
▶ Other disorders associated with familial disease (MEN)
▶ About 50% at 5 years, stage and familial disease dependent

Gender, Race and Age Distribution
▶ Female > Male
▶ Fifth and sixth decades for sporadic; third decade for familial types

Clinical Features
▶ Sporadic cases usually have a unilateral, solitary thyroid mass
▶ Familial cases have multicentric and bilateral thyroid gland enlargement
▶ Frequently discovered as part of evaluation of parathyroid, adrenal, pituitary, pancreas and gastrointestinal disease (MEN syndrome), in which thyroid symptoms may be sub-clinical
▶ Lymphadenopathy is common (about 50% of patients at clinical presentation)
▶ Serum calcitonin levels elevated in both types

Radiologic Features
▶ ^{131}I-meta-iodobenzylguanidine (MIBG) positive mass

Prognosis and Therapy
▶ Clinical stage and inherited type dependent
▶ Excellent prognosis for small tumors confined to the thyroid, incidentally discovered and without lymph node metastases (100%)
▶ Women, <40 years, calcitonin rich, and abundant amyloid tumors have better prognosis
▶ Overall about 70–80% 10-year survival
▶ Total thyroidectomy and central lymph node dissection
▶ Chemotherapy and radiation usually not employed
▶ Screening identifies a 10–15% familial incidence

---

with nearly 50% having cervical lymphadenopathy at presentation. Serum calcitonin levels are almost invariably elevated, a finding not usually seen in other types of neuroendocrine carcinomas.

Familial medullary carcinoma may be found while the diseases of the MEN syndromes are being evaluated in the parathyroid, adrenal, pituitary, pancreas and gastrointestinal tract. These syndromes have an autosomal dominant mode of inheritance. MEN 2A is most frequently associated with familial medullary carcinoma. The patients usually present at a young age (mean, third decade) with multicentric and bilateral thyroid lobe nodules/enlargement. If there is an association with

MEN 2B, the patients are even younger, with the mucosal neuromas often bringing the patient to clinical attention. Neuromas of the oral cavity, lips, tongue, and gastrointestinal tract may present with clinical findings which are similar to Hirshsprung's disease, but a rectal biopsy will reveal the distinction. It is important to note that the signs and symptoms of the MEN syndrome may dominate the clinical presentation, with none of the findings referable to calcitonin increase. Diarrhea and flushing is more common in patients with very high levels of calcitonin (for which there is no medical treatment). Therefore, a careful and complete evaluation is necessary to make this determination. Non-MEN related, but still inherited forms of medullary carcinoma are less common and often present at the same age as the sporadic cases.

RADIOLOGIC FEATURES

CT and ultrasound often show only a mass lesion. However, ^{131}I-meta-iodobenzylguanidine (MIBG) scintigraphy will greatly aid in the diagnosis. This radiopharmaceutical and guanethidine analog, is a radiocompound that shows a remarkable affinity for neural crest derived tissues and tumors that belong to the dispersed neuroendocrine system (DNES), where it is taken up by neurotransmitter vesicles. Therefore, medullary carcinoma will 'light-up' with this technique, confirming the neuroendocrine nature of the neoplasm.

PATHOLOGIC FEATURES

GROSS FINDINGS

Sporadic tumors are usually unilateral, solitary masses, while familial tumors are multifocal and bilateral, usually located in the middle to upper third of each lobe. Depending upon the symptoms and whether familial or not, the tumor can be 'microscopic' to completely replacing the thyroid lobe. Tumors are usually circumscribed, but infiltration can be seen. The cut section is tan, yellow to pink, and is soft to rubbery or firm. A gritty cut surface represents the calcifications that may be seen.

MICROSCOPIC FINDINGS

Normal C-cells are difficult to identify on routine light microscopy. They are small polygonal to spindle shaped cells identified immediately adjacent to or within thyroid follicles. The nuclei are pale and the cytoplasm is often clear or slightly granular (Figure 3-56). Solid cells nests are thought to be remnants of the ultimobranchial body (Figure 3-57), and are nests of pavemented cells without intercellular bridges. They are found in the

---

MEDULLARY CARCINOMA PATHOLOGIC FEATURES

Gross Findings
▸ Sporadic tumors are unilateral and solitary
▸ Familial tumors are multifocal and bilateral
▸ Usually encapsulated with a tan-yellow soft to firm cut surface
▸ Calcifications can be seen

Microscopic Findings
▸ Pre-neoplastic C-cell hyperplasia has bilateral nodules of >50 cells per aggregate
▸ Multitude of patterns of growth
▸ Entrapment of benign follicular epithelial cells common
▸ Round to oval, spindled to plasmacytoid cells
▸ Round to oval nuclei with stippled, 'salt-and-pepper' nuclear chromatin
▸ Intranuclear cytoplasmic inclusions common
▸ Mitotic figures and necrosis is uncommon
▸ Amyloid is present in up to 80 % of tumors

Immunohistochemical Results
▸ Chromogranin, calcitonin, keratin, and CEA positive
▸ TTF-1 positive and thyroglobulin non-reactive
▸ Amyloid positive (although Congo red apple-green birefringence is easier to interpret)

Fine Needle Aspiration
▸ Cellular aspirates with single cells and small, loosely cohesive clusters
▸ Colloid absent but amyloid present
▸ Round to oval, spindle to polygonal cells
▸ Bi- and multinucleated cells with moderate pleomorphism
▸ Plasmacytoid appearance with eccentric nucleus placement
▸ Stippled to coarse nuclear chromatin
▸ Metachromatic red cytoplasmic granules on air-dried preparations

Pathologic Differential Diagnosis
▸ C-cell hyperplasia can mimic intraglandular spread, solid cell nests and palpation thyroiditis
▸ Follicular adenoma/carcinoma, paraganglioma, hyalinizing trabecular tumor, amyloid goiter and lymphoma

---

upper and outer lobes of the thyroid gland, frequently found incidentally in thyroid glands removed for different reasons.

- *Precursor lesion:* C-cell hyperplasia is thought to be either reactive (physiologic or secondary; Figure 3-58) or pre-neoplastic, with the pre-neoplastic hyperplasia considered the precursor of heritable medullary carcinoma (Figure 3-59). Many subjective points of separation exist. However, if there are aggregations of more than 50 C-cells, and especially if identified in nodules, bilaterally, or diffusely, pre-neoplastic C-cell hyperplasia is diagnosed. This form will have germline mutations in the *RET* proto-oncogene. These small aggregates are often noted adjacent to medullary carcinoma (Figure 3-60). Furthermore, if the tumor is <1 cm, the term 'microcarcinoma' may be employed. Physiologic C-cell hyperplasia usually is

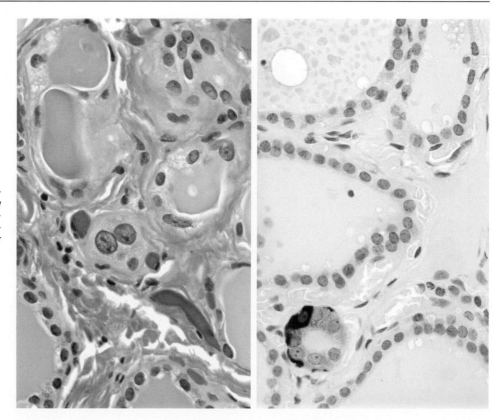

FIGURE 3-56

Left: Normal C-cells have a parafollicular distribution with slightly basophilic cytoplasm. Right: Individual C-cells are calcitonin immunoreactive (heavy, dark, granular cytoplasmic immunoreactivity).

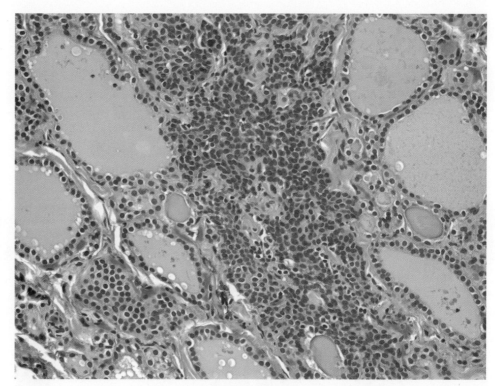

FIGURE 3-57

Solid cell nests with oval nuclei with coarse nuclear chromatin and a lack of intercellular borders.

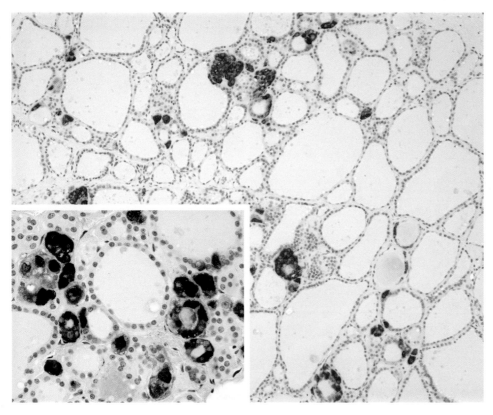

FIGURE 3-58
The small aggregates of C-cells are part of a physiologic response to chronic disease, aging or other abnormalities. No nest contains >50 cells, the nodules do not coalesce, and there is no associated fibrosis or amyloid. Inset demonstrates small groups of cells, but usually still in a parafollicular distribution without destruction of the parenchyma (calcitonin immunohistochemistry).

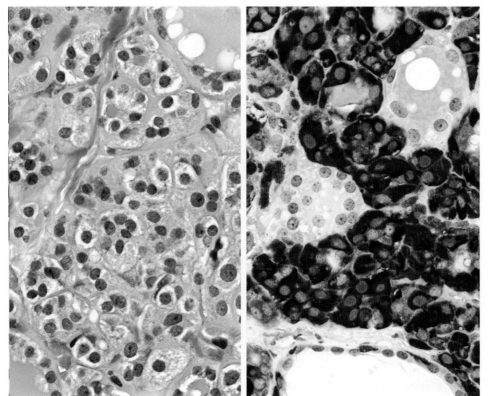

FIGURE 3-59
Left: Pre-neoplastic C-cell hyperplasia shows aggregates of >50 C-cells with associated fibrosis. A small uninvolved thyroid follicle is present (upper right). Right: Calcitonin immunohistochemistry accentuates the cells around the thyroid follicles.

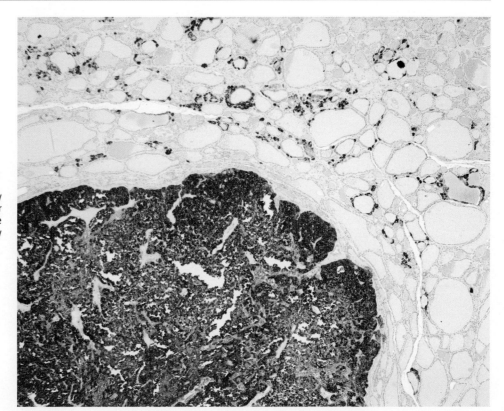

FIGURE 3-60
The medullary carcinoma is strongly and diffusely immunoreactive for calcitonin. Groups of C-cells are highlighted around the medullary carcinoma.

not identified by standard H&E, and is composed of normal appearing C-cells of <50 cells per aggregate. With increased experience, physiologic C-cells can be seen by H&E, with calcitonin used as confirmation. This type of response is seen in aging, chronic disease, renal disorders, hyperparathyroidism, and lymphocytic thyroiditis, just to name a few.

• *Medullary carcinoma*: The borders are irregular, circumscribed to encapsulated, with tumor cells extending out into the thyroid parenchyma, entrapping benign, uninvolved follicular epithelium (Figure 3-61). In very large tumors, extension into adjacent soft tissues and neck organs may be present. A host of different patterns of growth are observed in medullary carcinoma and include solid sheets, organoid, lobular, trabecular, insular, glandular, tubular and papillary patterns; cell types include spindle, oncocytic, clear and amphicrine (Figures 3-62 and 3-63). The various patterns of growth are separated by a fibrovascular stroma. The cells are round to oval, spindled to plasmacytoid cells. The nuclei are usually round to oval and are surrounding by ill-defined eosinophilic or amphophilic, granular cytoplasm. Bi- and multinucleation is common, with moderate nuclear pleomorphism present. The chromatin is coarse to stippled and 'salt-and-pepper' in distribution. Nucleoli are not prominent. Intranuclear cytoplasmic inclusions can be identified. An increased mitotic index and necrosis is usually identified only in large tumors. Amyloid, a homogenous, acellular, eosinophilic, extracellular matrix material is seen in most cases (up to 80%; Figure 3-64). Mucin production is occasionally noted, but is of limited amount.

ANCILLARY STUDIES

IMMUNOHISTOCHEMICAL RESULTS

C-cells are easily accentuated by calcitonin (Figure 3-60) or chromogranin (synaptophysin too), while keratin and polyclonal carcinoembryonic antigen (CEA) are also reactive.

Argyrophilic stains (Grimelius stain) can be employed, but calcitonin, chromogranin and CEA are easier to interpret in medullary carcinoma. It is important to know that medullary carcinoma is also TTF-1 reactive although not positive with thyroglobulin (Figure 3-65). Polarization of a Congo red stain will give the characteristic apple-green birefringence when amyloid is present. Crystal violet can be used as an alternate stain. Occasionally, amyloid immunohistochemistry may be performed, but it is a difficult stain to interpret due to diffusion artifact.

FINE NEEDLE ASPIRATION

There is significant cytologic variability from case to case. Most aspirates are cellular with single cells or small, loosely cohesive clusters of cells (Figure 3-66).

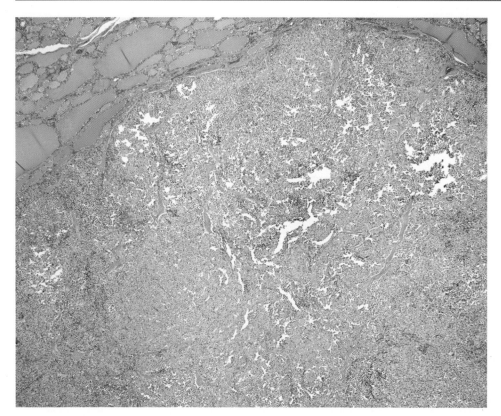

FIGURE 3-61

A predominantly solid growth pattern is noted in this medullary carcinoma. The interface between the tumor and the adjacent thyroid is irregular. Small wisps of pink amyloid are noted.

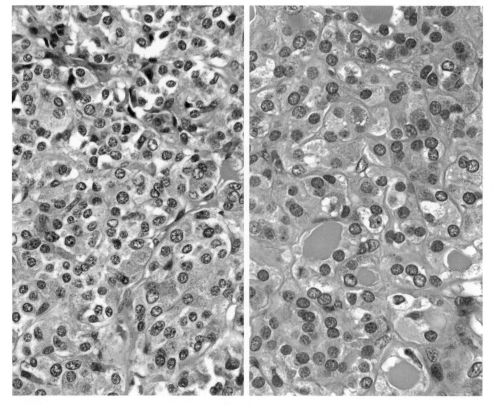

FIGURE 3-62

Left: Organoid pattern of growth with basophilic granular cytoplasm noted around nuclei with coarse, salt-and-pepper nuclear chromatin distribution. Right: Follicular growth may mimic a follicular epithelial neoplasm. Entrapment of benign follicular epithelium is common at the periphery.

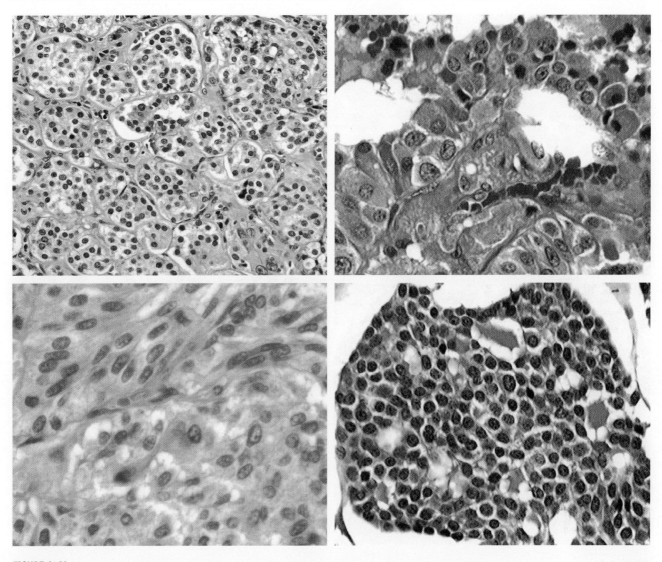

FIGURE 3-63

Patterns of growth and cell types in medullary carcinoma. Left upper: Organoid. Left lower: Tumor spindling. Right upper: Papillary architecture with basophilic, granular cytoplasm. Right lower: Lobular architectural with amphicrine cells and inspissated material.

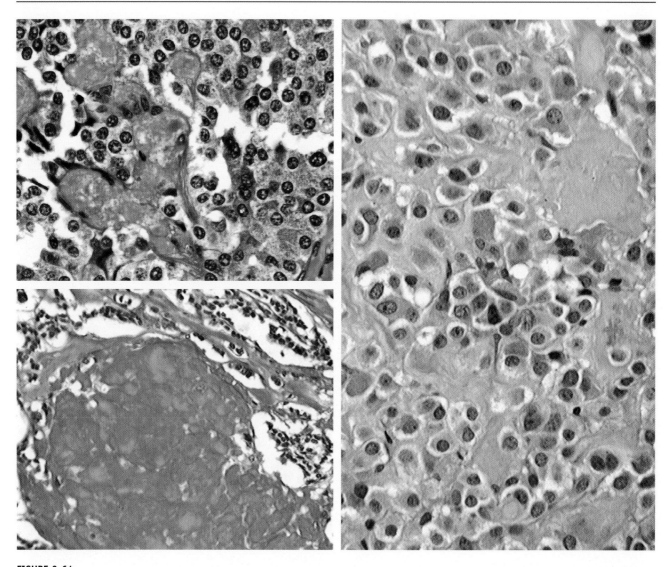

FIGURE 3-64

Amyloid is common. Left upper: Pink amyloid blending with surrounding tumor cells. Left lower: An aggregation of acellular, eosinophilic, extracellular amyloid matrix material. Right: The plasmacytoid cells with basophilic cytoplasm contrast with the pale, eosinophilic amyloid material.

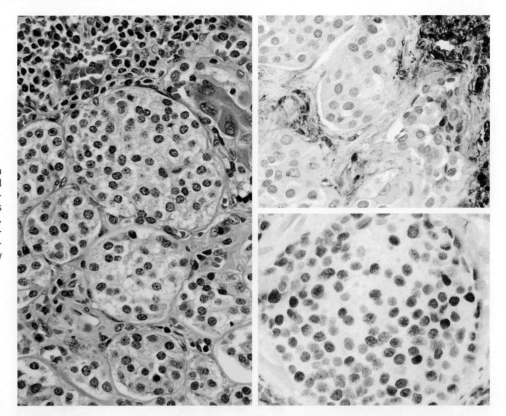

FIGURE 3-65

Left: Small nests of tumor cells with pale cytoplasm surrounding round nuclei with delicate nuclear chromatin. Right upper: Thyroglobulin is non-reactive in the tumor cells, although there is a diffusion artifact in the stroma. Right lower: TTF-1 stains the nuclei of a medullary carcinoma.

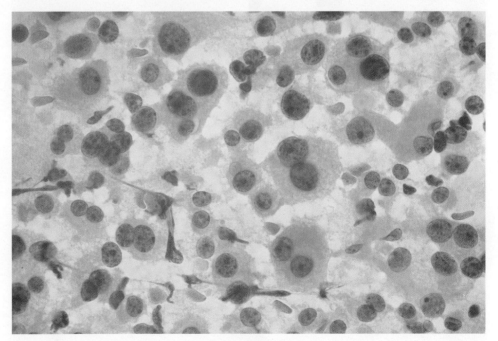

FIGURE 3-66

A cellular aspirate with loosely cohesive tumor cells. Plasmacytoid architecture is prominent. There is slight nuclear pleomorphism (FNA, alcohol fixed, Papanicolau stained).

Colloid is absent; however, the extracellular, homogenous, amorphous eosinophilic clumps or spheres of amyloid (seen in about 60% of aspirates) may sometimes be misinterpreted as colloid (Figure 3-67). The tumor cells vary from round to oval, spindle-shaped (Figure 3-68) and polygonal. Bi- and multinucleation can be seen, along with moderate pleomorphism. The nuclear chromatin is stippled or coarsely granular ('salt-and-pepper') with abundant, eosinophilic cytoplasm often eccentrically surrounding the nucleus. This plasmacytoid appearance is quite characteristic (Figure 3-66). Intranuclear cytoplasmic inclusions may be seen.

Air-dried preparations often highlight the distinctive metachromatic red cytoplasmic granules.

MOLECULAR ANALYSIS

Somatic *RET* mutations, most commonly the M918T mutation, have been shown to occur in 20–80% of sporadic medullary thyroid carcinoma, a wide range because of different detection techniques. Germline *RET* oncogene mutations are identified in all hereditary forms, although the mutations occur in different codons and with different degrees of penetrance.

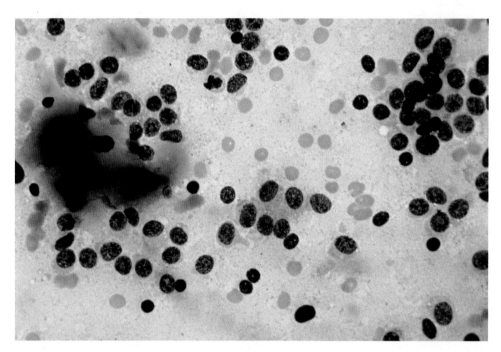

FIGURE 3-67

Small cells arranged in slightly cohesive clusters with an amorphous aggregate of amyloid associated with the clusters (FNA, alcohol fixed, Papanicolau stained).

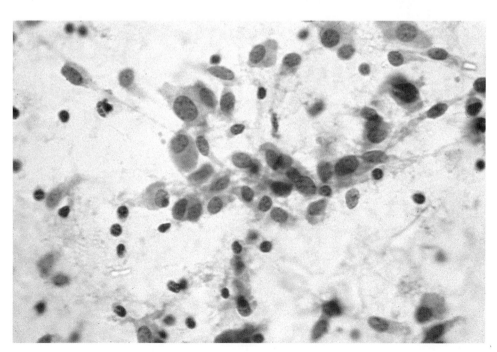

FIGURE 3-68

Tumor cell spindling is common in medullary carcinoma (FNA, alcohol fixed, Papanicolau stained).

DIFFERENTIAL DIAGNOSIS

Pre-neoplastic C-cell hyperplasia may be mistaken for intraglandular spread of medullary carcinoma, although C-cell hyperplasia usually doesn't have fibrosis and the cells tend to have a more intense calcitonin immunoreactivity. Solid cell nests and palpation thyroiditis can usually be separated by histology alone.

The differential diagnosis of medullary carcinoma includes most of the primary tumors of the thyroid gland. Hyalinizing trabecular tumor, follicular carcinoma, paraganglioma, amyloid goiter and lymphoma may mimic medullary carcinoma. Direct extension into the thyroid by laryngeal neuroendocrine carcinomas may occasionally cause diagnostic difficulty. Metastatic foci of medullary carcinoma may be difficult to separate from other carcinomas, although immunohistochemical analysis for calcitonin, CEA and chromogranin aid in this distinction.

PROGNOSIS AND THERAPY

Clinical stage is important in determining the patient prognosis. If there is no metastatic disease, patients can enjoy nearly 100% cure rates following surgery. This is especially true in tumors found incidentally (usually small and without metastasis) during screening for familial disease. Metastatic disease to cervical lymph nodes is common, with metastases to liver, lungs and bone less commonly identified. However, if there is metastatic disease or elevated calcitonin and/or CEA levels, the prognosis is more guarded and difficult to predict. Overall, there is between a 70–80% 10-year survival. Survival is best for familial non-MEN related, followed by sporadic and MEN 2A, which is better than MEN 2B patients. Women and patients <40 years tend to have a better prognosis, as do tumors which are rich in calcitonin (>75% of cells) and with abundant amyloid.

Total thyroidectomy is the treatment of choice, with central lymph node dissection as clinically or radiographically indicated. Parathyroid gland disease may also be present, especially if the medullary carcinoma is familial, necessitating parathyroidectomy. There is no effective chemotherapy and radiation is used only as a palliative measure. ^{131}I radioablative therapy is useless since there is no thyroid hormone production. Follow-up of the patient's serum calcitonin and CEA levels, especially if elevated pre-operatively, may help to assess disease progression.

Whenever medullary carcinoma is found, the incidence of discovering a genetic form when evaluating relatives of the proband is about 10–15%, a valuable screening tool, irrespective of the specific technique employed (biochemical or molecular).

PRIMARY THYROID LYMPHOMA

A primary lymphoma arising within the confines of the thyroid gland and usually associated with lymphocytic thyroiditis. An uncommon neoplasm, the understanding of the 'mucosa-associated lymphoid tissue' (MALT) concept, suggests that previous plasmacytomas may be within the spectrum of extranodal marginal zone B-cell lymphoma (EMZBCL).

CLINICAL FEATURES

Primary thyroid lymphomas account for about 2% of all thyroid gland neoplasms and about 5% of all extra-

---

**PRIMARY THYROID LYMPHOMA
DISEASE FACT SHEET**

Definition
▶ Primary lymphoma arising within the thyroid gland and usually associated with lymphocytic thyroiditis

Incidence and Location
▶ About 2% of thyroid neoplasms
▶ About 5% of extranodal lymphomas

Morbidity and Mortality
▶ Most arise within the setting of lymphocytic thyroiditis and/or Hashimoto's disease
▶ Mortality is grade and stage dependent

Gender, Race and Age Distribution
▶ Female >> Male (5:1)
▶ Mean age is in the seventh decade

Clinical Features
▶ Mass (often rapidly enlarging) with associated pain, dysphagia and hoarseness
▶ Hypothyroidism may develop
▶ Associated cervical adenopathy in some cases

Prognosis and Therapy
▶ Overall, approximately 60% 5-year survival, although grade and stage dependent
▶ Chemotherapy and radiation employed, dependent on grade and stage

nodal lymphomas. Primarily a disease of older individuals (mean, 65 years), there is a strong female predilection (3–5 : 1, F:M). Patients often have a history of lymphocytic thyroiditis (Hashimoto's thyroiditis), the MALT setting considered essential for the development of this lymphoma. Lymph node lymphomas directly extending into the thyroid are not considered primary thyroid lymphomas. Patients symptoms are non-specific, with a mass in the thyroid gland the most common, with pain, dysphagia and/or hoarseness reported in about 30% of patients. In diffuse large B-cell lymphomas, a rapidly enlarging mass is reported. The duration of symptoms is usually short (mean, 4 months). Patients are occasionally hypothyroid, perhaps due to the underlying autoimmune character of Hashimoto's thyroiditis. Staging is the same as that used for lymphomas in general, with 'E' added for extranodal. The perithyroidal lymph nodes may be involved, followed by other lymph nodes or bone marrow.

PATHOLOGIC FEATURES

GROSS FINDINGS

The lymphomas are often large (mean, 7 cm), firm to soft, lobulated and may be either a solid or cystic mass involving one or both thyroid lobes. The cut surface is often bulging, pale, with a 'fish-flesh', uniform, homogeneous to mottled appearance (Figure 3-69). Foci of hemorrhage and necrosis are frequently noted. Extension into the surrounding soft tissues is common.

MICROSCOPIC FINDINGS

Lymphomas of the thyroid gland occur in the setting of lymphocytic thyroiditis in almost all cases (Figure 3-70). There is a vaguely nodular to diffuse heterogeneous effacement of the thyroid gland (Figure 3-71). Perithyroidal extension is common, while lymphvascular invasion is more common in higher grade tumors. The B-cell infiltrate is composed of atypical small lymphocytes, centrocyte-like (cleaved) cells, monocytoid B-cells, scat-

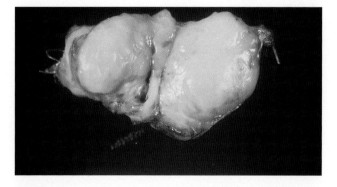

FIGURE 3-69
Malignant lymphoma with a characteristic 'fish-flesh' appearance.

PRIMARY THYROID LYMPHOMA PATHOLOGIC FEATURES

Gross Findings
▸ Wide variation in size
▸ Soft to firm, lobular and multinodular
▸ Effacement of the normal thyroid
▸ Cut surface is bulging, tan, and 'fish-flesh'
▸ Usually homogeneous or mottled
▸ Extension into perithyroidal soft tissues

Microscopic Findings
▸ Extranodal marginal zone B-cell lymphoma and diffuse large B-cell lymphoma with transitions between the two
▸ Constant background of lymphocytic thyroiditis
▸ Extension into fat and skeletal muscle
▸ Atypical small lymphocytes, centrocytes, monocytoid B-cell cells, and plasma cells
▸ Dutcher bodies and Russell bodies
▸ Lymphoepithelial lesions (atypical lymphoid cells within the follicular epithelium) are diagnostic
▸ Diffuse, large, atypical cells with increased mitotic figures suggests transformation into a diffuse large B-cell lymphoma

Immunohistochemical Results
▸ CD20 (co-expressed with CD43 occasionally)
▸ CD79a
▸ Kappa or Lambda light chain restriction
▸ Keratin highlights the lymphoepithelial lesions

Fine Needle Aspiration
▸ Marginal zone B-cell lymphomas are a dispersed, non-cohesive admixture of lymphocytes, centrocytes, monocytoid B cells, immunoblasts, plasma cells and histiocytes – perhaps indistinguishable from a lymphocytic thyroiditis
▸ Diffuse large B-cell lymphoma aspirates are hypercellular with dyscohesive, large, atypical neoplastic cells

Pathologic Differential Diagnosis
▸ Lymphocytic thyroiditis; undifferentiated carcinoma, myeloid sarcoma and melanoma

---

tered large immunoblasts and plasma cells in areas of extranodal marginal zone B-cell lymphoma (Figures 3-72 and 3-73). Reactive germinal centers, which may often demonstrate colonization by neoplastic cells, are invariably present. However, the follicular architecture may recapitulate a follicle center lymphoma. Lymphoepithelial lesions, which represent infiltration of epithelial follicular structures by neoplastic B cells, are a consistent feature. Rounded balls or masses, filling and distending the lumen of the thyroid follicles ('MALT balls') are unique (Figure 3-74). Plasma cells (Figure 3-75) and plasmacytoid cells (Figure 3-76) with Dutcher bodies or cytoplasmic immunoglobulin (Figure 3-77) are also seen, occasionally simulating a plasmacytoma. There may be single or multifocal areas of large cell transformation adjacent to the low-grade component, suggesting a transformation or 'dedifferentiation'.

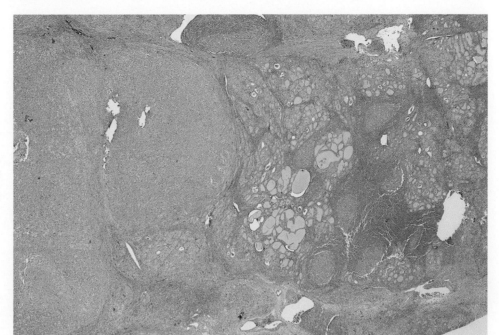

FIGURE 3-70

The left portion of the field demonstrates nodular effacement of the thyroid parenchyma by lymphoma, while the right shows lymphocytic thyroiditis.

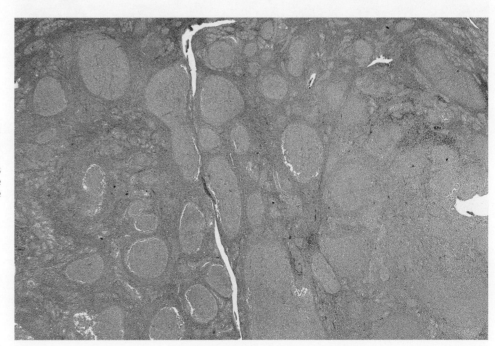

FIGURE 3-71

A pseudofollicular architecture is seen in this MALT lymphoma. Notice the large 'spaces' created by the dilated lymphatic channels.

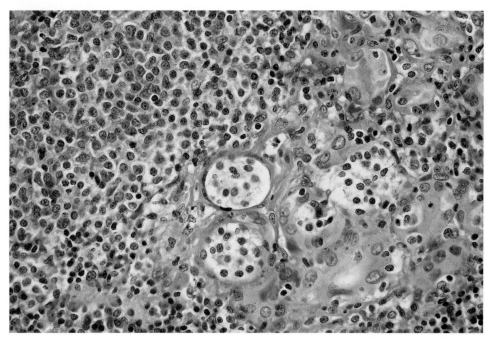

FIGURE 3-72

Atypical small lymphocytes, centrocyte-like cells, and monocytoid B-cells are arranged in sheets and small clusters, growing into the follicular epithelium of the thyroid gland (right side).

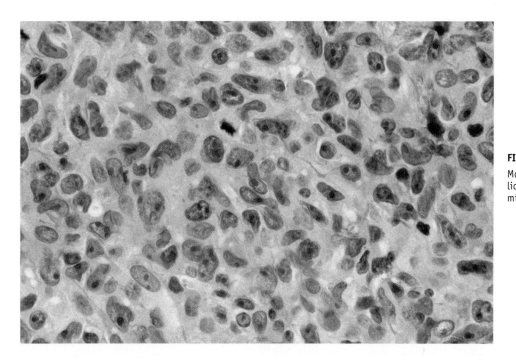

FIGURE 3-73

Monocytoid B-cells have an 'epithelioid' appearance. Nucleoli and mitotic figures are present.

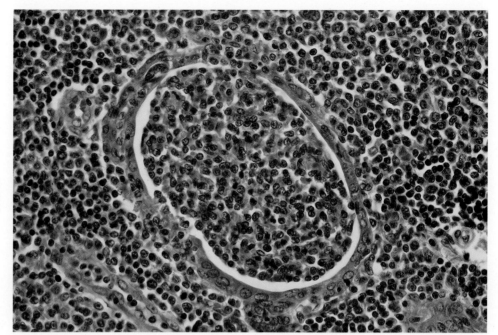

FIGURE 3-74

Masses of lymphoid cells are noted distending a thyroid follicle. This type of lymphoepithelial lesion is referred to as a 'MALT ball'.

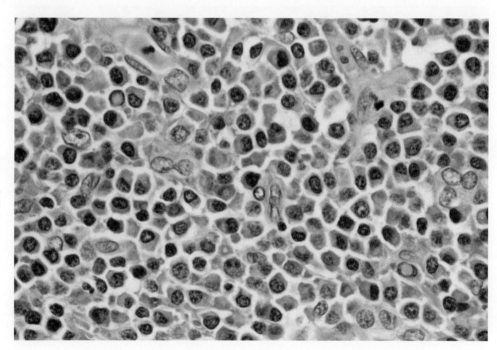

FIGURE 3-75

A prominent plasmacytoid differentiation is noted with Dutcher bodies (intranuclear cytoplasmic inclusions) in this MALT lymphoma.

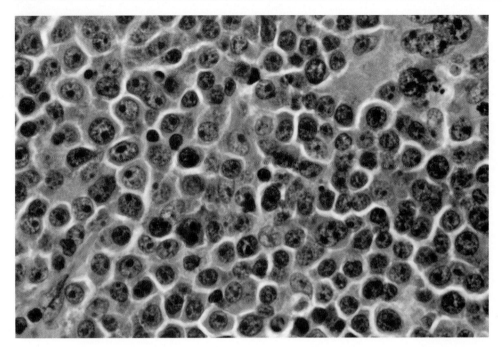

FIGURE 3-76
Plasmacytic cells in this MALT lymphoma have prominent nucleoli within eccentrically located nuclei.

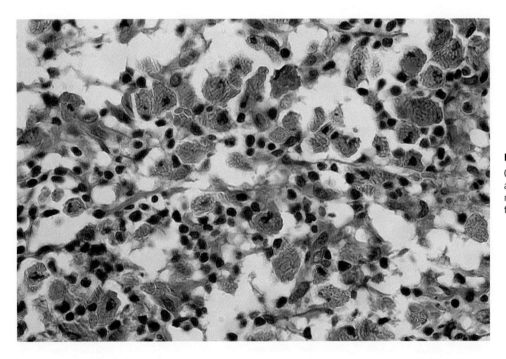

FIGURE 3-77
Crystalline type immunoglobulins are seen filling the cytoplasm of the neoplastic plasmacytoid cells of this MALT lymphoma.

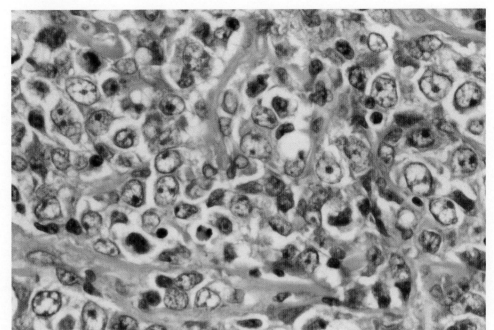

FIGURE 3-78

A diffuse, large cell population of centroblastic-like B-cells comprises this diffuse large B-cell lymphoma.

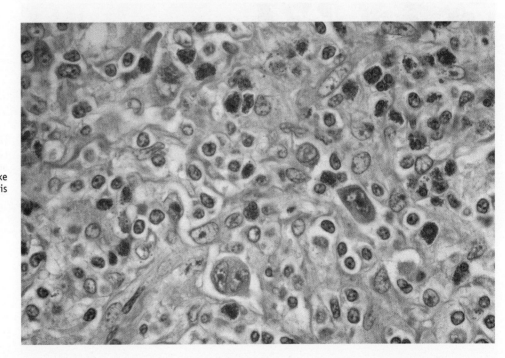

FIGURE 3-79

Eosinophils and Reed-Sternberg-like cells are focally identified in this diffuse large B-cell lymphoma.

Alternatively, areas of diffuse large B-cell lymphoma may occur in the absence of any recognizable low-grade areas. The large cells show a spectrum of cytologic features that resemble centroblasts, immunoblasts, monocytoid B cells and plasmacytoid cells (Figure 3-78). DLBCL is seen more commonly than EMZBCL. Focal Reed-Sternberg-like (Figure 3-79) or Burkitt-like cells may be noted that are associated with brisk mitotic activity, apoptosis and a starry sky pattern (Figure 3-80). Atrophy of residual thyroid parenchyma and fibrosis are often noted.

ANCILLARY STUDIES

IMMUNOHISTOCHEMICAL RESULTS

The B-cell immunophenotype of EMZBCL and DLBCL are confirmed by immunoreactivity for CD20 and/or CD79a. Bcl-2 reactivity in the neoplastic, colonizing B cells (but not in the residual, reactive germinal center cells) is also characteristic. Immunoglobulin light chain restriction for either kappa or lambda may

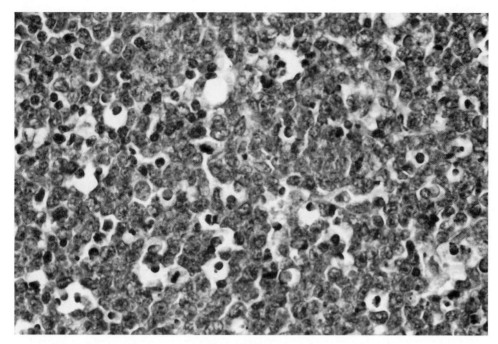

FIGURE 3-80
A Burkitt-like pattern shows brisk mitotic activity, apoptosis, and a 'starry-sky' pattern with numerous tingible body macrophages in this diffuse large B-cell lymphoma.

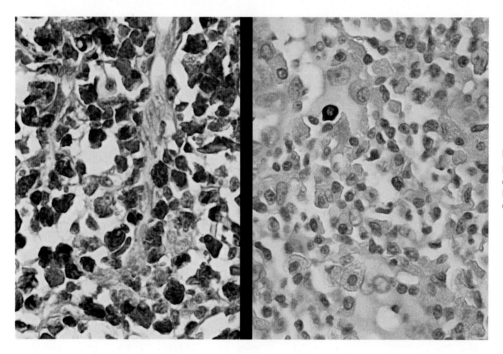

FIGURE 3-81
Left: A kappa restricted population of atypical lymphoid cells. Right: Lambda highlights only a plasma cell.

be demonstrated (Figure 3-81), especially in the plasma cell or plasmacytoid component. Co-expression of CD43 with CD20 may be seen in a small percentage of EMZBCL. An antibody to cytokeratin will highlight the epithelial remnants in the lymphoepithelial lesions (Figure 3-82).

FINE NEEDLE ASPIRATION

The full spectrum of lymphoid elements will often be present within the cellular aspirates from an EMZBCL, making separation from lymphocytic thyroiditis nearly impossible. However, the dyscohsive, monotonous pop-ulation of large atypical cells with scant cytoplasm and large nuclei with vesicular nuclear chromatin and back-ground lymphoglandular bodies suggest a diagnosis of DLBCL.

DIFFERENTIAL DIAGNOSIS

The distinction between EMZBCL and lymphocytic thyroiditis may be difficult at times. In EMZBCL, the diffuse pattern, colonization of the benign germinal center, Dutcher bodies, and lymphoepithelial cells

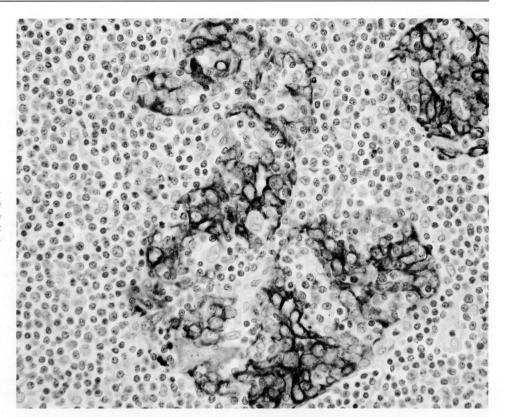

FIGURE 3-82
A malignant lymphoma immuno-stained for keratin highlights the residual thyroid follicles which are extensively infiltrated by neoplastic lymphoid cells, creating lymphoepithelial lesions.

should help make the diagnosis. In a few cases, however, immunohistochemical, flow cytometric or molecular genetic analyses may be required. DLBCL may be indistinguishable from undifferentiated carcinoma, melanoma or myeloid sarcoma by histology alone and may require a more thorough antibody panel, including CD45RB, CD20, cytokeratin, S-100 protein and myelomonocytic markers to make the correct diagnosis.

PROGNOSIS AND THERAPY

The prognosis of thyroid MALT type lymphomas is very favorable in general, although the prognosis is stage and histology dependent. In general, localized (stage IE or IIE) tumors with a low grade histology have an excellent prognosis (>95% disease specific 5-year survival) whereas those with either a large cell component or diffuse large B-cell type, have a worse overall survival (approximately 50–70% disease specific 5-year survival) and are much more likely to die of disease. Poor prognostic features include high stage, extrathyroidal extension, vascular invasion, and a high mitotic rate. Nearly all patients with stage IVE die with disease. While surgery is used to debulk or decompress and obtain tissue for the diagnosis, chemotherapy and radiation are standard, the regimen determined by the histologic grade and stage.

THYMIC AND RELATED BRANCHIAL POUCH NEOPLASMS

CLINICAL FEATURES

This is a rare group of tumors which have spindle cells and thymic-like areas of differentiation. Spindle cell tumor with thymus-like differentiation (SETTLE) occurs in young patients (mean, 15–20 years) without a significant gender predilection. Patients usually have an asymptomatic neck mass. Carcinoma showing thymus-like differentiation (CASTLE) is slightly more common in women than men and tends to develop in adults in the fifth decade. An asymptomatic neck or thyroid mass, which may or may not be invasive at the time of presentation, is the most common clinical presentation. Metastatic disease can be seen in about 30% of patients.

PATHOLOGIC FEATURES

GROSS FINDINGS

The tumors are usually well circumscribed and may be encapsulated, although infiltration may be seen. The tumors are firm to hard, white-tan, up to 6 cm in greatest

THYMIC-LIKE NEOPLASMS
DISEASE FACT SHEET

Definition

▶ Tumors which have thymic-like areas of differentiation including spindle cell tumor with thymus-like differentiation (SETTLE) and carcinoma showing thymus-like differentiation (CASTLE)

Incidence and Location

▶ Rare
▶ CASTLE often involves the lower thyroid lobes

Gender, Race and Age Distribution

▶ SETTLE occurs in young patients (mean, 15–20 years) with an equal gender distribution
▶ CASTLE is slightly more common in women and usually in the fifth decade

Clinical Features

▶ Asymptomatic neck or thyroid mass
▶ Metastatic disease at presentation in about 30 % of CASTLE patients

Prognosis and Therapy

▶ Prolonged, indolent course
▶ Surgery for both tumor types
▶ Radiation is often used for CASTLE

THYMIC-LIKE NEOPLASMS
PATHOLOGIC FEATURES

Gross Findings

▶ Well circumscribed and may be encapsulated, although infiltration may be seen (especially in CASTLE)
▶ Firm to hard, white-tan and fleshy, up to 6 cm
▶ Cysts are more common in SETTLE

Microscopic Findings

SETTLE

▶ Highly cellular biphasic tumor
▶ Spindle shaped cells merging with epithelial cells separated into lobules by dense fibrosis
▶ Delicate nuclear chromatin in both cell types
▶ Epithelial cells are arranged in glands, tubules, papillae or sheets
▶ Abrupt keratinization can be seen
▶ Mucinous or ciliated cells are seen within glands
▶ Calcifications are noted

CASTLE

▶ Solid, nests and lobules, infiltrative growth
▶ Epithelioid cells with large vesicular-appearing nuclei, pleomorphism and prominent nucleoli
▶ Syncytial arrangement
▶ Squamous differentiation is noted, often abrupt
▶ Dense fibrosis frequently associated with lymphocytes and plasma cells

Immunohistochemical Results

▶ Spindle and epithelial cells in SETTLE are keratin positive
▶ CASTLE cells are keratin and CD5 positive
▶ Both tumors are negative for thyroglobulin, TTF-1, calcitonin, CEA and S-100 protein

Pathologic Differential Diagnosis

▶ Thymic carcinoma, ectopic thymoma, synovial sarcoma, solitary fibrous tumor, teratoma, spindle cell carcinoma, squamous cell carcinoma, medullary carcinoma

---

dimension and may have small cysts present within a vaguely whorled mass.

Microscopic Findings

- *Spindle cell tumor with thymus-like differentiation:* This is a highly cellular biphasic tumor characterized by an admixture of spindle-shaped cells which merge with epithelial cells (Figure 3-83). Sclerotic fibrosis abruptly separates the spindle cell component into a lobular pattern (Figure 3-84). The elongated nuclei have delicate nuclear chromatin and small nucleoli (Figure 3-85) The epithelial cells are more polygonal and are arranged in glands, tubules, trabeculae, papillae and sheets (Figure 3-86). Sometimes, abrupt keratinization may be seen. Branching cystic glands can occasionally be identified, lined by mucinous or ciliated cells. Calcifications can be seen in the stroma. It is important to note the often abrupt transition between the two components of this tumor (Figure 3-87).

- *Carcinoma showing thymus-like differentiation:* The tumor is arranged in solid nests or lobules with an expansive or infiltrative growth of epithelioid cells into the surrounding thyroid parenchyma (Figure 3-88). There is often dense fibrosis separating the bands of neoplastic cells into vague lobules. Lymphocytes and plasma cells may be present. The epithelioid cells have a resemblence to thymomas or thymic carcinomas with epithelioid to spindle-shaped cells arranged in sheets and nests (Figure 3-89). The cells show mild to moderate nuclear pleomorphism, with large, round to oval nuclei with pale to vesicular-appearing chromatin, distinct nucleoli, and abundant eosinophilic cytoplasm with indistinct cell borders (syncytial arrangement; Figure 3-90). Mitotic figures are usually limited. Squamous differentiation may be present including keratinization and intercellular bridges.

Ancillary Studies

In SETTLE both the spindle cells and epithelial cells are cytokeratin positive (Figure 3-91), while in CASTLE the tumor cells are keratin and CD5 positive (Figure 3-92). In both tumors, the cells are negative for thyroglobulin, TTF-1, calcitonin, carcinoembryonic antigen and S-100 protein.

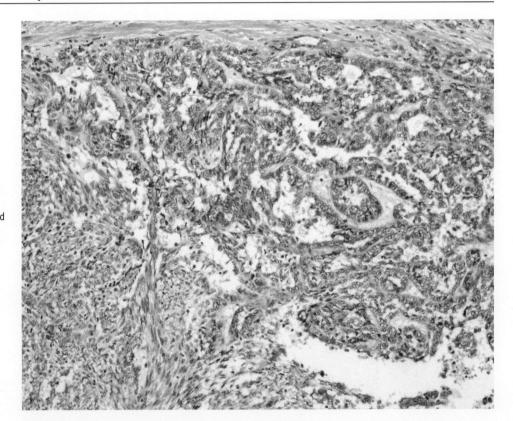

FIGURE 3-83
There is a blending of spindled and
epithelial cells in this SETTLE.

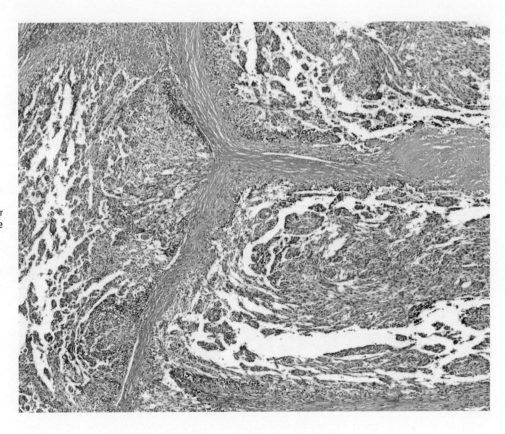

FIGURE 3-84
Bands of fibrosis separate the tumor
in the thyroid into lobules of spindle
and epithelial cells in SETTLE.

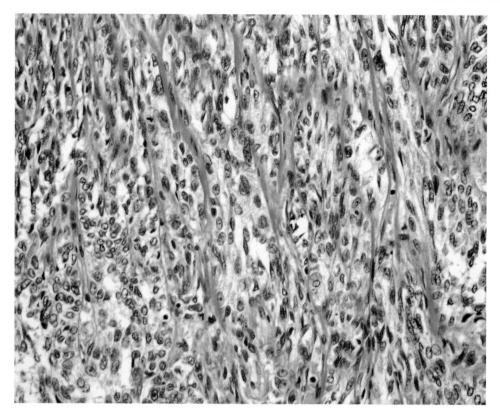

FIGURE 3-85
The spindled and epithelioid cells have delicate nuclei with small nucleoli. Note the wisps of fibrosis separating the tumor cells.

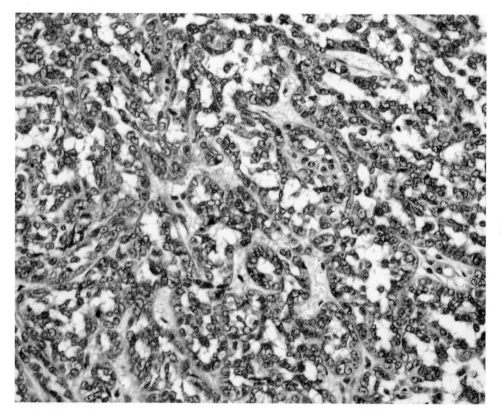

FIGURE 3-86
Epithelioid cells are arranged in tubules, glands and papillary projections. Note the 'optical' clearing of the nuclei.

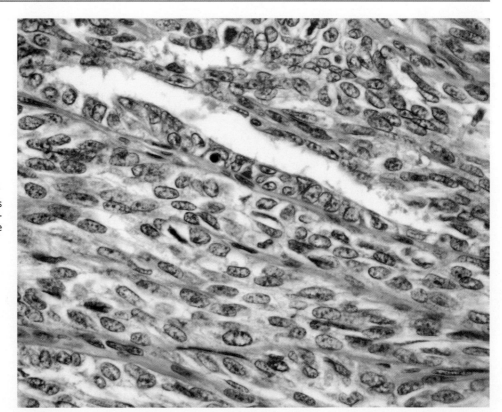

FIGURE 3-87

A SETTLE shows spindled cells immediately juxtaposed to the epithelioid cells. This finding is quite characteristic.

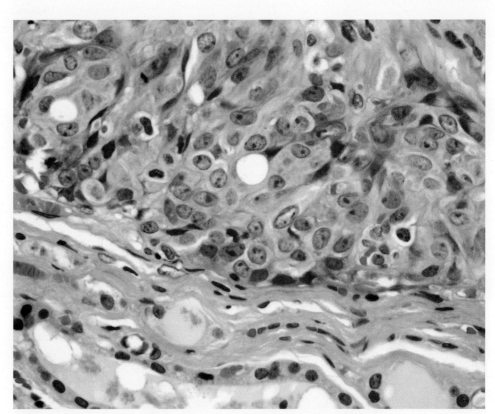

FIGURE 3-88

The thyroid epithelium is noted at the bottom of the image, separated from the neoplastic cells by fibrosis. Note the mitotic figure in the upper left quadrant in this CASTLE, comprised of large, polygonal, epithelioid cells with vesicular nuclear chromatin distribution.

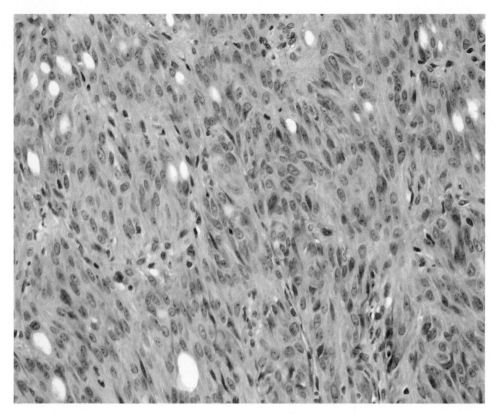

FIGURE 3-89
This CASTLE shows a syncytial arrangement of spindled cells. The nuclei are pale with small, but distinct nucleoli.

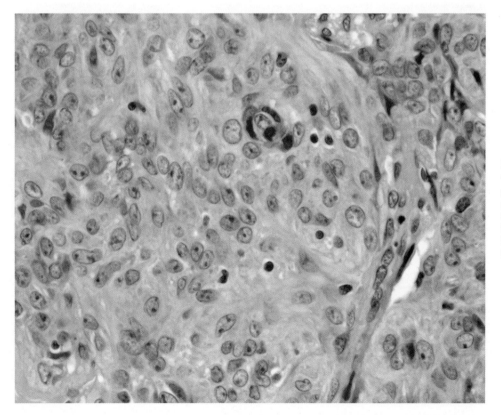

FIGURE 3-90
This CASTLE shows the syncytial arrangement of epithelial cells with open, pale to vesicular nuclear chromatin distribution. There is a hint of 'squamous pearl' formation. Nucleoli are easily identified, but are not prominent.

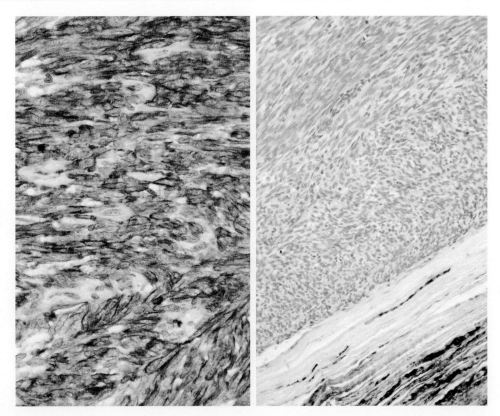

FIGURE 3-91

Keratin is strongly and diffusely immunoreactive in the neoplastic cells of a SETTLE (left), while thyroglobulin is non-reactive (right).

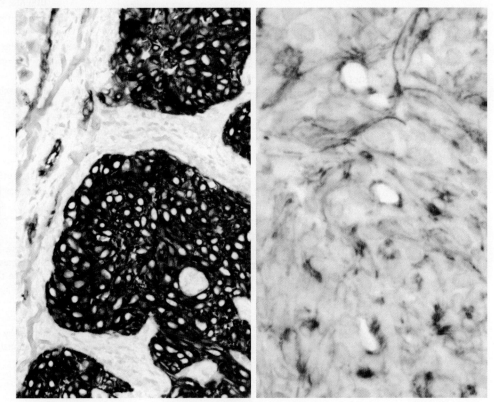

FIGURE 3-92

A CASTLE shows strong keratin immunoreactive (left), with a delicate immunoreaction with CD5 (right), confirming the thymic-like differentiation.

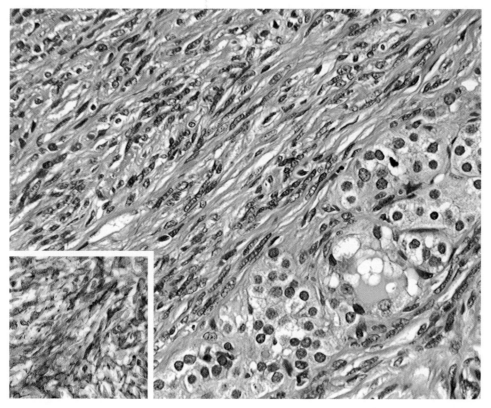

FIGURE 3-93
A solitary fibrous tumor infiltrates around the uninvolved thyroid follicles (lower right). The spindle cell population is separated by bands of collagen. Inset demonstrates positivity with bcl-2.

DIFFERENTIAL DIAGNOSIS

Thymic carcinoma, ectopic thymoma, synovial sarcoma, solitary fibrous tumor (Figure 3-93), teratoma, spindle cell carcinoma, squamous cell carcinoma and medullary carcinoma are all considered in the differential diagnosis. However, the distinct histology of the tumor and the immunohistochemical profile help with separation.

PROGNOSIS AND THERAPY

Due to the rare nature of these tumors, a definitive prognosis is difficult to predict, although most pursue a prolonged indolent course. Local recurrence and regional metastases have been reported more often in CASTLE than in SETTLE with delayed metastases seen more often in SETTLE. Surgical excision is the treatment of choice, with radiation occasionally employed for CASTLE.

METASTATIC NEOPLASMS

Tumors that occur in the thyroid as a result of lymph-vascular spread from distant sites are considered as metastatic disease. While not covered in this section, it

---

**METASTATIC NEOPLASMS
DISEASE FACT SHEET**

Definition
▶ Lymph-vascular spread from distant sites to the thyroid gland

Incidence and Location
▶ Up to 25 % in autopsied patients, but less common in clinically series

Morbidity and Mortality
▶ Usually poor clinically outcome, although exceptions occur

Gender, Race and Age Distribution
▶ Female > Male, although tumor type specific
▶ Usually older patients

Clinical Features
▶ Rapidly enlarging thyroid mass, although sometimes a thyroid disorder may be the clinical presentation
▶ In up to 40 % of patients, the thyroid presentation is the initial manifestation of an occult primary

Prognosis and Therapy
▶ Usually poor and determined by the underlying primary
▶ When limited to the thyroid gland, surgery may yield a prolonged survival

is should be noted that direct extension into the thyroid from the adjacent organs (larynx [squamous cell carcinoma], trachea, esophagus, lymph nodes [lymphoma], soft tissues) may sometimes need to be included in the differential diagnosis of thyroid masses.

CLINICAL FEATURES

While not as common in clinical patients, up to 25% of autopsied patients with disseminated malignancies will have thyroid gland metastases. In clinical series, metastatic deposits are identified at a higher frequency in abnormal glands: those with adenomatoid nodules, thyroiditis and follicular neoplasms. Further, the metastatic deposits may be found within primary thyroid tumors (i.e., metastatic renal cell carcinoma to a thyroid papillary carcinoma). A rapidly enlarging thyroid mass may be the presenting sign, although more often the underlying thyroid disease may result in the clinical presentation. In a number of patients (up to 40%), the thyroid gland metastatic deposit is the initial presentation of the occult primary tumor. The most common primary sites in order of frequency are kidney (Figure 3-94), lung, breast (Figure 3-95), stomach, and skin (melanoma).

PATHOLOGIC FEATURES

GROSS FINDINGS

Multifocal and bilateral disease is more common, but in clinically significant metastatic deposits, a unilateral solitary mass is more likely to result in clinical evaluation. They can be large, up to 15 cm in maximum dimension.

MICROSCOPIC FINDINGS

The thyroid gland is a richly vascularized endocrine organ, susceptible to metastatic deposits. For the most part, the metastatic deposits morphologically resemble the primary site, with rare examples of more poorly differentiated tumor in the thyroid. Close examination of the periphery of the thyroid gland, immediately adjacent to the capsule where the vasculature is the most dense, will help to identify intravascular metastatic deposits. When the tumor deposits form a mass lesion, they usually have an architecture and cytomorphology distinct from thyroid primaries. Metastatic clear cell renal cell carcinoma is an exception (Figure 3-94). Metastatic neuroendocrine (small cell) carcinomas may also pose some difficulty, as they may resemble a medullary thyroid carcinoma; or they may also be TTF-1 immunoreactive if they are from the lung.

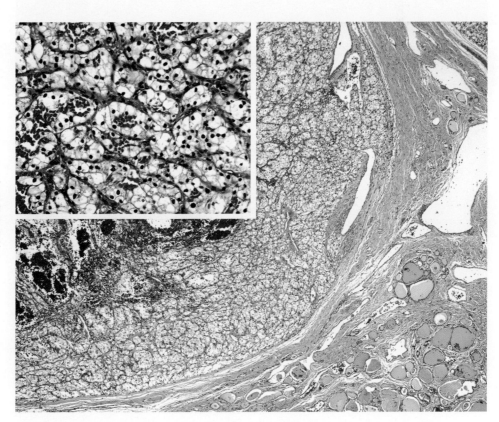

FIGURE 3-94

An encapsulated metastatic clear cell renal cell carcinoma to the thyroid gland may mimic a primary thyroid neoplasm with clear cells. Inset shows erythrocytes in the center of pseudoglands. Prominent cell borders and small hyperchromatic nuclei are present.

METASTATIC NEOPLASMS
PATHOLOGIC FEATURES

Gross Findings

▸ Usually multifocal and bilateral
▸ Can metastasize to pre-existing thyroid lesions

Microscopic Findings

▸ Usually resemble the primary tumor although dedifferentiation can occur
▸ Lymph-vascular channels at the periphery of the thyroid gland shows tumor most frequently
▸ Distinctly different architecture and histology from primary thyroid neoplasms (although clear cell metastatic renal cell carcinoma and metastatic neuroendocrine carcinomas may cause difficulty)

Immunohistochemical Results

▸ Metastatic tumors have unique immunohistochemical profiles, distinctly different from thyroid primaries

Pathologic Differential Diagnosis

▸ Clear cell adenoma/carcinoma, medullary carcinoma, lymphoma

ANCILLARY STUDIES

Primary thyroid follicular tumors will usually be thyroglobulin, CK7 and TTF-1 immunoreactive, while C-cell derived tumors will be calcitonin and chromogranin reactive. While there are exceptions, metastatic tumors will not be thyroglobulin reactive (Figures 3-96 and 3-97), and only rare examples of calcitonin immunoreactivity in metastatic neuroendocrine neoplasms are known.

DIFFERENTIAL DIAGNOSIS

A solitary metastatic renal cell carcinoma may be difficult to separate from the clear cell change seen in follicular adenomas or carcinomas, and more rarely in papillary and medullary carcinoma. The prominent vascularity, glandular lumina filled with erythrocytes, sharp intercellular borders and small, hyperchromatic nuclei favor a renal cells carcinoma. The neoplastic cells are RCC, CD10, and EMA immunoreactive, while nonreactive for TTF-1 or thyroglobulin. The latter can have diffusion artifacts from the surrounding thyroid parenchyma, requiring careful interpretation.

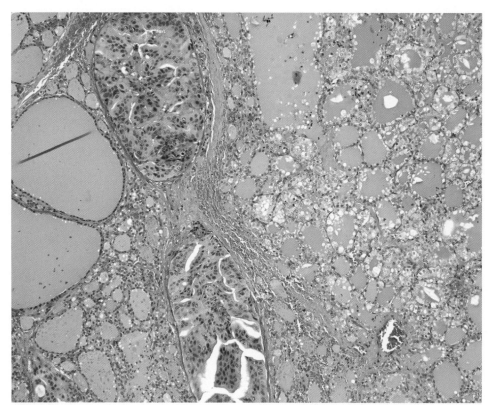

FIGURE 3-95

The vascular spaces are filled with neoplastic cells that have a different appearance from the adenomatoid nodules (left) and the papillary thyroid carcinoma (right). This is a metastatic breast carcinoma.

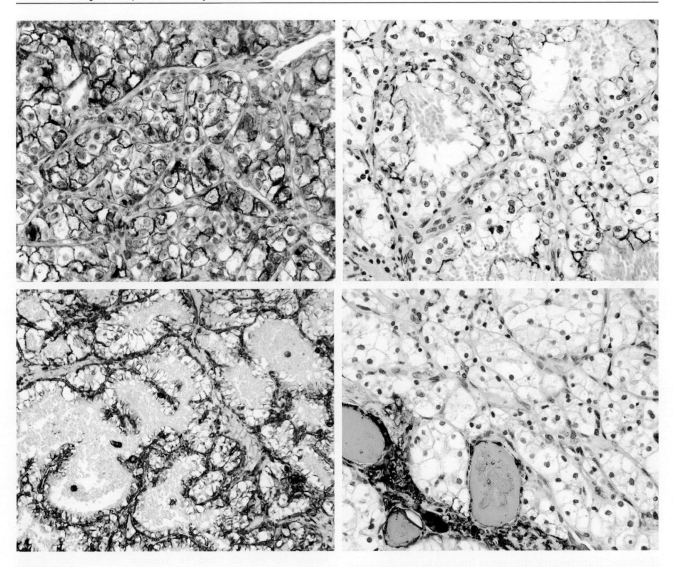

FIGURE 3-96

An immunohistochemical panel can help to separate metastatic from primary neoplasms. This renal cell carcinoma is CD10 (left upper), vimentin (left lower) and EMA (right upper) positive, while there is no reactivity with thyroglobulin (right lower).

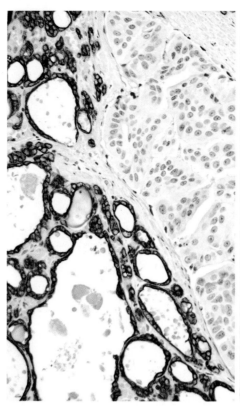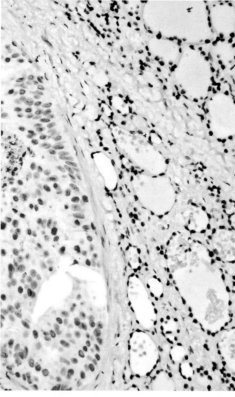

FIGURE 3-97

A metastatic breast carcinoma is non-reactive with thyroglobulin (left) and TTF-1 (right). The tumor cells are within a vascular space.

PROGNOSIS AND THERAPY

For the most part, the prognosis is determined by the underlying primary, and almost by dint of metastases to the thyroid gland correlates with a poor prognosis. However, if metastatic disease is limited to the thyroid, surgery can result in prolonged survival, especially for renal cell carcinoma, a primary tumor known for capricious behavior.

SUGGESTED READING

Papillary Carcinoma (Including Variants)

Albores-Saavedra J, Gould E, Vardaman C, Vuitch F. The macrofollicular variant of papillary thyroid carcinoma: a study of 17 cases. Am J Clin Pathol 1990;94:442–445.

Baloch ZW, LiVolsi VA. Etiology and significance of the optically clear nucleus. Endocr Pathol 2002;13:289–299.

Baloch ZW, Livolsi VA. Follicular-patterned lesions of the thyroid: the bane of the pathologist. Am J Clin Pathol 2002;117:143–150.

Beckner M, Heffess CS, Oertel JE. Oxyphilic papillary thyroid carcinomas. Am J Clin Pathol 1995;103:180–187.

Bennedbaek FN, Hegedus L. Management of the solitary thyroid nodule: results of a North American survey. J Clin Endocrinol Metab 2000;85:2493–2498.

Berho M, Suster S. The oncocytic variant of papillary carcinoma of the thyroid: a clinicopathologic study of 15 cases. Hum Pathol 1997;28:47–53.

Carcangiu ML, Bianchi S. Diffuse sclerosing variant of papillary thyroid carcinoma: clinicopathologic study of 15 cases. Am J Surg Pathol 1989;13:1041–1049.

Carcangiu ML, Sibley RK, Rosai J. Clear cell changes in primary thyroid tumors: a study of 38 cases. Am J Surg Pathol 1985;9:705–722.

Chan JK. Papillary carcinoma of thyroid: classical and variants. Histol Histopathol 1990;5:241–257.

Chow SM, Chan JK, Law SC, et al. Diffuse sclerosing variant of papillary thyroid carcinoma–clinical features and outcome. Eur J Surg Oncol 2003;29:446–449.

Ferreiro JA, Hay ID, Lloyd RV. Columnar cell carcinoma of the thyroid: report of three additional cases. Hum Pathol 1996;27:1156–1160.

Gamboa-Dominguez A, Vieitez-Martinez I, Barredo-Prieto BA, et al. Macrofollicular variant of papillary thyroid carcinoma: A case and control analysis. Endocr Pathol 1996;7:303–308.

Gharib H, Goellner JR, Johnson DA. Fine-needle aspiration cytology of the thyroid. A 12-year experience with 11,000 biopsies. Clin Lab Med 1993;13:699–709.

Lang W, Borrusch H, Bauer L. Occult carcinomas of the thyroid: evaluation of 1020 sequential autopsies. Am J Clin Pathol 1988;90:72–76.

LiVolsi VA, Albores-Saavedra J, Asa SL, et al. Papillary carcinoma. In: DeLellis RA, Lloyd RV, Heitz PU, Eng C (eds). Pathology and Genetics of Tumours of Endocrine Organs. Kleihues P, Sobin LH, series eds. World Health Organization Classification of Tumours. Lyon, France: IARC Press, 2004:57–66.

Lloyd RV, Erickson LA, Casey MB, et al. Observer variation in the diagnosis of follicular variant of papillary thyroid carcinoma. Am J Surg Pathol. 2004;28:1336–1340.

Nardone HC, Ziober AF, LiVolsi VA, et al. c-Met expression in tall cell variant papillary carcinoma of the thyroid. Cancer 2003;98:1386–1393.

Nikiforov YE. RET/PTC rearrangement in thyroid tumors. Endocr Pathol 2002;13:3–16.

Piersanti M, Ezzat S, Asa SL. Controversies in papillary microcarcinoma of the thyroid. Endocr Pathol 2003;14:183–191.

Prendiville S, Burman KD, Ringel MD, et al. Tall cell variant: an aggressive form of papillary thyroid carcinoma. Otolaryngol Head Neck Surg 2000;122:352–257.

Rassael H, Thompson LDR, Heffess CS. Microscopic papillary carcinoma of the thyroid gland: a non-surgical entity. A clinicopathologic correlation of 90 cases. Eur Arch Otorhinolaryngol 1998;225:462–467.

Rosai J, Carcangiu ML, DeLellis RA. Papillary carcinoma. Tumors of the Thyroid gland. Atlas of Tumor Pathology, Third Series, Fascicle 5. Washington, DC: Armed Forces Institute of Pathology, 1992:65–95.

Rosai J, Carcangiu ML, DeLellis RA. Papillary carcinoma variants. Tumors of the Thyroid gland. Atlas of Tumor Pathology, Third Series, Fascicle 5. Washington, DC: Armed Forces Institute of Pathology, 1992:96–122.

Rosai J, Zampi G, Carcangiu ML. Papillary carcinoma of the thyroid: a discussion of its several morphologic expressions, with particular emphasis on the follicular variant. Am J Surg Pathol 1983;7:809–817.

Schroder S, Bocker W. Clear-cell carcinomas of thyroid gland: a clinicopathological study of 13 cases.Histopathology 1986;10:75–89.

Thompson LDR, Wieneke JA, Heffess CS. Diffuse sclerosing papillary thyroid carcinoma. A clinicopathologic and immunophenotypic analysis of 22 cases. Endo Pathol 2006;16:331–348.

Wenig BM, Thompson LD, Adair CF, et al. Thyroid papillary carcinoma of columnar cell type: a clinicopathologic study of 16 cases. Cancer 1998;82:740–753.

Follicular Carcinoma

Akslen LA, Myking AO. Differentiated thyroid carcinomas: the relevance of various pathological features for tumour classification and predictiion of tumour progress. Virch Arc A Pathol Anat Histopathol 1992;421:17–23.

Brennan MD, Bregstralh EJ, van Heerden JA, McConahey WM. Follicular thyroid cancer treated at the Mayo Clinic, 1946 through 1970: initial manifestations, pathologic features, therapy, and outcome. Mayo Clin Proc 1991;66:11–22.

Carcangiu ML, Bianchi S, Savino D, et al. Hürthle cell neoplasms of the thyroid gland. A study of 153 cases. Cancer 1991;68:1944–1953.

Baloch ZW, LiVolsi VA. Intraoperative assessment of thyroid and parathyroid lesions. Semin Diagn Pathol 2002:19:219–226.

Evans HL, Vassilopoulou-Sellin R. Follicular and Hürthle cell carcinomas of the thyroid: a comparative study. Am J Surg Pathol 1998;22:1512–1520.

Hundahl SA, Fleming ID, Fremgen AM, Menck HR. A National Cancer Data Base report on 53,856 cases of thyroid carcinoma treated in the U.S., 1985–1995. Cancer 1998;83:2638–2648.

Nikiforova MN, Biddinger PW, Caudill CM, et al. PAX8-PPAR gamma rearrangement in thyroid tumors: RT-PCR and immunohistochemical analyses. Am J Surg Pathol 2002;26:1016–1023.

Rosai J, Carcangiu ML, DeLellis RA. Follicular carcinoma. Tumors of the Thyroid gland. Atlas of Tumor Pathology, Third Series, Fascicle 5. Washington, DC: Armed Forces Institute of Pathology, 1992:49–64.

Sobrinho Simões M, Asa SL, Kroll TG, et al. Follicular carcinoma. In: DeLellis RA, Lloyd RV, Heitz PU, Eng C (eds). Pathology and Genetics of Tumours of Endocrine Organs. Kleihues P, Sobin LH, series eds. World Health Organization Classification of Tumours. Lyon, France: IARC Press, 2004:67–72.

Thompson LDR, Wieneke JA, Frommelt RA, et al. Minimally invasive follicular carcinoma of the thyroid gland: a clinicopathologic study of 130 cases. Cancer 2001;91:505–524.

Undifferentiated (Anaplastic) Carcinoma

Carcangiu ML, Steeper T, Zampi G, Rosai J. Anaplastic thyroid carcinoma. A study of 70 cases. Am J Clin Pathol 1985;83:135–158.

Miettinen M, Franssila KO. Variable expression of keratins and nearly uniform lack of thyroid transcription factor 1 in thyroid anaplastic carcinoma. Hum Pathol 2000;31:1139–1145.

Ordóñez NG, Baloch Z, Matias-Guiu X. Undifferentiated (anaplastic) carcinoma. In: DeLellis RA, Lloyd RV, Heitz PU, Eng C (eds). Pathology and Genetics of Tumours of Endocrine Organs. Kleihues P, Sobin LH, series eds. World Health Organization Classification of Tumours. Lyon, France: IARC Press, 2004:77–80.

Ordóñez NG, El-Naggar AK, Hickey RC, Samaan NA. Anaplastic thyroid carcinoma: immunocytochemical study of 32 cases. Am J Clin Pathol 1991;96:15–24.

Rosai J, Carcangiu ML, DeLellis RA. Undifferentiated (Anaplastic) Carcinoma. Tumors of the Thyroid gland. Atlas of Tumor Pathology, Third Series, Fascicle 5. Washington, DC: Armed Forces Institute of Pathology, 1992:135–160.

Venkatesh YS, Ordóñez NG, Schultz PN, et al. Anaplastic carcinoma of the thyroid. A clinicopathologic study of 121 cases. Cancer 1990;66:321–330.

Medullary Thyroid Carcinoma

Albores-Saavedra JA, Krueger JE. C-cell hyperplasia and medullary thyroid microcarcinoma. Endocr Pathol 2001;12:365–377.

Block MA. Surgical treatment of medullary carcinoma of the thyroid. Otolaryngol Clin North Am 1990;23:453–473.

Bose S, Kapila K, Verma K. Medullary carcinoma of the thyroid: A cytological, immunocytochemical, and ultrastructural study. Diagn Cytopathol 1992;8:28–32.

Matias-Guiu X, DeLellis R, Moley JF, et al. Medullary thyroid carcinoma. In: DeLellis RA, Lloyd RV, Heitz PU, Eng C (eds). Pathology and Genetics of Tumours of Endocrine Organs. Kleihues P, Sobin LH, series eds. World Health Organization Classification of Tumours. Lyon, France: IARC Press, 2004:86–91.

Rosai J, Carcangiu ML, DeLellis RA. Medullary carcinoma. Tumors of the Thyroid gland. Atlas of Tumor Pathology, Third Series, Fascicle 5. Washington, DC: Armed Forces Institute of Pathology, 1992:207–246.

Saad MF, Ordóñez NA, Rashid RK, et al. Medullary carcinoma of the thyroid: a study of the clinical features and prognostic factors in 161 patients. Medicine 1984;63:319–342.

Schröder S, Böcker W, Baisch H, et al. Prognostic factors in medullary thyroid carcinoma: survival in relation to sex, stage, histology, immunocytochemistry, and DNA content. Cancer 1988;61:806–816.

Thomas CC, Cowan RJ, Albertson DA, Cooper MR. Detection of medullary carcinoma of the thyroid with I-131 MIBG. Clin Nucl Med 1994;19:1066–1068.

Primary Thyroid Lymphoma

Abbondanzo SL, Aozasa K, Boerner S, Thompson LDR. Primary lymphoma and plasmacytoma. In: DeLellis RA, Lloyd RV, Heitz PU, Eng C (eds). Pathology and Genetics of Tumours of Endocrine Organs. Kleihues P, Sobin LH, series eds. World Health Organization Classification of Tumours. Lyon, France: IARC Press, 2004:109–111.

Anscombe AM, Wright DH. Primary malignant lymphoma of the thyroid: a tumour of mucosa-associated lymphoid tissue: review of seventy-six cases. Histopathology 1985;9:81–97.

Compagno J, Oertel JE. Malignant lymphoma and other lymphoproliferative disorders of the thyroid gland. A clinicopathologic study of 245 cases. Am J Clin Pathol 1980;74:1–11.

Derringer GA, Thompson LDR, Frommelt RA, et al. Malignant lymphoma of the thyroid gland: a clinicopathologic study of 108 cases. Am J Surg Pathol 2000;24:623–639.

Isaacson PG. Lymphoma of the thyroid gland. Curr Top Pathol 1997;91:1–14.

Isaacson PG, Müller-Hermelink HK, Piris MA, et al. Extranodal marginal zone B-cell lymphoma of mucosa-associated lymphoid tissue (MALT lymphoma). In: Jaffe ES, Harris NL, Stein H, Vardiman JW, eds. Pathology and Genetics Tumors of Haematopoietic and Lymphoid Tissues. World Health Organization Classification of Tumours. Lyon, France: IARC Press, 2001;157–160.

Oertel JE, Heffess CS. Lymphoma of the thyroid and related disorders. Semin Oncol 1987;14:333–342.

Pedersen RK, Pedersen NT. Primary non-Hodgkin's lymphoma of the thyroid gland: a population based study. Histopathology 1996;28:25–32.

Spindle Cell Tumor with Thymus-Like Differentiation

Cheuk W, Chan JKC, Dorfman DM, Giordano T. Spindle cell tumour with thymus-like differentiation. In: DeLellis RA, Lloyd RV, Heitz PU, Eng C (eds). Pathology and Genetics of Tumours of Endocrine Organs. Kleihues P, Sobin LH, series eds. World Health Organization Classification of Tumours. Lyon, France: IARC Press, 2004:94–95.

Cheuk W, Jacobson AA, Chan JK. Spindle epithelial tumor with thymus-like differentiation (SETTLE): a distinctive malignant thyroid neoplasm with significant metastatic potential. Mod Pathol 2000;13:1150–1155.

Iwasa K, Imai MA, Noguchi M, et al. Spindle epithelial tumor with thymus-like differentiation (SETTLE) of the thyroid. Head Neck 2002;24:888–893.

Rosai J, Carcangiu ML, DeLellis RA. Tumors with Thymic or Related Branchial Pouch Differentiation. Tumors of the Thyroid gland. Atlas of Tumor Pathology, Third Series, Fascicle 5. Washington, DC: Armed Forces Institute of Pathology, 1992:282–284.

Weigensberg C, Hubert D, Asa SL, et al. Thyroid thymoma in childhood. Endocr Pathol 1990;1:123–127.

Carcinoma Showing Thymus-like Differentiation

Asa SL, Dardick I, van Nostrand AW, et al. Primary thyroid thymoma: a distinct clinicopathologic entity. Hum Pathol 1988;19:1463–1467.

Chan JK, Rosai J. Tumors of the neck showing thymic or related branchial pouch differentiation: a unifying concept. Hum Pathol 1991;22:349–367.

Cheuk W, Chan JKC, Dorfman DM, Giordano T. Carcinoma showing thymus-like differentiation. *In*: DeLellis RA, Lloyd RV, Heitz PU, Eng C (eds). Pathology and Genetics of Tumours of Endocrine Organs. Kleihues P, Sobin LH, series eds. World Health Organization Classification of Tumours. Lyon, France: IARC Press, 2004:96–97.

Rosai J, Carcangiu ML, DeLellis RA. Tumors with Thymic or Related Branchial Pouch Differentiation. Tumors of the Thyroid gland. Atlas of Tumor Pathology, Third Series, Fascicle 5. Washington, DC: Armed Forces Institute of Pathology, 1992:282–284.

Metastatic Neoplasms

Czech JM, Lichtor TR, Carney JA, van Heerden JA. Neoplasms metastatic to the thyroid gland. Surg Gynecol Obstet 1982;155:503–505.

DeLellis R. Secondary tumours of the thyroid. *In*: DeLellis RA, Lloyd RV, Heitz PU, Eng C (eds). Pathology and Genetics of Tumours of Endocrine Organs. Kleihues P, Sobin LH, series eds. World Health Organization Classification of Tumours. Lyon, France: IARC Press, 2004:122–123.

Halbauer M, Kardum-Skelin I, Vranesic D, Crepinko I. Aspiration cytology of renal-cell carcinoma metastatic to the thyroid. Acta Cytol 1991;35:443–446.

Heffess CS, Wenig BM, Thompson LDR. Metastatic renal cell carcinoma to the thyroid gland: A clinicopathologic study of 36 cases. Cancer 2002;95:1869–1878.

Nakhjavani MK, Gharib H, Goellner JR, van Heerden JA. Metastasis to the thyroid gland. A report of 43 cases. Cancer 1997;79:574–578.

Rosai J, Carcangiu ML, DeLellis RA. Secondary Tumors. Tumors of the Thyroid gland. Atlas of Tumor Pathology, Third Series, Fascicle 5. Washington, DC: Armed Forces Institute of Pathology, 1992:289–296.

4

Non-neoplastic Lesions of the Parathyroid Gland

Lester DR Thompson

GENERAL CONSIDERATIONS

There are a variable number of glands (2–10), but usually four are present, symmetrically arranged. About 5% of people have more than four glands. They are usually soft, pliable, and measure <0.5 cm (5 mm) with a combined weight of about 120–140 mg. It is agreed that no one gland should be more than 60 mg, although the lower glands are often slightly larger than the upper glands. Embryologically, the upper pair arise from the 4th branchial pouch, while the lower pair arise from the 3rd branchial pouch. Glands can be found anywhere along the normal route of migration, resulting in glands embedded within the thyroid gland, thymus, pericardium, esophagus, and mediastinum.

The parathyroid gland is comprised of four cell types:

- The chief cell is the basic functional cell usually involved in hypersecretory processes;
- The oxyphilic cell, which has abundant granular cytoplasm and increases in number as the patient ages;
- The water-clear cell which is quite rare; and
- Adipocytes, which also increase with age, comprising up to 50% of the cellular mass.

The cells can be arranged in cords, sheets, and pseudo-glandular or pseudoacinar patterns.

Spatial constraints limit the discussion of parathyroid gland function, but calcium homeostasis is the principle function. Disorders of calcium metabolism are the usual clinical manifestations. Calcium homeostasis is maintained by dietary intake, intestinal absorption and bone resorption of calcium balanced by bone accretion of calcium and its excretion in urine, sweat and other fluids. Nearly 99% of calcium is stored in the skeletal system, and osteoclastic resorption is most important. The three most important hormones are parathyroid hormone (PTH), calcitonin, and Vitamin D. PTH is a polypeptide hormone (84 amino acid residues; the n-terminal is active, while the c-terminal is assayed) that stimulates osteoclastic resorption of bone, increasing blood calcium levels and renal phosphate excretion. This results in hypophosphatemia, and can cause metabolic acidosis due to inhibition of HCO_3. PTH also stimulates production of 1,25 dihydroxy-cholecalciferol. The half-life of PTH is 20–30 minutes.

Parathyroid non-neoplastic disorders include aplasia, cysts, parathyroiditis and hyperplasia. This discussion will be limited to hyperplasia and parathyroiditis.

Hyperparathyroidism is separated into primary, secondary and tertiary, with primary hyperparathyroidism caused by adenoma (80%), hyperplasia (15%), and carcinoma (5%) most commonly. Most hyperplasia results from secondary hyperparathyroidism as a result of renal disease.

PRIMARY CHIEF CELL HYPERPLASIA

Primary chief cell hyperplasia is a non-neoplastic increase in the parenchymal cell mass within all of the

---

PRIMARY CHIEF CELL HYPERPLASIA DISEASE FACT SHEET

Definition
- Non-neoplastic increase in parathyroid parenchymal cell mass within all parathyroid tissue without a known stimulus

Incidence and Location
- Approximately 17/million population

Morbidity and Mortality
- Calcium metabolism abnormality
- Cardiovascular disease may cause death

Gender, Race and Age Distribution
- Female > Male (3:1)
- Adults, 50–70 years

Clinical Features
- 20% may be familial
- Asymptomatic, discovered during multichannel analyzer studies
- If symptomatic, fatigue, lethargy, anorexia, weakness, vomiting, depression, polyuria, polydipsia, hypertension
- 'Bones, stones, abdominal moans' not seen often
- Nephrolithiasis, nephrocalcinosis
- Biochemical findings include elevated calcium, decreased inorganic phosphorus and increased parathyroid hormone levels

Prognosis and Therapy
- Excellent, although recurrences occur (about 15%)
- Surgery with autotransplantation

parathyroid tissue without a known clinical stimulus for increased parathyroid hormone secretion.

CLINICAL FEATURES

About 15% of all primary hyperparathyroidism is caused by primary chief cell hyperplasia. Women are affected much more commonly than men (3:1), with the overall incidence increasing with age. Most patients present with sporadic disease, although about 20% of patients have familial disease (most commonly multiple endocrine neoplasia [MEN] syndromes). MEN1 (Wermer's syndrome) is the most common syndrome, with nearly 90% of patient's having parathyroid hyperplasia.

A fair number of patients are asymptomatic, the disorder discovered incidentally during routine multiphasic screening for other reasons. The presentation is vague, including fatigue, lethargy, anorexia, weakness, nausea, vomiting, constipation, depression, polyuria, polydipsia, hypertension and arthralgias. The classic triad of 'bones, stones, and abdominal moans' is not commonly seen in modern care, but refers to osteitis fibrosa cystica (brown tumor of bone), kidney stones, and peptic ulcer disease. Patients will have polyuria, nephrocalcinosis, nephrolithiasis and metastatic calcifications. Emotional instability, depression, psychosis, and confusion are frequent. The symptoms relate specifically to the level and to the duration of serum calcium elevation. Rarely, patient's will present with a neck mass.

Biochemical findings include an elevation of serum ionized calcium levels, with associated decrease in serum inorganic phosphorus concentrations and a high serum alkaline phosphatase. Serum parathyroid hormone levels, utilizing the intact hormone assay, will usually be increased above the normal range of 210–310 pg/ml. There will be a high urine calcium, cAMP, hydroxproline and phosphate.

RADIOLOGIC FEATURES

Technetium sestamibi imaging has gained significant favor as the preferred technique for detecting the topographic location of parathyroid tissue (Figure 4-1). However, the technique is limited in detecting hyperplasia, and has greater clinical utility in detecting adenoma or carcinoma. Surgery is successful in parathyroid disease without imaging in about 95% of patients. However, radiographic studies are generally used in the setting of recurrent disease after failed surgery. Unusual locations of parathyroid tissue may be found with MR imaging with gadolinium and fat suppression techniques. Hyperplasia, however, does not enhance as much with gadolinium as does an adenoma.

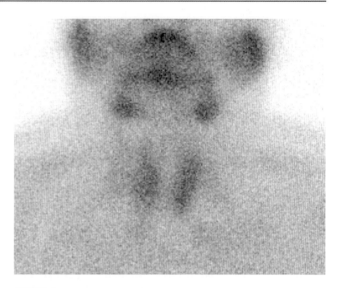

FIGURE 4-1

A delayed technetium-99 sestamibi image demonstrates uneven, increased uptake in all glands, consistent with hyperplasia (Courtesy Dr W Chen).

PATHOLOGIC FEATURES

GROSS FINDINGS

All of the glands will be affected, although sometimes the glands are not affected to the same degree, creating uneven hyperplasia or asymmetric enlargement. At least two glands *must* be sampled, including a 'normal' gland to accurately separate adenoma and hyperplasia. Radiographic studies and intraoperative laboratory assessments are insufficiently reliable to allow for accurate separation. Diffuse or nodular enlargement is noted, with cystic change occasionally identified. The glands

---

PRIMARY CHIEF CELL HYPERPLASIA PATHOLOGIC FEATURES

Gross Findings
- All glands affected, although not equally (at least 2 glands sampled for accurate diagnosis)
- Diffuse or nodular enlargement
- Soft, tan-brown glands

Microscopic Findings
- Variance between glands is common, but all are affected
- Parenchyma increased with decreased fat content
- Cellularity increased
- Chief and oncocytic cells are increased
- Solid, follicular and cord-like patterns can be seen
- Secondary changes are common

Pathologic Differential Diagnosis
- Parathyroid adenoma, parathyroid carcinoma, metastatic renal cell carcinoma

are usually <1 g in total weight, although about 40 % are >1 g. The glands are soft and tan-brown.

MICROSCOPIC FINDINGS

Primary Chief Cell Hyperplasia

The histology of all of the glands is similar, although variance is common. The parenchymal component is increased with a commensurate decrease in fat (Figure 4-2). The process can appear nodular, multinodular or diffuse depending on the proportion of the gland involved (Figure 4-3). The process may extend into the soft tissue surrounding the parathyroid gland, and should not be over-interpreted as 'invasive'. Overall, the cellularity is increased, even if it is different between glands. In general, both a chief and oncocytic cell components will be increased and there is a variety of different architectures and varying degrees of cellularity (Figure 4-4). Solid, follicular (Figure 4-5), and cord-like patterns (Figure 4-6) are noted in addition to a vaguely nodular appearance (Figure 4-7). Cellular atypia can be seen (Figure 4-8), but it is usually not widespread or profound. Secondary changes including fibrosis, hemorrhage and hemosiderin laden macrophages are common findings (Figure 4-9). Intracellular glycogen is often increased in hyperplastic glands above what is seen in atrophy or adenoma.

Water-Clear Cell Hyperplasia

This is a very uncommon type of hyperplasia seen slightly more commonly in men, most commonly in the fifth decade of life. The upper glands tends to be preferentially involved, and all reported cases have a combined gland weight of >1 g. The large cells have cytoplasm which is completely clear on H&E (Figure 4-10). The feature is usually present on frozen section material, while usual processing may cause the artifact to be lost, resulting in a finely reticulated cytoplasm composed of numerous small vacuoles. Cell borders are prominent. The nuclei tend to be basal oriented. There is no adipose tissue present. Neutral fat stains are negative, but glycogen is present in the cytoplasm.

ANCILLARY STUDIES

Fine needle aspiration (FNA) does not reliably separate between adenoma and hyperplasia, and so is not of value. Ultrastructural findings usually show abundant mitochondria and endoplasmic reticulum with interdigitating cell membranes, but is not useful in diagnosis. The chief cells with be positive for keratin and chromogranin, but immunohistochemical studies do not help with the principle differential diagnostic consideration: adenoma. Fat staining of cryostat sections may help to discriminate between normal and slightly hyperplastic glands, but is not always helpful.

The use of intraoperative parathyroid hormone assays has profoundly altered the management of parathyroid disease. An intraoperative decline of parathyroid hormone to normal levels at 10 minutes and greater than 50 % of the initial baseline value suggests surgical cure.

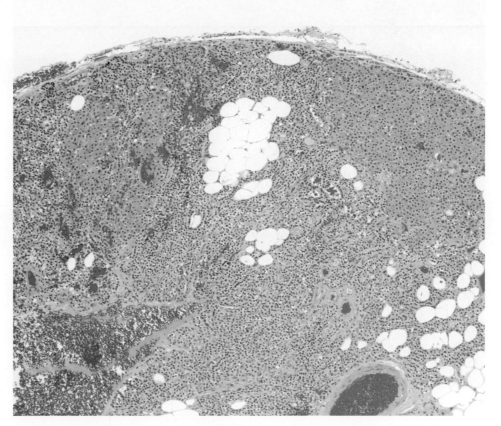

FIGURE 4-2

The entire gland has an increased parenchymal cellularity with a decrease in the amount of adipose tissue in this hyperplastic parathyroid gland.

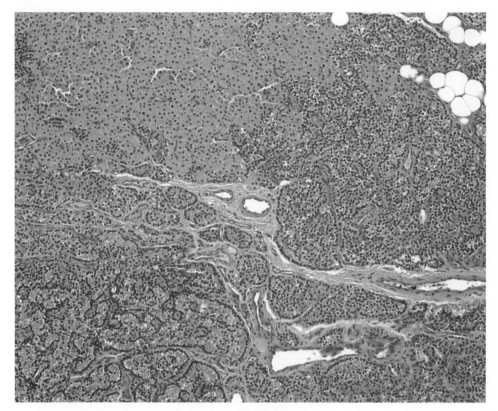

FIGURE 4-3
Increased parenchymal cellularity and decreased fat in this example of hyperplasia. Both chief and oxyphilic cell increase is noted.

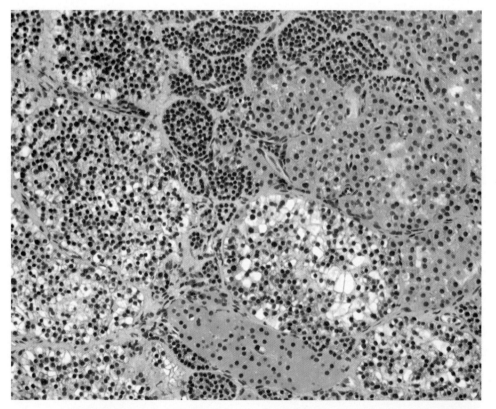

FIGURE 4-4
Nodules of different cellular components are seen, but intracellular fat is not present.

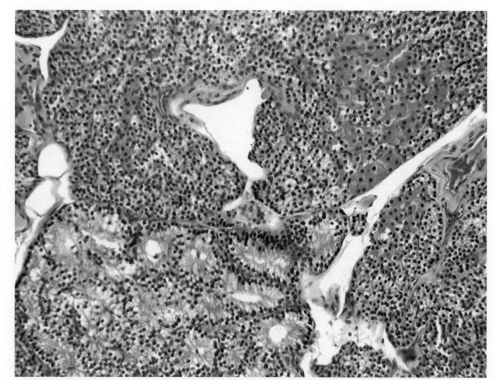

FIGURE 4-5

Solid and follicular patterns of growth are identified. A few onco-cytic cells are also identified in the predominantly chief cell hyperplasia.

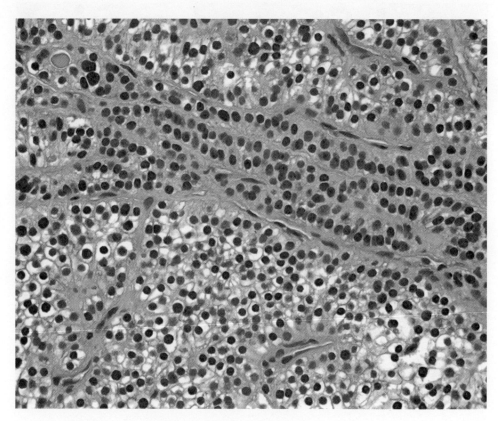

FIGURE 4-6

Cord and 'follicular' growth is present within areas of sheet-like growth in this example of para-thyroid hyperplasia.

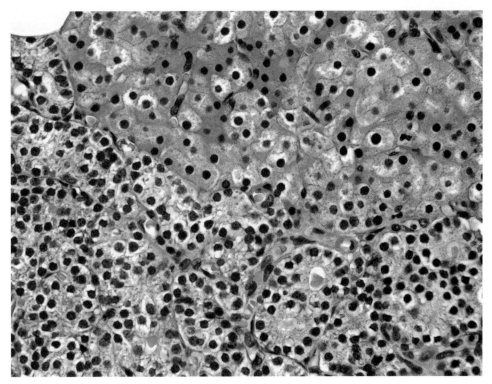

FIGURE 4-7
A nodule of oncocytic cells is noted in this sample of hyperplasia. Note the follicular architecture immediately below the nodule of oxyphilic cells.

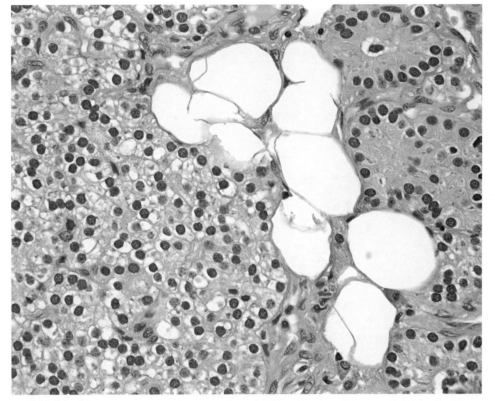

FIGURE 4-8
Fat can be seen within hyperplastic tissue. Slight nuclear atypia is present in the far right of the field.

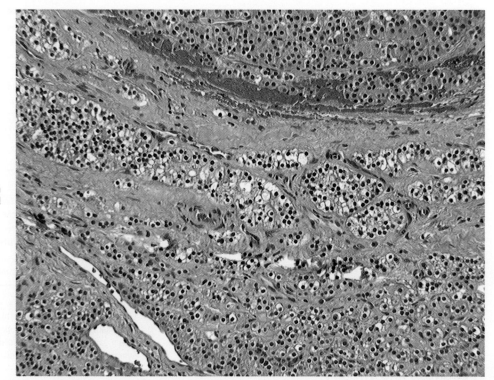

FIGURE 4-9

Fibrosis and hemorrhage are seen within this example of parathyroid hyperplasia.

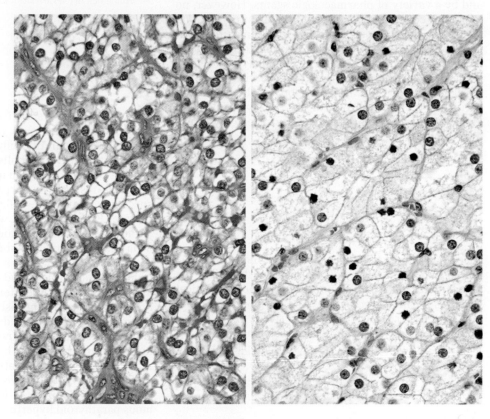

FIGURE 4-10

Water-clear cell hyperplasia presents with optically clear cytoplasm on frozen section material (left), but standard processing yields a finely reticulated cytoplasm on routine processing (right). The cell borders are prominent and the nuclei tend to be basally oriented.

DIFFERENTIAL DIAGNOSIS

The principle differential is with parathyroid adenoma, although sometimes in recurrent disease, separation from parathyroid carcinoma may be more difficult. Tiny glandular biopsies from normal associated glands are difficult to interpret since the distribution of parenchymal and fat cells are often irregular. Identification of a capsule, a single cell population, pseudoacinar growth, secretions, and cellular monotony are features seen more commonly in adenoma. While not diagnostic, pleomorphism when seen in multiple foci suggests an adenoma. Reactive fibrosis is seen in recurrent hyperplasia, while dense, acellular, perivascular fibrosis is seen in carcinoma. Lithium has been known to produce hyperparathyroidism, but it resolves with drug discontinuance. Bony metastasis may result in hypercalcemia due to the osteolytic effect, but these patients do not have hyperparathyroidism per se. Clear cell hyperplasia may be confused with metastatic renal cell carcinoma, especially if there is renal disease.

PROGNOSIS AND THERAPY

The serum calcium level can be lowered by hydration and by a variety of pharmacologic agents. However, no long-term correction is achieved without surgery. Complete removal of three glands, while leaving a remnant of the fourth gland is the most widely employed surgery. Auto-transplantation into the forearm may also be performed in order to avoid neck dissection if recurrence develops. Recurrence may develop in about 15% of patients. Hypoparathyroidism may rarely result if all glands are removed. Subtotal parathyroidectomy is preferred for water clear-cell hyperplasia.

SECONDARY AND TERTIARY PARATHYROID HYPERPLASIA

Secondary hyperparathyroidism is a non-neoplastic increase in the parenchymal cell mass within all of the parathyroid tissue in response to a known clinical stimulus for increased parathyroid hormone secretion. Tertiary hyperparathyroidism is when there is an increased parathyroid parenchyma cell mass associated with an autonomous hyperfunction in patients who have had secondary hyperparathyroidism and now are on dialysis or have had a renal transplant.

CLINICAL FEATURES

The most common cause of secondary hyperparathyroidism is chronic renal failure, the clinical stimulus

---

SECONDARY AND TERTIARY PARATHYROID HYPERPLASIA DISEASE FACT SHEET

Definition
▶ Non-neoplastic increase in parathyroid parenchymal cell mass within all parathyroid tissue with a known stimulus

Incidence and location
▶ Especially common in patients with renal failure and/or on dialysis

Morbidity and Mortality
▶ Control of calcium level may be difficult, leading to skeletal deformities and vessel calcification

Gender, Race and Age Distribution
▶ Female > Male (about 3:1)
▶ Older patients in general, but renal disease occurs in all ages

Clinical Features
▶ Chronic renal failure, malabsorption, Vitamin D metabolism abnormalities and pseudohypoparathyroidism can all cause disease
▶ Serum calcium level is decreased
▶ Symptoms reflect underlying disease

Prognosis and Therapy
▶ Depends on underlying renal disease
▶ Subtotal parathyroidectomy performed early to avoid skeletal deformities and vessel calcification

---

that results in the adaptive increase in production of parathyroid hormone. A variety of other causes may result in hyperparathyroidism, and include abnormalities of vitamin D metabolism, calcium deficiency, malabsorption and low serum magnesium. Lithium therapy may also result in hyperparathyroidism. A broad age spectrum is affected, reflecting the underlying renal disease. Patients present with symptoms of increased parathyroid hormone, which often results in osteomalacia and periarticular abnormal calcium deposition. The serum calcium level is usually decreased. In renal failure, parathyroid glands seem to expand diffusely and polyclonally, while later developing areas of nodular hyperplasia with diminished expression of both the vitamin D receptor and calcium-sensing receptor. When more than one parathyroid gland progresses to nodular hyperplasia, the hyperparathyroidism is often refractory to medical treatment.

Tertiary hyperparathyroidism usually occurs after years of renal failure and is preported to be an autonomous parathyroid hyperfunction occuring in a setting of known secondary hyperparathyroidism. Most cases result from diffuse or nodular chief cell hyperplasia affecting multiple glands. The hypercalcemia which can result often threatens a kidney transplant graft function, requiring prompt treatment.

PATHOLOGIC FEATURES

GROSS FINDINGS

The findings are no different from primary hyperplasia, with all of the glands affected, whether it is uniform, nodular or asymmetric. The glands are yellow to tan-brown. In tertiary disease, asymmetry can be quite star-tling, with glands often reaching up to 40 times the size of normal glands.

MICROSCOPIC FINDINGS

There is an overall increase of parenchymal cells, including chief, oxyphilic and transitional types (Figure 4-11), while there is a decrease in the amount of adipocytes. The adipocyte decrease seems more pronounced if the disease has been present for a long duration. Nodular or diffuse growth is present, with sheets, cords and acinar structures noted. The cells are quite enlarged in comparison to normal cells. Oxyphilic cells tend to be increased more than chief cells. However, in tertiary hyperparathyroidism, the chief cells are more frequently affected. Fibrosis, calcification and hemorrhage are seen in many cases.

SECONDARY AND TERTIARY PARATHYROID HYPERPLASIA PATHOLOGIC FEATURES

Gross Findings
▶ Identical to primary hyperplasia although gland enlargement may be huge

Microscopic Findings
▶ Increased parenchyma with decreased adipocytes
▶ Nodular or diffuse growth
▶ Oncocytic cell increase may be more noticeable than chief cell
▶ Secondary changes are common

Pathologic Differential Diagnosis
▶ Primary chief cell hyperplasia, parathyroid adenoma, parathyroid carcinoma

---

DIFFERENTIAL DIAGNOSIS

Primary chief cell hyperplasia is the main differential diagnostic consideration, although this is a clinical separation in most cases. Parathyroid adenoma and carcinoma are also considered in the differential diagnosis, but are usually eliminated with clinical information. With recurrence of hyperparathyroidism, small islands of residual parenchyma within the fat may take on an atypical and 'invasive' appearance which should not be over-interpreted as carcinoma.

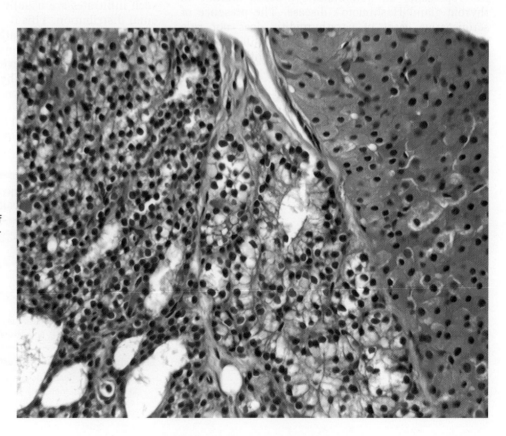

FIGURE 4-11
Hyperplasia is shows with chief cell, transitional cells and oncocytic cells.

PROGNOSIS AND THERAPY

Prevention and treatment of secondary hyperparathyroidism is a continual management predicament for the nephrologist and endocrinologist. Subtotal parathyroidectomy is the treatment of choice, with a small remnant of tissue left or auto-transplanted. However, it is important to perform surgery early to avoid skeletal deformities and vessel calcifications which will not involute after surgery. Recurrence of hyperparathyroidism is an ongoing management problem with renal failure patients. Likewise, the autonomous hyperfunction of the parathyroid glands results in an alteration of the 'set-point' of serum calcium levels, which causes stimulation of the parathyroid tissue in spite of 'normal' calcium levels.

PARATHYROIDITIS

CLINICAL FEATURES

Parathyroiditis is a rare and poorly understood condition. Chronic parathyroiditis may occur in patients with hypoparathyroidism as well as those with primary chief cell hyperplasia. Most patients are asymptomatic. Antibodies to parathyroid tissue are seen in only a few cases of parathyroiditis. It is thought that parathyroiditis represents an autoimmune process, similar to thyroid gland Hashimoto's disease. The presence of seronegative cases of parathyroiditis does not rule against an autoimmune etiology, as a similar phenomenon is observed in Hashimoto's thyroiditis. Based on this assumption, it is believed that the lymphocytic infiltration is an ongoing destructive process.

PATHOLOGIC FEATURES

Parathyroiditis is characterized by a slightly enlarged gland, although the macroscopic appearance is not specific. Histologically, there are aggregates of mature lymphocytes infiltrating otherwise normal parathyroid tissue (Figure 4-12). There is often lymphoid follicle formation with prominent germinal centers (Figure 4-13). Plasma cells and fibrosis (often heavy) may be identified, and destruction of the parenchyma has been reported. Atrophy of the residual parathyroid tissue may also be seen. The histologic picture of the lymphoid infiltration closely resembles the lymphoid infiltration identified in thyroid gland Hashimoto's thyroiditis. More than one parathyroid gland may be involved, although multifocal disease is seen in the presence of autoimmune disorders, such as Sjögren's disease.

DIFFERENTIAL DIAGNOSIS

A chronic inflammatory proliferation composed predominantly of mature lymphocytes may occur in the parathyroid glands as a non-specific reaction in patients with various infectious disease processes; however, such infiltrates are usually sparse and have a perivascular distribution. This is in contrast to the exuberant proliferation seen in parathyroiditis. The distribution and extent of the fibrosis may be mis-diagnosed as parathyroid carcinoma. However, the lack of other cytomorphologic features of parathyroid carcinoma should help with this distinction. Lymphoma involving the parathyroid glands (as part of systemic disease) is reported, but is vanishingly rare. The cytomorphologic features of lymphoma are usually distinct.

**PARATHYROIDITIS
DISEASE FACT SHEET**

Definition
▶ Inflammatory infiltrate within the parathyroid parenchyma, possibly related to autoimmunity

Incidence and Location
▶ Extremely rare

Gender, Race and Age Distribution
▶ Female > Male
▶ Older age patients

Clinical Features
▶ Most patients are asymptomatic

Prognosis and Therapy
▶ Unknown
▶ Supportive management, if necessary

**PARATHYROIDITIS
PATHOLOGIC FEATURES**

Gross Findings
▶ Slightly enlarged gland

Microscopic Findings
▶ Aggregates of mature lymphocytes within parathyroid parenchyma
▶ Lymphoid follicle formation may be seen, with germinal centers
▶ Plasma cells, fibrosis and atrophy may be seen

Pathologic Differential Diagnosis
▶ Non-specific inflammation related to infectious etiology, parathyroid carcinoma

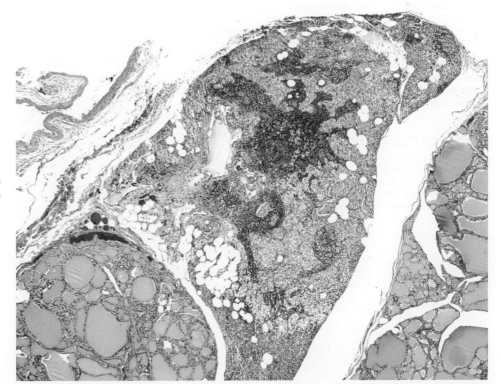

FIGURE 4-12

A parathyroid gland, adjacent to benign thyroid parenchyma, shows an infiltrate of lymphoid cells.

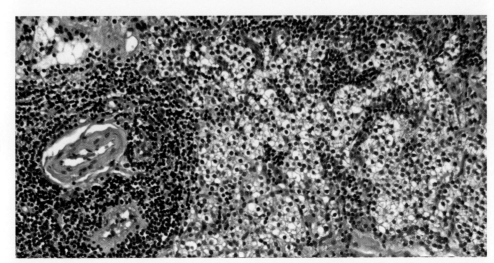

FIGURE 4–13

Lymphocytes are sprinkled throughout the parathyroid gland in this example of parathyroiditis.

PROGNOSIS AND THERAPY

The significance is unknown and management is supportive, if clinically necessary.

SUGGESTED READING

Primary Chief Cell Hyperplasia

Bombi JA, Nadal A, Munoz J, et al. Ultrastructural pathology of parathyroid glands in hyperparathyroidism: a report of 69 cases. Ultrastruct Pathol 1993;17:567–582.

Bondeson L, Bondeson AG, Nissborg A, Thompson NW. Cytopathological variables in parathyroid lesions: a study based on 1,600 cases of hyperparathyroidism. Diagn Cytopathol 1997;16:476–482.

Bondeson AG, Bondeson L, Ljungberg O, Tibblin S. Fat staining in parathyroid disease – diagnostic value and impact on surgical strategy: clinicopathologic analysis of 191 cases. Hum Pathol 1985;16:1255–1263.

Dedeurwaerdere F, Van Damme B. Histopathology of the parathyroid glands. Acta Otorhinolaryngol Belg 2001;55:95–101.

DeLellis RA. Primary chief cell hyperpplasia. Tumors of the Parathyroid gland. Atlas of Tumor Pathology, Third Series,, Fascicle 6. Washington, DC: Armed Forces Institute of Pathology, 1993:65–78.

Fitko R, Roth SI, Hines JR, Roxe DM, Cahill E. Parathyromatosis in hyperparathyroidism. Hum Pathol. 1990;21:234–237.

Grimelius L, Bondeson L. Histopathological diagnosis of parathyroid diseases. Pathol Res Pract 1995;191:353–365.

Lloyd RV, Douglas BR, Young WF Jr. Parathyroid gland. Endocrine Diseases. Atlas of Nontumor Pathology, First Series, Fascicle 1. Washington, DC: Armed Forces Institute of Pathology, 2002:45–90.

Udelsman R. Primary hyperparathyroidism. Curr Treat Options Oncol 2001;2:365–372.

Weber AL, Randolph G, Aksoy FG. The thyroid and parathyroid glands. CT and MR imaging and correlation with pathology and clinical findings. Radiol Clin North Am 2000;38:1105–1129.

Secondary and Tertiary Parathyroid Hyperplasia

Fukagawa M. Cell biology of parathyroid hyperplasia in uremia. Am J Med Sci 1999;317:377–382.

Lloyd RV, Douglas BR, Young WF Jr. Parathyroid gland. Endocrine Diseases. Atlas of Nontumor Pathology, First Series, Fascicle 1. Washington, DC: Armed Forces Institute of Pathology, 2002:45–90.

Tominaga Y. Management of renal hyperparathyroidism. Biomed Pharmacother 2000;54 Suppl 1:25s-31s.

Parathyroiditis

Bondeson AG, Bondeson L, Ljüngberg O. Chronic parathyroiditis associated with parathyroid hyperplasia and hyperparathyroidism. Am J Surg Pathol 1984;8:211–215.

Boyce BF, Doherty, VR, Mortimer, G. Hyperplastic parathyroiditis-a new autoimmune disease? J Clin Pathol 1982;35:812–814.

Lloyd RV, Douglas BR, Young WF Jr. Parathyroid gland. Endocrine Diseases. Atlas of Nontumor Pathology, First Series, Fascicle 1. Washington, DC: Armed Forces Institute of Pathology, 2002:45–90.

5 Benign Neoplasms of the Parathyroid Gland

Lester DR Thompson

PARATHYROID ADENOMA

An encapsulated benign neoplasm of either chief or oncocytic cells. Parathyroid disease is separated into primary, secondary or tertiary, based on whether the parathyroid gland is primarily the source of the disease or if the gland is reacting to exogenous stimulation (such as renal disease). This distinction is sometimes quite difficult on histology alone, and even more so if only a single gland is sampled. Intra-operative selective venous parathyroid hormone assay is a clinical parameter which may assist with the distinction.

**PARATHYROID ADENOMA
DISEASE FACT SHEET**

Definition
▶ An encapsulated benign neoplasm of either the chief or the oncocytic cells

Incidence and Location
▶ Approximately 1 per 1000 persons

Morbidity and Mortality
▶ Associated with excess calcium, with cardiovascular abnormalities the most significant
▶ No mortality

Gender, Race and Age Distribution
▶ Female ≫ Male (3:1)
▶ Mean age at presentation: 50–60 years

Clinical Features
▶ Non-specific findings of fatigue, weakness and pain related to hypercalcemia
▶ Polydipsia, polyuria and nephrolithiasis
▶ Pancreatitis and peptic ulcer disease are less common
▶ Mass lesion may be palpated
▶ Rarely associated with inherited syndromes

Prognosis and Therapy
▶ Excellent without recurrence (by definition)
▶ Surgery is treatment of choice

CLINICAL FEATURES

Early detection of parathyroid disease has improved dramatically with increased use of multichannel autoanalyzers, with calcium levels determined as part of routine blood chemistries. Therefore, a true incidence is difficult to determine, although 1 per 1000 is considered an approximate incidence. Parathyroid adenomas account for approximately 80% of primary hyperparathyroidism. Women are affected more frequently than men (about 3:1), with a peak incidence in the sixth and seventh decades. There is a rare association with inherited syndromes (MEN1, MEN2 and hyperparathyroidism-jaw tumor syndrome). Two simultaneous adenomas are quite uncommon, but have been reported. The sites of involvement are usually perithyroidal, but mediastinal and esophageal tumors are recognized along with intrathyroidal neoplasms. Symptoms of excess calcium and/or parathyroid hormone may yield a non-specific clinical presentation which includes fatigue, malaise, abdominal pain, depression, constipation, peptic ulcer disease, kidney stones and/or pancreatitis.

RADIOGRAPHIC FEATURES

A variety of techniques can be utilized to detect and localize abnormal parathyroid glands, including ultrasonography, computed tomography, magnetic resonance imaging and nuclear scintigraphy, specifically with technetium 99 sestamibi. Technetium is concentrated by parathyroid tissue (Figure 5-1), effectively identifying adenomas in 40–90% of cases, suggesting it cannot be used in isolation.

PATHOLOGIC FEATURES

GROSS FINDINGS

The gland is typically enlarged, with a mean weight of about 1g. The surface is smooth and surrounded by a thin capsule, although multinodularity and multilobularity may develop. The cut surface is soft and reddish-brown, often distinct from the yellowish-brown surrounding parathyroid parenchyma. If the adenoma is large, degenerative changes are noted.

**PARATHYROID ADENOMA
PATHOLOGIC FEATURES**

Gross Findings

▶ A single enlarged parathyroid gland (rarely 2 adenomas may occur)
▶ Smooth, encapsulated mass
▶ Reddish brown, with rim of uninvolved parenchyma adjacent to proliferation
▶ Usually <1g

Microscopic Findings

▶ Single mass
▶ Encapsulated (although often a thin, irregular capsule)
▶ Fatless nodule
▶ Distinct histology within the neoplasm different from remaining gland
▶ Atrophy or compression of parathyroid parenchyma
▶ Usually a single histologic population of enlarged cells
▶ Glandular architecture with 'secretions' more common in adenoma than hyperplasia

Immunohistochemical Results

▶ Parathyroid hormone and chromogranin positive
▶ TTF-1 and calcitonin negative

Fine Needle Aspiration

▶ Similar to thyroid follicular lesions
▶ Clear cytoplasm and distinct cell borders are helpful

Pathologic Differential Diagnosis

▶ Parathyroid hyperplasia, thyroid adenoma, medullary thyroid carcinoma, metastatic renal cell carcinoma

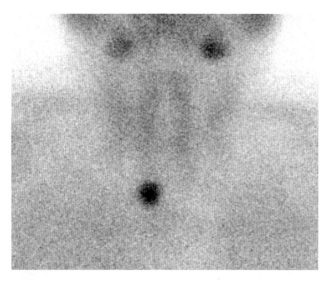

FIGURE 5-1

A technetium-99 sestamibi scan shows increased uptake disproportionate to the other parathyroid glands, a finding consistent with adenoma (Courtesy Dr. W Chen).

MICROSCOPIC FINDINGS

A single gland is usually affected by a well circumscribed and usually encapsulated mass with a fatless population of cells within the tumor, distinct from the uninvolved, compressed or atrophic parathyroid parenchyma (Figures 5-2 and 5-3). The capsule is sometimes extremely thin and attenuated (Figures 5-4 to 5-6). The tumor is usually comprised of a single cell proliferation of enlarged chief (Figure 5-7) or oncocytic cells (Figure 5-8), although occasionally a mixture of both can be seen. The cells are often arranged in a solid or acinar-glandular (follicular) distribution, a finding uncommon in hyperplasia (Figures 5-9 and 5-10). Peritheliomatous palisading is occasionally identified. The chief cells have ample cleared to slightly eosinophilic cytoplasm surrounding nuclei which are round to oval with heavy nuclear chromatin distribution (Figure 5-11). Lipid within the cytoplasm is limited if present at all.

Nuclear pleomorphism can be seen, although it is usually focal or arranged in clusters. Mitotic figures are inconspicuous, with usually 1 or fewer mitotic figures per 10 high power fields. Eosinophilic 'secretions' may sometimes be mistaken for colloid and may occasionally calcify, simulating a psammoma body. Amyloid may occasionally be identified between the neoplastic cells. Stroma is scant, but delicate fibrovascular bands separate the neoplastic cells. Hemosiderin laden macrophages, inflammation and fibrosis may be part of degenerative changes, especially in large tumors. Oncocytic cell adenomas are composed of cells with abundant eosinophilic, granular cytoplasm and may have prominent, centrally placed eosinophilic nucleoli (Figure 5-12); otherwise there is no difference from chief cell adenomas. Clear-cell adenoma and lipoadenoma are recognized, but are exceedingly uncommon.

ANCILLARY STUDIES

IMMUNOHISTOCHEMICAL RESULTS

The parenchymal cells will be chromogranin and parathyroid hormone immunoreactive, although the interpretation of the parathyroid hormone reaction is fraught with diffusion artifacts and serum reactions. TTF-1 and thyroglobulin are non-reactive, while specific keratins may be positive.

FINE NEEDLE ASPIRATION

Separation of a thyroid follicular neoplasm from a parathyroid proliferation is difficult. Papillary and follicular arrangements are common. Secretions and 'colloid-like' substances may suggest a thyroid lesion. Cleared cytoplasm may be noted, but separation from a metastatic renal cell tumor or a thyroid gland neoplasm may be difficult. Fluid parathyroid hormone levels may help, but only if fluid is obtained from a cystic lesion.

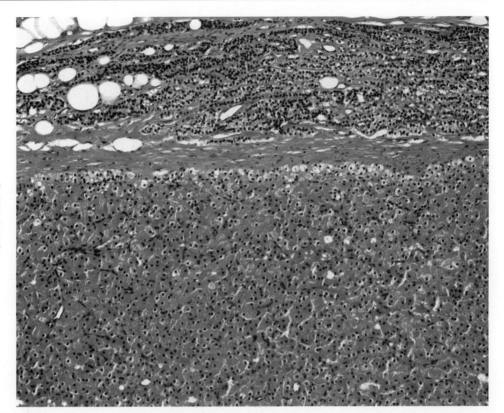

FIGURE 5-2

A well-formed capsule separates the oncocytic neoplasm from the surrounding, compressed uninvolved parathyroid parenchyma which contains fat. The cells of the neoplasm are oncocytic with a monotonous appearance.

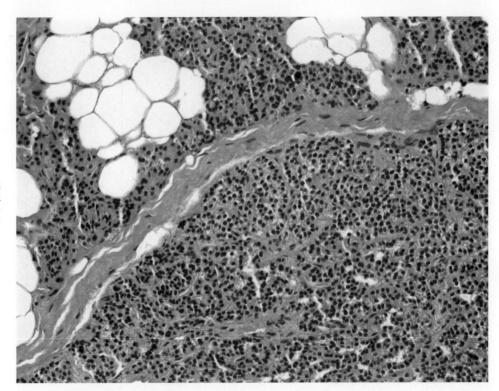

FIGURE 5-3

A thin, but well-formed fibrous capsule separates this chief cell adenoma from the surrounding non-atrophic parenchyma. Fat is seen in the uninvolved parenchyma.

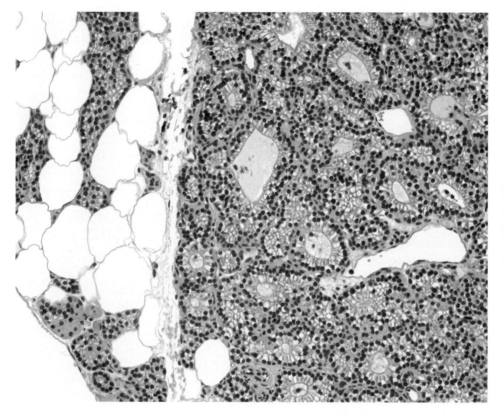

FIGURE 5-4

A nearly non-existent capsule separates the adenoma from the surrounding parenchyma. The parenchyma contains cells which are smaller than the neoplasm and has fat. The neoplastic cells are arranged in a pseudoglandular distribution.

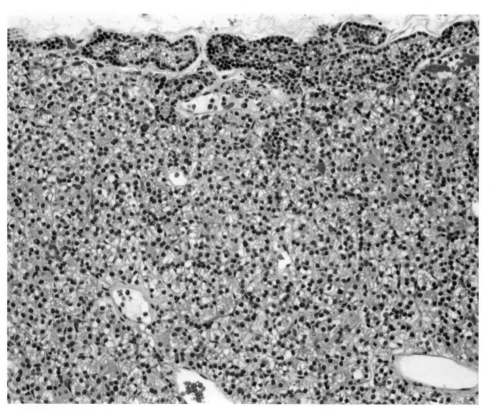

FIGURE 5-5

Compressed parenchyma is noted at the superior portion of the field. A true capsule is not present in this example of an adenoma.

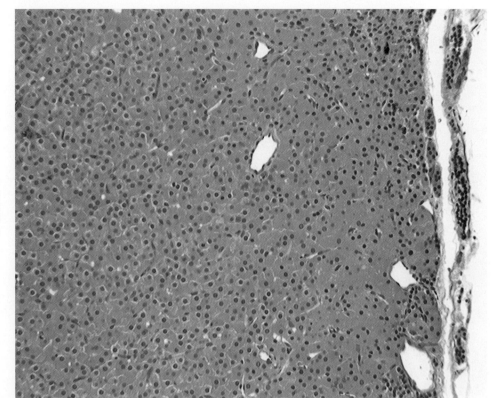

FIGURE 5-6

Sometimes the compressed parenchyma looks like lymphocytes at the
periphery (right side). However, a
delicate capsule separates this
adenoma from the surrounding atrophic parenchyma.

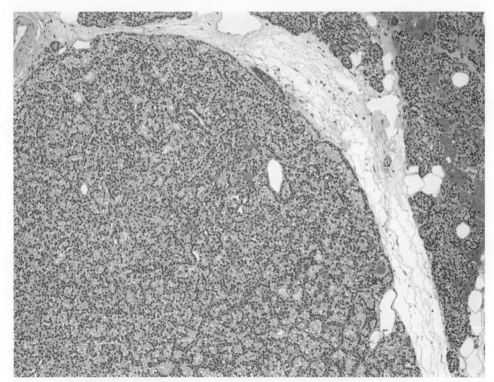

FIGURE 5-7

Chief cells compose this adenoma
without any fat cells present. There
is a thin, edematous capsule separating the tumor from uninvolved
parenchyma which still contains
adipocytes.

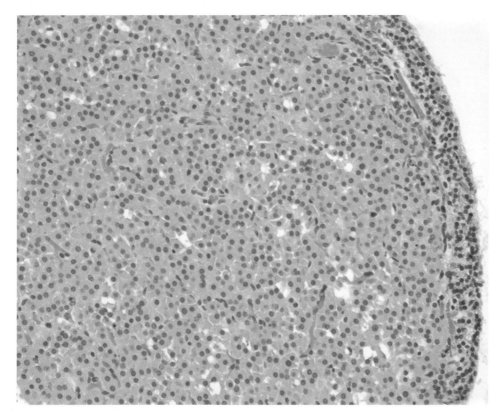

FIGURE 5-8

This oncocytic adenoma shows a rim of atrophic parenchyma at the periphery (right sided), with only an attenuated capsule noted.

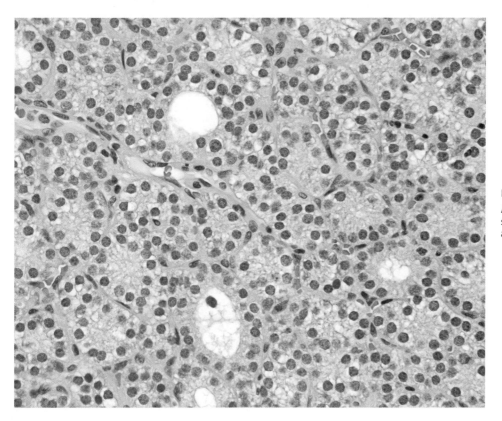

FIGURE 5-9

A glandular pattern is commonly seen in adenomas, with cells arranged around a lumen.

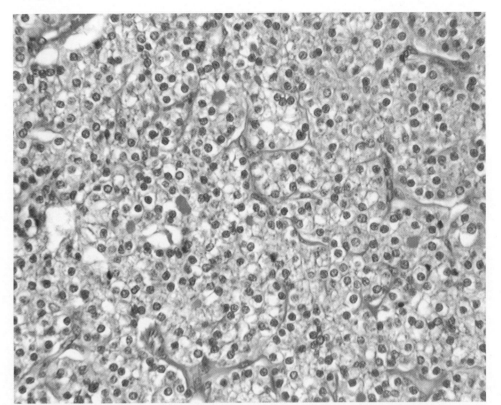

FIGURE 5-10

A pseudofollicular pattern of growth is present in this adenoma. Inspissated 'colloid-like' material is noted.

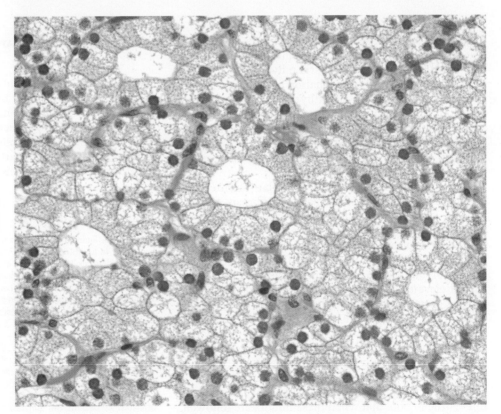

FIGURE 5-11

Cytoplasmic clearing can be seen in parathyroid adenoma, although a slightly granular or vacuolated appearance may remain.

DIFFERENTIAL DIAGNOSIS

Parathyroid hyperplasia and carcinoma are occasionally difficult to separate from an adenoma, while thyroid neoplasms and metastatic renal cell carcinoma may also occasionally enter the differential diagnosis. Uneven, nodular hyperplasia will mimic an adenoma, especially if only a single gland is sampled. A 'remnant' can be seen in both lesions. The easiest way to separate hyperplasia and adenoma is to sample more than one gland. If more than one gland is enlarged or abnormal,

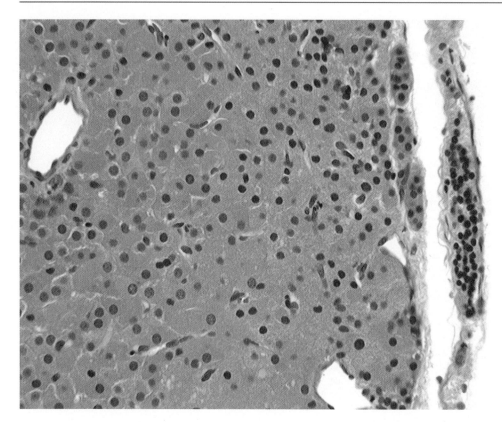

FIGURE 5-12

Granular, oncocytic or oxyphilic cytoplasm may be seen in adenoma (compressed uninvolved parathyroid is present at the right).

if there is an increase in the parenchyma to fat ratio (age variability considered), and nodular distribution of both chief and oncocytic cells, then hyperplasia should be considered. Clinical information about renal status, serum calcium and/or parathyroid hormone levels and condition of the remaining '*in situ*' glands will help to make the separation. Intraoperative changes in the serum parathyroid hormone levels may also serve to confirm the diagnosis of adenoma versus hyperplasia.

Carcinoma usually has a trabecular architecture, demonstrates thick, acellular bands of fibrosis, a thick capsule, capsular, vascular or perineural invasion, profound nuclear pleomorphism, increased mitotic figures, including atypical forms, and the presence of necrosis. Adherence to the thyroid gland, difficulty in removing the tumor, and extremely elevated serum calcium levels should elevate the suspicion of parathyroid carcinoma. In sites of previous surgery, the reactive changes in the stroma may also simulate invasive growth or result in attachment to the surrounding tissues, factors which should be weighed carefully in determining the final diagnosis. Occasionally, in cases which cannot be definitively separated, the term 'atypical adenoma' can be used, detailing the histologic features of concern. It is interesting to note that when these tumors are followed, there is usually a benign clinical outcome.

Thyroid lesions which can cause diagnostic difficult, do not have a rim of uninvolved parathyroid tissue, may have birefringent oxalate crystals, and will be TTF-1 or thyroglobulin immunoreactive.

PROGNOSIS AND THERAPY

Surgery is the treatment of choice if there is significant calcium elevation, other complications of hyperparathyroidism or if the patient is <50 years. Surgery ameliorates the calcium effects of hyperparathyroidism, specifically those of the cardiovascular system. Rarely parathyromatosis (ruptured, implanted or remnant parathyroid adenoma tissue) may occur.

SUGGESTED READING

Akerstrom G, Rudberg C, Grimelius L, et al. Histologic parathyroid abnormalities in an autopsy series. Hum Pathol 1986;17: 520–527.

Arnold A, Shattuck TM, Mallya SM, et al. Molecular pathogenesis of primary hyperparathyroidism. J Bone Miner Res 2002;17 Suppl 2: N30–N36.

Bondeson AG, Bondeson L, Ljungberg O, Tibblin S. Fat staining in parathyroid disease–diagnostic value and impact on surgical strategy: clinicopathologic analysis of 191 cases. Hum Pathol 1985;16:1255–1263.

DeLellis RA. Parathyroid adenoma. Tumors of the Parathyroid Gland. Atlas of Tumor Pathology, Third Series, Fascicle 6. Washington, DC: Armed Forces Institute of Pathology, 1993:25–52.

Gotthardt M, Lohmann B, Behr TM, et al. Clinical value of parathyroid scintigraphy with technetium-99m methoxyisobutylisonitrile: discrepancies in clinical data and a systematic metaanalysis of the literature. World J Surg 2004;28:100–107.

Grimelius L, DeLellis RA, Bondeson L, et al. Parathyroid adenoma. *In*: DeLellis RA, Lloyd R, Heitz PU, Eng C (eds) Pathology and Genetics of Tumours of the Endocrine Organs. World Health Organization Classification of Tumours. Lyon, France: IARC Press, 2004:128–132.

Vasef MA, Brynes RK, Sturm M, et al. Expression of cyclin D1 in parathyroid carcinomas, adenomas, and hyperplasias: a paraffin immunohistochemical study. Mod Pathol 1999;12:412–416.

6 Malignant Neoplasms of the Parathyroid Glands

Lester DR Thompson

PARATHYROID CARCINOMA

Parathyroid carcinoma comprises <5% of all primary hyperparathyroidism cases and is a rare tumor. This is a malignant neoplasm of parathyroid parenchymal cells (no malignant adipose tumors are recognized in the parathyroid). Secondary parathyroid hyperplasia and neck irradiation are suggested as etiologic factors. There are no well accepted histologic features which are used alone to diagnose carcinoma, but a constellation of features can help to secure the diagnosis.

CLINICAL FEATURES

Parathyroid carcinoma occurs in all ages without a gender bias. The clinical features are due primarily to the effects of excessive parathyroid hormone secretion (PTH) and hypercalcemia. The non-specific symptoms (weakness, fatigue, anorexia, weight loss, nausea) overlap with adenoma, but excessively high serum calcium levels (>16 mg/dL) are associated with nephrolithiasis, renal insufficiency and bone 'brown tumors'. A palpable neck mass, often difficult to remove at surgery due to adherence to the soft tissues, nerves (recurrent laryngeal nerve) and/or thyroid gland, suggests carcinoma. Interestingly, there are recurrent losses of chromosome 13q in parathyroid carcinomas, the region known to contain the retinoblastoma (RB1) and BRCA2 tumor suppressor genes. A genomic region frequently lost in parathyroid adenomas is 11q, the location of MEN1, but it is almost never identified in carcinoma, supporting the contention that parathyroid carcinomas arise *de novo* rather than from preexisting adenomas. Carcinoma is a suggested component of hyperparathyroidism-jaw tumor syndrome.

PARATHYROID CARCINOMA
DISEASE FACT SHEET

Definition
▸ A malignant neoplasm derived from parathyroid parenchymal cells

Incidence and Location
▸ Accounts for <5% of primary hyperparathyroidism

Morbidity and Mortality
▸ Calcium metabolism adverse effects on the cardiovascular system
▸ Indolent tumor with recurrences and metastases, about 15–25% mortality at 5 years

Gender, Race and Age Distribution
▸ Equal gender distribution
▸ Wide age range, although predominantly older patients

Clinical Features
▸ Symptoms referable to excess calcium and parathyroid hormone
▸ Nephrolithiasis and bone 'brown tumors'
▸ Palpable neck mass, often difficult to remove surgically
▸ Hoarseness is common with recurrent laryngeal nerve involvement

Prognosis and Therapy
▸ Indolent with recurrences common (about 50%)
▸ About 50% 10-year survival
▸ Surgery

PATHOLOGIC FEATURES

GROSS FINDINGS

Carcinoma is usually large and adherent to the surrounding soft tissues, nerves and thyroid gland. If there has been previous surgery, scarring and hemorrhage may simulate 'invasion'. The cut surface is firm, white-tan and may have areas of necrosis.

MICROSCOPIC FINDINGS

No one histologic feature, other than metastatic disease, is considered diagnostic for parathyroid carcinoma. However, a constellation of features can usually be used to support the diagnosis. Definitive vascular invasion (endothelial lined space with attachment to the wall by the neoplastic cells; Figure 6-1), capsular invasion (Figure 6-2), extension into the uninvolved periparathyroidal adipose tissue (Figure 6-3) and/or invasion-attachment to the thyroid parenchyma (Figures 6-4 and 6-5) are reliable features of malignancy. Perineural invasion is almost diagnostic of carcinoma (Figure 6-6), although this feature is not commonly identified. Epithelial entrapment in fibrosis (usually secondary to degenerative changes) can mimic invasion and may be neigh unto impossible to separate from true invasion in

PARATHYROID CARCINOMA
PATHOLOGIC FEATURES

Gross Findings

▸ Large tumors
▸ Adherent to soft tissues and thyroid gland
▸ Firm, gray-white cut surface
▸ Central necrosis may be present

Microscopic Findings

▸ Adherence to the thyroid gland
▸ Capsular, vascular or perineural invasion
▸ Soft tissue extension
▸ Tumor cell necrosis (comedonecrosis)
▸ Trabecular growth with thick, acellular bands of fibrosis
▸ Tumor cell monotony, although profound pleomorphism can be seen
▸ High nuclear to cytoplasmic ratio
▸ Spindling of tumor cells
▸ Prominent, eosinophilic, irregular macronucleoli
▸ Increased mitotic figures, including atypical forms

Immunohistochemical Results

▸ Chromogranin and parathyroid hormone, along with keratins

Pathologic Differential Diagnosis

▸ Parathyroid adenoma, medullary carcinoma, thyroid follicular neoplasms, metastatic renal cell carcinoma

some cases. A thick capsule is frequently associated with band-forming, acellular, dense fibrosis, occasionally associated with hemosiderin laden macrophages or hemorrhage (Figure 6-7). The fibrosis often shows a perivascular distribution, with collagen expanding into the tumor. Small compartments are often formed by the fibrosis (Figure 6-8). True tumor necrosis, often in a central, comedonecrosis pattern, suggests malignancy (Figure 6-9). The tumor cells are arranged in solid, diffuse (Figure 6-10) or organoid groups, with a trabecular pattern noted in a number of cases (Figure 6-11). Many different patterns of growth can be seen in parathyroid carcinoma, including glandular, pseudoacinar, spindle cell, perivascular palisade and papillary (Figure 6-12). Chief cell neoplasms are more common than oncocytic neoplasms, although the cytoplasmic quality does not influence patient outcome (Figure 6-13). Tumor cell spindling, 'watermelon seeds' and pyknosis are seen more frequently in carcinoma, but not exclusively (Figure 6-14). A monotonous cellular population (in which the cells may be atypical or not) suggests malignancy. There is an increased nuclear to cytoplasmic ratio, cellular enlargement, profound pleomorphism and prominent, irregular, eosinophilic macronucleoli (Figure 6-15). Remarkably increased mitotic activity, including atypical forms, is more likely in carcinoma (Figure 6-16), but mitotic figures alone cannot separate between adenoma and carcinoma. Frozen section is discouraged, especially if it is an incisional biopsy, as it results in

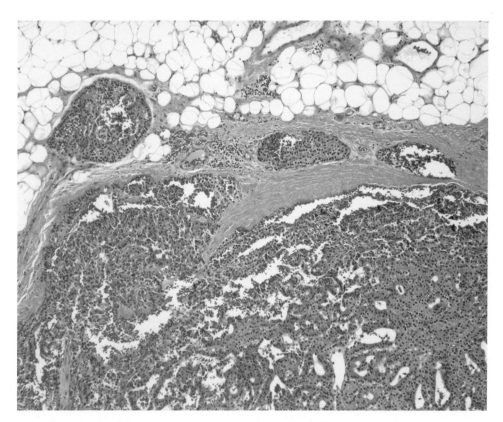

FIGURE 6-1

Neoplastic cells are identified within vascular spaces of the fibrous connective tissue capsule of this parathyroid carcinoma.

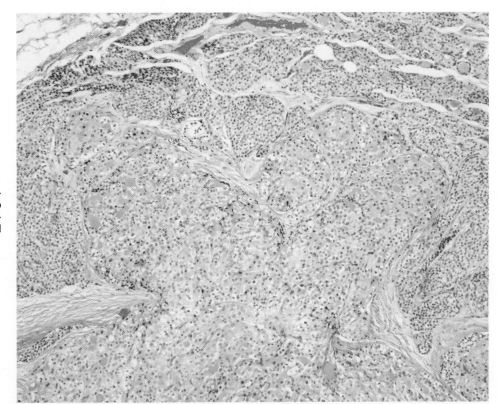

FIGURE 6-2

A 'mushroom' projection of neoplastic cells through the capsule into the surrounding parathyroid parenchyma is seen in this parathyroid carcinoma.

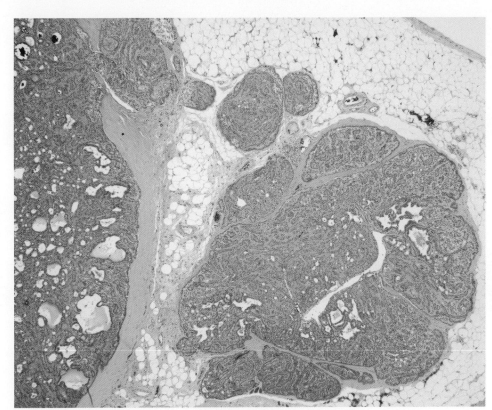

FIGURE 6-3

A thick capsule surrounding the neoplasm, with areas of invasion and direct extension into the surrounding periparathyroidal adipose tissue.

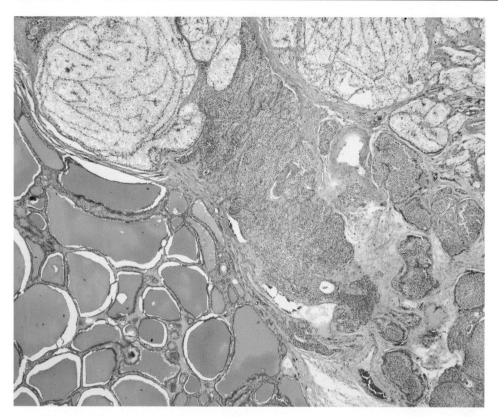

FIGURE 6-4
Different morphologic patterns of parathyroid carcinoma are identified immediately adjacent to thyroid parenchyma (lower left quadrant).

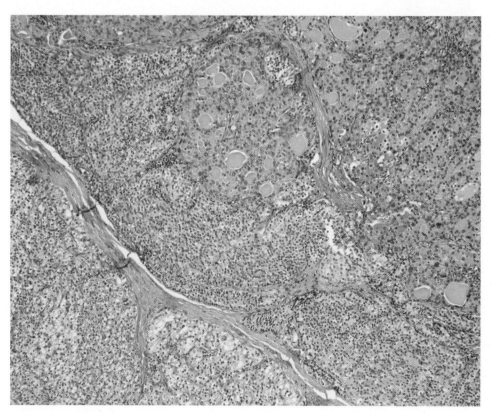

FIGURE 6-5
The neoplastic parathyroid cells are intimately associated with thyroid tissue. Thyroid tissue is on the upper right. Bands of fibrosis are dissecting between the parathyroid neoplasm.

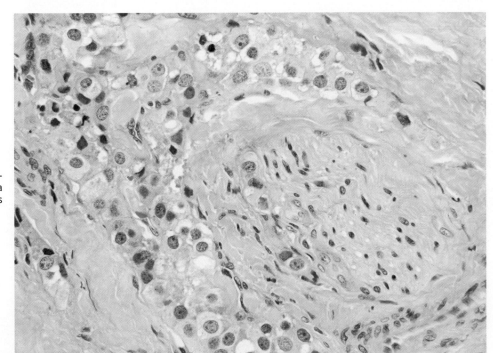

FIGURE 6-6
Perineural invasion, including intraneural invasion, is diagnostic of a parathyroid carcinoma in this example.

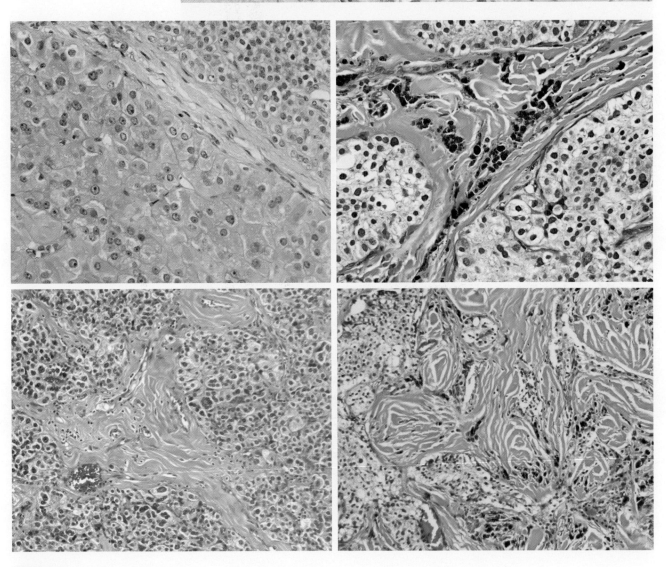

FIGURE 6-7
Fibrosis is common in parathyroid carcinoma. Scant fibrosis (left upper) to dense, acellular, eosinophilic perivascular fibrosis (left lower) is seen in parathyroid carcinoma. Hemosiderin may be deposited within the fibrosis to a variable degree (right upper and right lower).

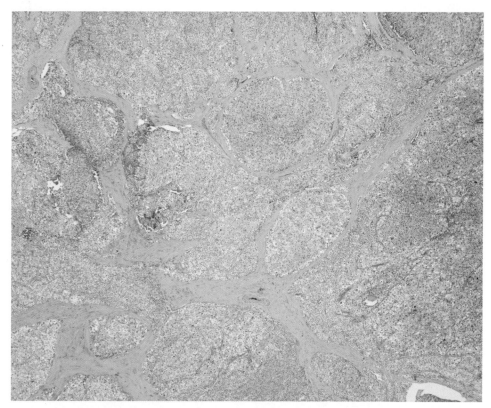

FIGURE 6-8
Multiple nodules of monotonous cells are separated by the dense fibrosis in this parathyroid carcinoma.

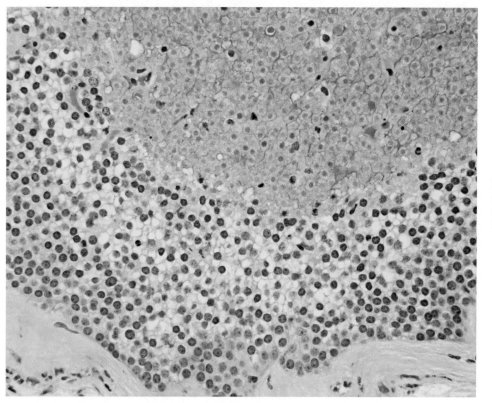

FIGURE 6-9
Comedonecrosis showing 'ghost-cell' outlines is not a feature of a benign condition.

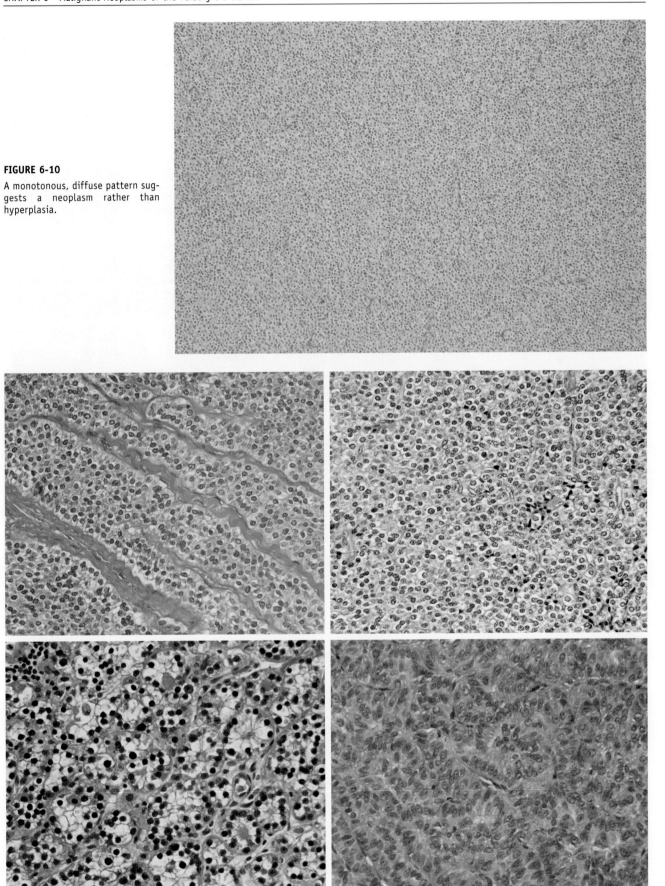

FIGURE 6-10

A monotonous, diffuse pattern suggests a neoplasm rather than hyperplasia.

FIGURE 6-11

Many patterns can be seen in carcinoma, including trabecular (left upper), follicular (left lower), solid (right upper), and festoons (right lower).

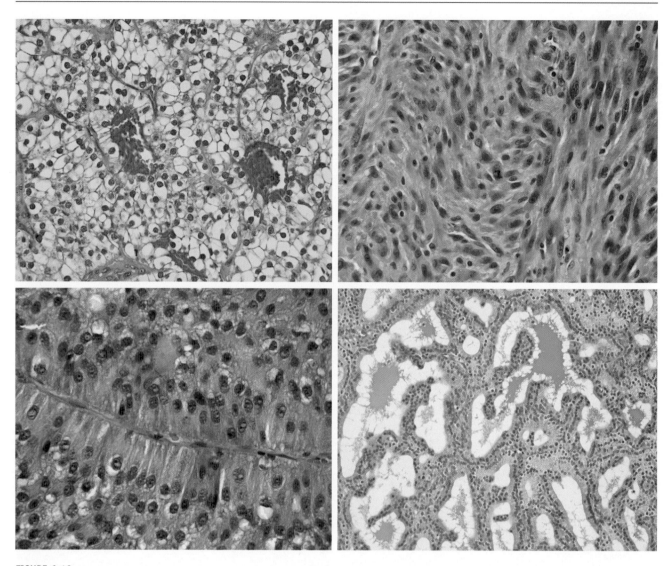

FIGURE 6-12
Many patterns can be seen in carcinoma, including pseudoglandular (left upper), perivascular palisade (left lower), spindled (right upper), and papillary (right lower).

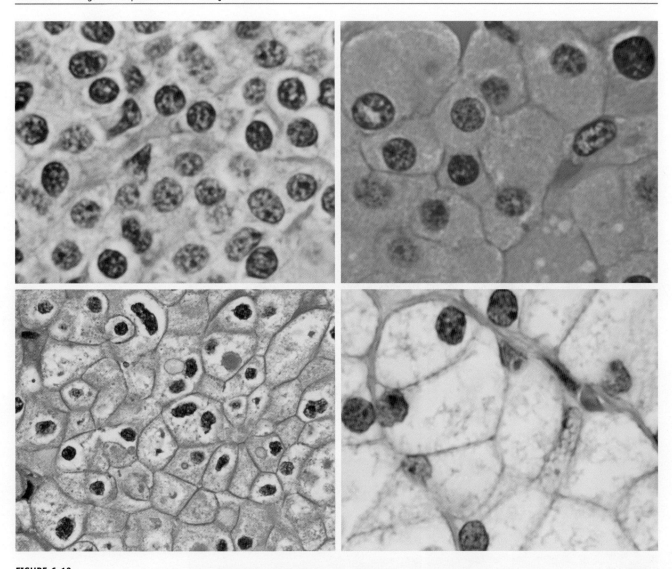

FIGURE 6-13
The cytoplasmic quality can range from amphophilic (left upper), to clearing (left lower), oxyphilic (right upper), to completely clear (right lower). Note how the cell membranes are prominent in all types of cytoplasm.

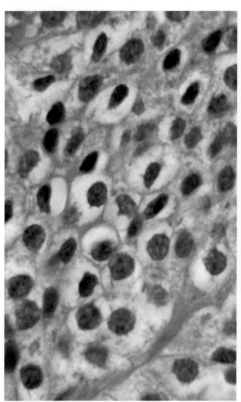
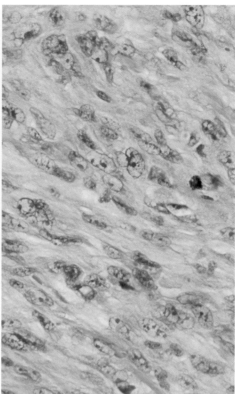

FIGURE 6-14

Left: Pyknotic, 'watermelon seed' appearance to the nuclei is common in carcinoma. Right: Tumor cell spindling and remarkably anaplasia is seen in this parathyroid carcinoma.

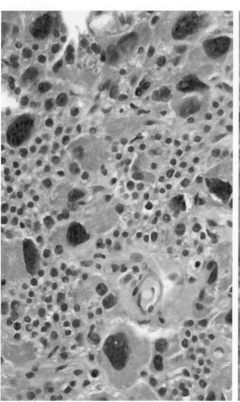
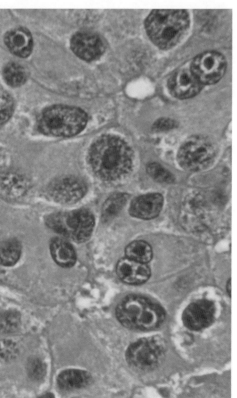

FIGURE 6-15

Left: Profound nuclear pleomorphism. Right: Prominent, irregular, macro, eosinophilic nucleoli with a perinucleolar halo are almost diagnostic of carcinoma.

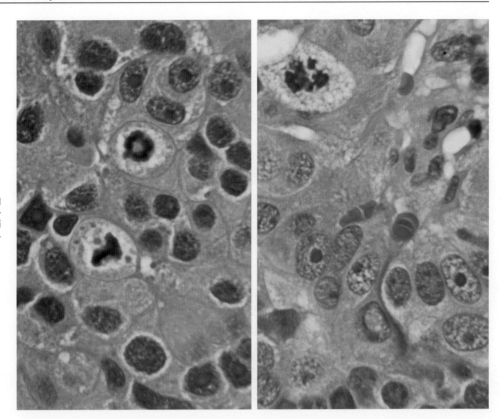

FIGURE 6-16
Left: Mitotic figures, including atypical forms are seen in carcinoma. Right: Prominent nucleoli and intranuclear cytoplasmic inclusions are common in carcinoma.

tumor cell seeding, with recurrent hyperparathyroidism, whether the original disease was benign or malignant.

ANCILLARY STUDIES

The neoplastic cells are chromogranin and parathyroid hormone immunoreactive (Figure 6-17), while nonreactive with TTF-1 and thyroglobulin. Increased Ki-67 (Figure 6-18) and cyclin-D1 overexpression are seen more commonly in parathyroid carcinoma. A variety of other markers may occasionally be expressed in parathyroid carcinoma, and include CK7, CK18, muc-1, epithelial membrane antigen, p16 and renal cell marker (RCC), among others (Figures 6-19 and 6-20). The clinical utility of these markers is limited at present.

DIFFERENTIAL DIAGNOSIS

The difficulty with the diagnosis of parathyroid carcinoma is the separation of parathyroid adenoma from carcinoma, especially in the setting of previous surgery or with 'neck manipulation'. Parathyroid carcinoma must be separated from parathyroid adenoma, thyroid conditions, and metastatic neoplasms. The most difficult separation is from parathyroid adenoma. Adeno-

mas are usually smaller, but with increased use of screening laboratory studies, this feature is not as useful in present medical practice. Unfortunately, large adenomas will frequently display fibrosis, hemosiderin deposits, and cystic degeneration. A rim of uninvolved parathyroid parenchyma is rarely seen in parathyroid carcinoma, but in large adenomas it may be more difficult to detect. When adenoma cells are arranged in acinar or glandular-type structures, eosinophilic material can be seen, a feature uncommon in carcinoma. The cells of an adenoma are enlarged, but do not usually have the increased N:C ratio of a carcinoma; nucleoli are usually small and inconspicuous. Mitotic activity is usually low in adenomas, but mitotic figures alone cannot be used to separate benign from malignant tumors.

A thyroid follicular neoplasm may be simulated by the 'follicular' pattern of growth and by inspissated material within the lumen in parathyroid carcinoma (Figure 6-21). Parathyroid tissue usually has clear cytoplasm and will display very prominent and easy to detect cell borders. Intrathyroidal parathyroid tissue often lacks a well-defined capsule and may show pseudoinvasive growth patterns. Immunohistochemistry will also help with separation. Medullary carcinoma may metastasize or directly invade into parathyroid tissue and will be chromogranin immunoreactive, but will be calcitonin and CEA positive. Metastatic renal cell carcinoma may present as a 'clear cell neoplasm' in the parathyroid gland (Figure 6-22). However, the vascular pattern, sinusoidal growth and immunoreactivity with

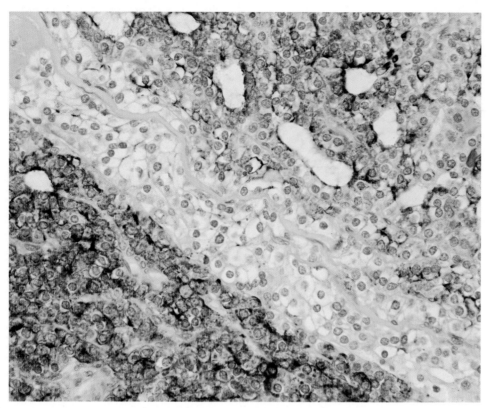

FIGURE 6-17
Variable expression of chromogranin is seen in this carcinoma, with heavy reaction in the lower left, focal reaction in the middle, while intermediate staining is present in the upper right.

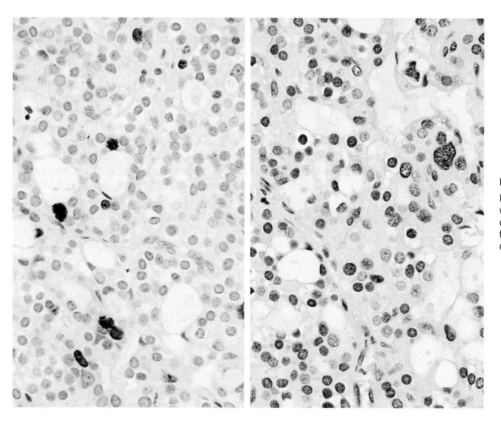

FIGURE 6-18
Left: Ki-67 is strongly reactive within the nuclei of a number of cells. Right: p16 is strongly and diffusely immunoreactive in nearly all of the neoplastic nuclei.

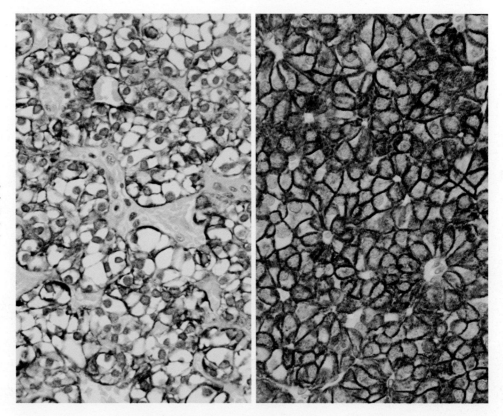

FIGURE 6-19
Left: CK7 shows a predominantly membrane reactivity in this clear cell parathyroid carcinoma. Right: CK18 has both membrane and cytoplasmic reactivity, with accentuation of the cell membranes.

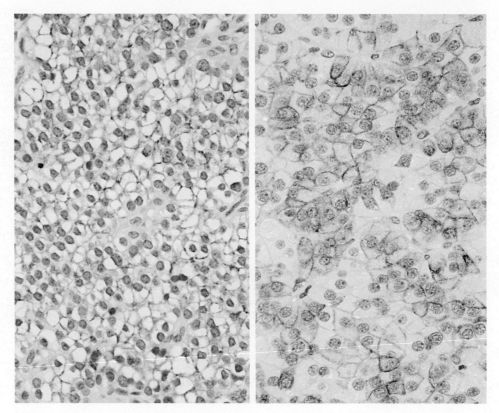

FIGURE 6-20
Renal cell marker reacts along the membranes of parathyroid carcinoma cells in some cases, while also yielding a positive reaction in the cytoplasm of other cells.

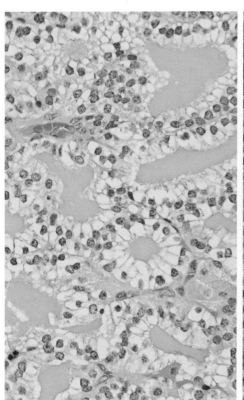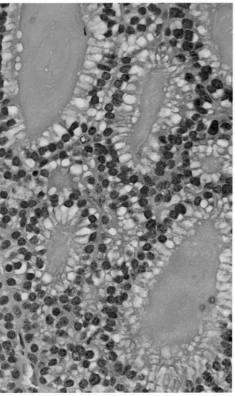

FIGURE 6-21

Parathyroid carcinoma can have inspissated secretions which can mimic a thyroid neoplasm (left). The prominent cell borders and clear cytoplasm (right) will help with the separation from a thyroid neoplasm.

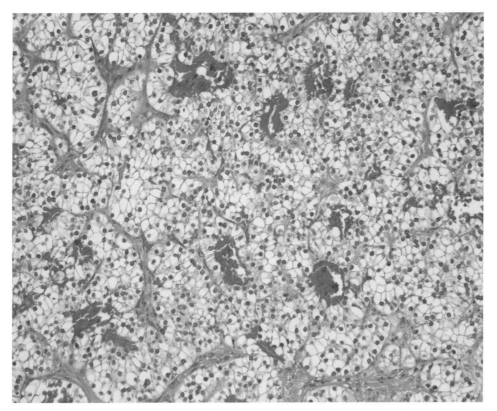

FIGURE 6-22

Parathyroid carcinoma may occasionally have a sinusoidal pattern of growth, including prominent cell borders, making separation from metastatic renal cell carcinoma a challenge. This renal cell carcinoma has prominent cell borders and a pseudoglandular pattern.

vimentin, CD10, and EMA without other markers will probably help to make this distinction in the correct clinical context.

As nice as it would be to have a definitive diagnosis in each case, the concept of an intermediate category must be addressed. The term 'atypical adenoma' is suggested for a parathyroid neoplasm lacking unequivocal evidence of invasiveness, even though it may be adherent to surrounding tissues, but showing some other feature(s) suspicious for malignancy. These tumors are considered of uncertain malignant potential, requiring close clinical follow-up. Curiously, this designation when applied to neoplasms which have clinical follow-up have enjoyed a benign outcome.

PROGNOSIS AND THERAPY

Overall, there is a 5-year survival up to 85% with a 10-year survival of approximately 50%. Local recurrence can occur in up to 70% of patients. Recurrences should be documented by localization studies in a patient with recurrent hypercalcemia, but a prolonged survival can still be expected after palliative surgery. Disruption of the capsule during surgery may cause seeding of parathyroid tissue and give rise to persistent or recurrent hyperparathyroidism, referred to as parathyromatosis. The best outcome for parathyroid carcinoma occurs when there is complete resection at the first surgery. Adjuvant therapy does not play much of a role in management, since it is the management of the metabolic effects of PTH and hypercalcemia which are important. When metastatic disease develops, lung, bone, cervical and mediastinal lymph nodes, and liver are most frequently affected. While axiomatic, benign 'brown tumors' caused by profound hyperparathyroidism may mimic bone metastases.

METASTATIC TUMORS

By definition, tumors which metastasize to or directly invade the parathyroid parenchyma or gland. While the glands are vascular, lymphatic spread is uncommon.

CLINICAL FEATURES

The vast majority of patients are asymptomatic, although occasionally a mass in the neck, hoarseness, and pain may be the presenting finding. Hypoparathyroidism is exceptionally rare. Women are affected slightly more frequently. The most common metastatic primary sites include breast, melanoma, lung, kidney and soft tissue primaries. Direct extension from a laryngeal or esophageal squamous cell carcinoma or lymphoma may also be identified.

PATHOLOGIC FEATURES

GROSS FINDINGS

The gland may be slightly enlarged, but metastases are usually not identified at macroscopic examination.

MICROSCOPIC FINDINGS

Lymphatic or vascular location of the tumor emboli will help to separate a primary lesion from metastatic disease. The histologic features of the primary site are usually maintained in the metastatic focus (Figure 6-23). When there is direct extension (Figures 6-24 and 6-25), the tumor is usually large, and the parathyroid gland involvement is incidental. Separation from thyroid gland (follicular or medullary) primary clear cell tumors

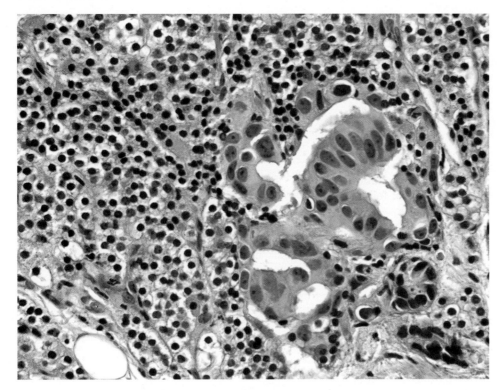

FIGURE 6-23
A neoplastic gland from a metastatic breast carcinoma is noted within the background parathyroid parenchyma.

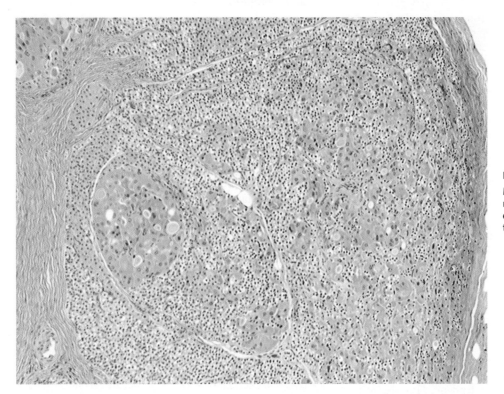

FIGURE 6-24
Metastatic thyroid follicular carcinoma creates nodules of oncocytic epithelium within a cellular parathyroid gland.

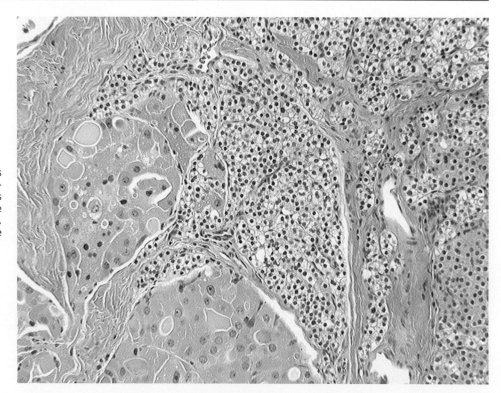

FIGURE 6-25

The follicular architecture of this metastatic oncocytic thyroid follicular carcinoma with colloid is quite distinctly different from the surrounding parenchyma. However, immunohistochemistry may be required to confirm the diagnosis.

and metastatic renal cell carcinoma may occasionally warrant the use of immunohistochemical studies to achieve the correct diagnosis.

PROGNOSIS AND THERAPY

The prognosis is usually guarded, with the nature of the underlying primary determining the overall outcome. In light of the metastatic nature of the disorder at time of presentation, the management is symptomatic or palliative.

SUGGESTED READING

Parathyroid Carcinoma

Bondeson L, Bondeson AG, Nissborg A, Thompson NW. Cytopathological variables in parathyroid lesions: a study based on 1,600 cases of hyperparathyroidism. Diagn Cytopathol 1997;16:476–482.

Bondeson L, Grimelius L, DeLellis RA, et al. Parathyroid carcinoma. *In:* DeLellis RA, Lloyd RV, Heitz PU, Eng C, eds. Pathology and Genetics of Tumours of Endocrine Organs. Kleihues P, Sobin LH, series eds. World Health Organization Classification of Tumours. Lyon, France: IARC Press, 2004:124–127.

DeLellis RA. Parathyroid carcinoma. Tumors of the Parathyroid gland. Atlas of Tumor Pathology, Third Series, Fascicle 6. Washington, DC: Armed Forces Institute of Pathology, 1993:53–64.

Erickson LA, Jin L, Papotti M, Lloyd RV. Oxyphil parathyroid carcinomas: a clinicopathologic and immunohistochemical study of 10 cases. Am J Surg Pathol 2002;26:344–349.

Evans HL. Criteria for diagnosis of parathyroid carcinoma. Surg Pathol 1991;4:244–265.

Hakaim AG, Esselstyn CB Jr. Parathyroid carcinoma: 50-year experience at The Cleveland Clinic Foundation. Cleve Clin J Med 1993;60:331–335.

Hundahl SA, Fleming ID, Fremgen AM, Menck HR. Two hundred eighty-six cases of parathyroid carcinoma treated in the U.S. between 1985–1995: a National Cancer Data Base Report. The American College of Surgeons Commission on Cancer and the American Cancer Society. Cancer 1999;86:538–544.

Sandelin K, Auer G, Bondeson L, et al. Prognostic factors in parathyroid cancer: a review of 95 cases. World J Surg 1992;16:724–731.

Schantz A, Castleman B. Parathyroid carcinoma. A study of 70 cases. Cancer 1973;31:600–605.

Shane E, Bilezikian JP. Parathyroid carcinoma: a review of 62 patients. Endocr Rev 1982;3:218–226.

Smith JF, Coombs RR. Histological diagnosis of carcinoma of the parathyroid gland. J Clin Pathol 1984;37:1370–1378.

Wynne AG, van Heerden J, Carney JA, Fitzpatrick LA. Parathyroid carcinoma: clinical and pathologic features in 43 patients. Medicine 1992;71:197–205.

Metastatic Tumors

de la Monte SM, Hutchins GM, Moore GW. Endocrine organ metastases from breast carcinoma. Am J Pathol 1984;114:131–136.

DeLellis RA. Secondary tumours of the parathyroid. *In:* DeLellis RA, Lloyd RV, Heitz PU, Eng C, eds. Pathology and Genetics of Tumours of Endocrine Organs. Kleihues P, Sobin LH, series eds. World Health Organization Classification of Tumours. Lyon, France: IARC Press, 2004:133–134.

DeLellis RA. Secondary tumors. Tumors of the Parathyroid gland. Atlas of Tumor Pathology, Third Series, Fascicle 6. Washington, DC: Armed Forces Institute of Pathology, 1993:94.

7 Non-neoplastic Lesions of the Adrenal Gland

Jacqueline A Wieneke • Lester DR Thompson

HETEROTOPIA AND ACCESSORY ADRENAL TISSUE

CLINICAL FEATURES

Heterotopic or accessory adrenal tissue results from the close spatial relationship of the embryologic development between gonadal structures and the adrenal primordium. Patients with such heterotopic/accessory tissue rarely have symptoms. 'Heterotopic adrenal tissue' refers to abnormal location of an otherwise normal adrenal gland (usually beneath the kidney capsule); 'accessory adrenal tissue' is adrenal cortical tissue found anywhere from the upper abdomen to sites along the descent of the gonads, including hernia sacs. The celiac axis is the most common site, followed by broad ligament (females) and spermatic cord, testicular hilum and epididymis (males). Rarely, adrenal cortical adenomas may develop within these rests.

PATHOLOGIC FEATURES

GROSS FINDINGS

Accessory adrenal cortical tissue typically presents as yellow, sharply circumscribed or encapsulated rounded nodules. Heterotopic adrenal glands are usually bilateral and often are flattened and smaller than adrenal glands located in a normal position.

MICROSCOPIC FINDINGS

Accessory adrenal rests are composed of benign lipid-rich adrenal cortical cells (Figure 7-1). Heterotopic tissue may be composed entirely of adrenal cortical tissue (Figure 7-2) or may be a mixture of adrenal cortical and medullary tissue.

**HETEROPTOPIA AND ACCESSORY ADRENAL GLANDS
DISEASE FACT SHEET**

Definition
▶ Normal adrenal tissue in an abnormal location

Incidence and Location
▶ Up to 32% of patients have ectopic adrenal tissue in the celiac axis, with reports in broad ligament, kidney, and spermatic cord

Morbidity and Mortality
▶ Typically not associated with endocrine abnormalities

Gender, Race and Age Distribution
▶ Slightly more common in males, especially if undescended testis

Clinical Features
▶ Incidental finding in surgical specimens removed for other reasons
▶ Rarely, ectopia may undergo hyperplasia secondary to ACTH stimulation
▶ Neoplasia is rare

Prognosis and Therapy
▶ Excellent
▶ No treatment necessary

**HETEROTOPIA AND ACCESSORY ADRENAL GLANDS
PATHOLOGIC FEATURES**

Gross Findings
▶ May be flattened or atrophic
▶ Small, round, well-demarcated nodules with yellow cut surface

Microscopic Findings
▶ Lipid-rich cells resembling zona fasciculata
▶ Zonation may be evident
▶ Medullary tissue may or may not be present

Immunohistochemical Features
▶ Inhibin variably reactive in cortical tissue
▶ Chromogranin, synaptophysin in medullary tissue

Pathologic Differential Diagnosis
▶ Renal cell carcinoma

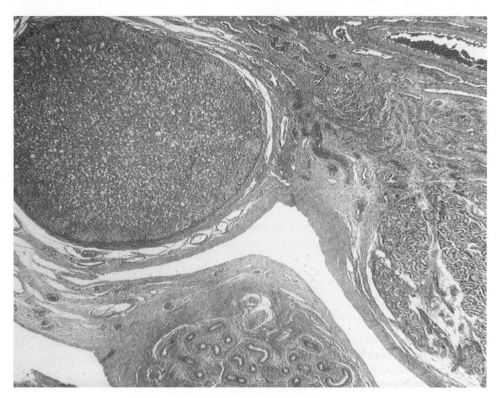

FIGURE 7-1
Ectopic adrenal gland tissue is present within the testis.

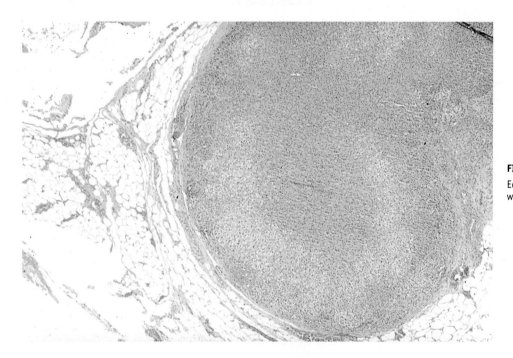

FIGURE 7-2
Ectopic adrenal cortical tissue within a hernia sac.

DIFFERENTIAL DIAGNOSIS

The diagnosis is usually made without difficulty, although rarely a renal cell carcinoma may arise near a focus of adrenal tissue.

PROGNOSIS AND THERAPY

Accessory adrenal tissue is benign and requires no specific therapy. It is typically non-functional without endocrine abnormality. Rarely, it is important to identify remaining adrenal gland tissue when heterotopic tissue is removed.

CONGENITAL HYPOPLASIA

CLINICAL FEATURES

Adrenal hypoplasia congenita (AHC) is a relatively uncommon condition characterized by reduced volume of adrenocortical tissue. It may occur sporadically or as part of a hereditary condition. Four forms are described:
- Sporadic associated with hypopituitarism;
- Autosomal recessive (affects both genders, 'miniature type')
- X-linked cytomegalic; and
- Association with glycerol kinase deficiency.

The most common is the X-linked cytomegalic form, characterized by adrenal insufficiency and hypogonadotropic hypogonadism, and associated with mutations of the X-linked gene DAX-1 (which encodes a novel orphan nuclear receptor). X-linked AHC and hypogonadotropic hypogonadism (HH) may result from inherited or de novo mutations of the DAX-1 gene. Adrenal hypoplasia congenita with glycerol kinase enzyme deficiency may be part of a contiguous gene deletion syndrome within the region Xp21, characterized by congenital adrenal hypoplasia, Duchenne muscular dystrophy, and glycerol kinase deficiency. In general, AHC patients present in infancy with signs of adrenal cortical insufficiency including weight loss, failure to thrive, vomiting, dehydration, hyponatremia and hyperkalemia. The severity of symptoms varies depending on the amount of functioning adrenal cortical tissue.

PATHOLOGIC FEATURES

GROSS FINDINGS

The adrenal glands are small and may appear atrophic (Figure 7-3); they may be dysmorphic (X-linked cytomegalic form) or extremely small (miniature type) (Figure 7-4).

MICROSCOPIC FINDINGS

The cytomegalic type shows distorted architecture with atypical cytomegalic cells. There is variable hyperchromasia and nuclear pleomorphism, frequent intranuclear cytoplasmic inclusions along with cytoplasmic vacuolization.

**CONGENITAL HYPOPLASIA
DISEASE FACT SHEET**

Definition
▸ Reduced volume of adrenocortical tissue often leading to adrenal cortical insufficiency

Incidence and Location
▸ Rare
▸ May be part of a familial/hereditary condition

Morbidity and Mortality
▸ Mortality is high if untreated

Gender, Race and Age Distribution
▸ Male predominance (often X-linked)
▸ Autosomal recessive form may affect both genders
▸ Usually in newborn to early infancy

Clinical Features
▸ Non-specific symptoms including weight loss, failure to thrive, vomiting, dehydration, hyponatremia and hyperkalemia
▸ Severity determined by amount of functional tissue
▸ Rarely, present with hypogonadotropic hypogonadism in adolescence

Prognosis and Therapy
▸ Used to be uniformly fatal, but glucocorticoid and mineralocorticoid replacement therapy yields good outcome

---

**CONGENITAL HYPOPLASIA
PATHOLOGIC FEATURES**

Gross Findings
▸ Bilateral, small, atrophic adrenal glands

Microscopic Findings
▸ Usually normal zonation and cytology
▸ X-linked type shows a distorted architecture with atypical cytology
▸ Changes in 'provisional' cortex in neonates and may be focal or diffuse

Pathologic Differential Diagnosis
▸ Adrenal cortical carcinoma

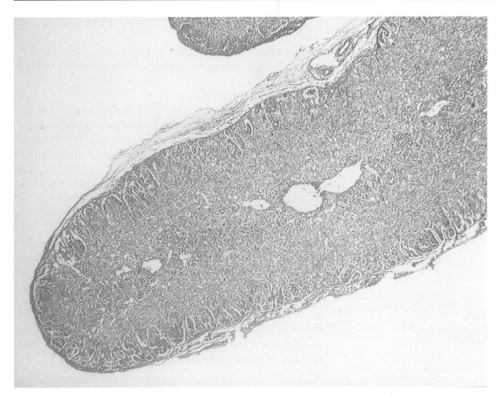

FIGURE 7-3
Congenital adrenal hypoplasia shows a thinned cortex with scant medullary component.

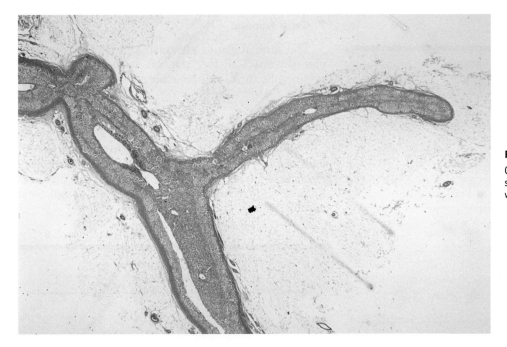

FIGURE 7-4
Congenital adrenal hypoplasia shows an extremely small cortex with a thin medullary portion.

ANCILLARY STUDIES

Molecular techniques (polymerase chain reaction, fluorescence in situ hybridization) can be used to identify mutations in the *DAX-1* gene when a clinical diagnosis of X-linked AHC and HH is suspected.

PROGNOSIS AND THERAPY

In the past AHC was uniformly fatal. However, with the availability of replacement glucocorticoids and mineralocorticoids, the prognosis is good. It is important to make an early diagnosis clinically before the onset of potentially life-threatening adrenal crisis or long-term effects of deficiency develop.

ADRENAL CYTOMEGALY

CLINICAL FEATURES

Adrenal cytomegaly can be an incidental finding in an otherwise grossly normal adrenal gland in neonates. It may be focal or diffuse and may involve one gland or both. It is reported in up to 3% of pediatric autopsies, but 6.5% of premature stillbirths. Adrenal cytomegaly is a characteristic feature of Beckwith-Wiedemann syndrome (BWS), in which both adrenal glands are enlarged. BWS is a rare congenital disorder (1 : 14 000 births), which is usually sporadic but may be inherited, resulting in overgrowth and neoplasia. The features include macroglossia, abdominal wall defects, macrosomia/hemihypertrophy and increased risk of developing certain malignancies. BWS may have epigenetic rather than genetic causes, although there is dysregulation of growth regulatory genes within the 11p15 region. Wilms tumor, hepatoblastoma, adrenocortical carcinoma, neuroblastoma, pancreatoblastoma and rhabdomyosarcoma have all been reported.

**ADRENAL CYTOMEGALY
DISEASE FACT SHEET**

Definition
▸ Marked nuclear and cytoplasmic atypia of adrenal cortical cells

Incidence and Location
▸ About 6.5% of premature stillbirths
▸ Frequent association with Beckwith-Wiedemann Syndrome (BWS; 1 : 14 000 births)

Morbidity and Mortality
▸ None; although mortality may be as a result of associated clinical manifestations of BWS

Gender, Race and Age Distribution
▸ Equal gender distribution
▸ Neonatal and pediatric patients

Clinical Features
▸ No specific clinical features
▸ If part of BWS, then macroglossia, macrosomia, abdominal wall defects, increased risk of hypoglycemia, predisposition for certain malignancies

Prognosis and Therapy
▸ No prognosis or treatment implications if incidental or isolated
▸ BWS may lead to decreased life expectancy

PATHOLOGIC FEATURES

GROSS FINDINGS

The adrenal glands are typically normal on gross examination when adrenal cytomegaly is an incidental finding. In BWS, the glands are typically enlarged, with redundant cortical folds that impart a cerebriform appearance to the large glands.

MICROSCOPIC FINDINGS

The cells of the provisional fetal cortex are typically affected and display significant nuclear pleomorphism with hyperchromasia, but still have abundant cytoplasm (Figures 7-5 and 7-6). Mitotic activity is characteristically absent. The changes may be focal or diffuse.

ANCILLARY STUDIES

Molecular and genetic studies of cases of BWS often indicate imprinting mutations in the chromosomal region 11p15 of the *LIT1* and *H19* genes.

DIFFERENTIAL DIAGNOSIS

Adrenal cytomegaly is fairly characteristic on histologic examination and once identified the most important diagnostic consideration is determining if the cytomegaly is an incidental finding or part of BWS. The risk of developing adrenal cortical carcinoma is increased in patients with BWS. Adrenal cortical carcinoma presents as a unilateral, discrete mass with increased mitotic activity, necrosis, vascular/capsular invasion, and broad fibrous bands.

**ADRENAL CYTOMEGALY
PATHOLOGIC FEATURES**

Gross Findings
▸ Usually unremarkable in incidental cases
▸ Cerebriform gland in cases associated with BWS

Microscopic Findings
▸ Marked cytoplasmic and nuclear atypia
▸ Cytomegalic cells with abundant eosinophilic cytoplasm
▸ Nuclear enlargement and pleomorphism, nuclear hyperchromasia, intranuclear cytoplasmic inclusions

Pathologic Differential Diagnosis
▸ Adrenal cortical carcinoma

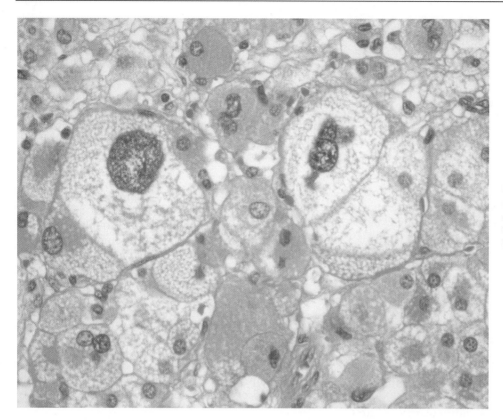

FIGURE 7-5
Extremely large cells have abundant cytoplasm (low nuclear to cytoplasmic ratio) containing remarkably pleomorphic nuclei.

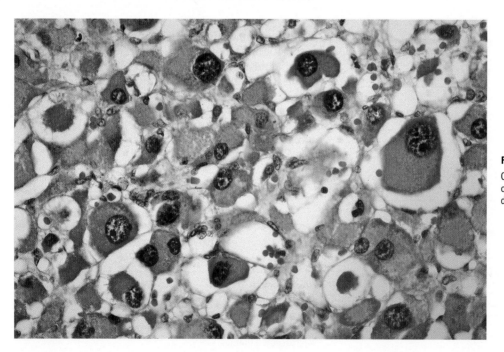

FIGURE 7-6
Cytomegaly may affect nearly all of the cells, or may be focal in distribution.

PROGNOSIS AND THERAPY

The cytomegaly has little clinical significance when discovered incidentally. If part of BWS, the increased risk of hypoglycemia and its complications, premature birth and predisposition for various neoplasms will determine prognosis and therapy.

CONGENITAL ADRENAL HYPERPLASIA

Congenital adrenal hyperplasia (CAH), also referred to as adrenogenital syndrome, is a complex group of auto-

somal recessive disorders that results from a deficiency of one of five enzymes involved in the biosynthesis of cortisol (Figure 7-7). Due to space limitations, discussion will be limited to the more common forms of the disease.

CAH is an inborn error of metabolism and is the most common cause of ambiguous genitalia in female infants. 21-Hydroxylase deficiency (21-OHD) and 11-β-hydroxylase deficiency are the most common deficiencies, with 21-OHD accounting for greater than 90% of the cases of CAH. The other deficiencies include 3-β-hydroxysteroid dehydrogenase, 17-hydroxylase and cholesterol desmolase. The enzyme deficiencies interfering with corticosteroid and/or mineralocorticoids synthesis lead to an accumulation of steroid precursors which spillover into the sex steroid pathway resulting in increased dehydroepiandrosterone (DHEA) and androstenedione, which causes virilization.

21-OHD has two well-described forms: the salt-wasting form (60–75%) and 'simple virilizing disease' (25–40%). In the salt-wasting form, the biosynthesis of aldosterone and cortisol is affected, which if unrecognized, may lead to potentially fatal 'salt-wasting' crisis. Affected females usually develop ambiguous genitalia in utero, sometimes to such an extreme as to be mistaken for a male. Internal organs develop normally. Male infants usually appear normal at birth and the disorder may not be recognized until they present in severe salt wasting crisis.

CONGENITAL ADRENAL HYPERPLASIA
DISEASE FACT SHEET

Definition
▶ Inherited disorder caused by deficiencies of enzymes required for biosynthesis of glucocorticoids and mineralocorticoids by the adrenal cortex

Incidence and Location
▶ 21-hydroxylase deficiency (classic from) accounts for >90% of CAH with 1:15000 live births
▶ 11-β-hydroxylase deficiency accounts for 5–8% of CAH with 1:100000 live births

Gender, Race and Age Distribution
▶ Genders affected equally, although clinical manifestations are gender dependent

Clinical Features
   Classic salt wasting form of 21–OHD
▶ Deficiencies of cortical and aldosterone secretion
▶ Genital ambiguity in females, but genital differentiation in males not affected
▶ Other signs of hyperandrogenism: facial and axillary hair; adult body odor; severe acne; penile enlargement (male)
▶ Infertility may develop in male patients
▶ Advanced bone growth with premature epiphyseal maturation and closure may lead to short adult stature
▶ Electrolyte disturbances, high plasma renin levels and fluid volume depletion ('salt wasting crisis')
   Classic simple virilizing form of 21-OHD
▶ Mineralocorticoid secretion is unaffected
▶ Features related to virilizing effects of excess androgen production: accelerated bone growth and advanced bone aging, ambiguous genitalia in female patients (as above)

Prognosis and Therapy
▶ Prognosis is dependent on severity of steroid deficiency
▶ Morbidity and mortality declined with early detection
▶ Glucocorticoid (suppresses androgens) and mineralocorticoid (normalizes electrolytes and plasma renin) replacement therapy
▶ Prenatal detection and treatment available
▶ Non-classic CAH requires no treatment

CLINICAL FEATURES

CLASSIC SALT WASTING FORM OF 21-OHD

In the classic salt wasting form, clinical signs and symptoms develop due to deficiencies of cortical and aldosterone secretion. Genital ambiguity in females results from excess androgens in utero. Female genital ambiguity may include clitoromegaly and fusion and scrotalization of the labial folds with a urogenital sinus. Genital differentiation in males is not affected and diagnosis often depends on screening. Other signs of hyperandrogenism include facial, axillary and pubic hair, adult body odor and severe acne. Infertility may develop in male patients. Premature epiphyseal maturation and closure may lead to short adult stature. In addition, due to the decreased levels of aldosterone, electrolyte disturbances, high plasma renin levels and fluid volume depletion may occur, leading to salt wasting crisis.

CLASSIC SIMPLE VIRILIZING FORM OF 21-OHD

Mineralocorticoid secretion is not affected and features are related to virilizing effects of excess androgen production with accelerated growth and advanced bone aging. Additionally, females patients present with ambiguous genitalia as described above (Figure 7-8).

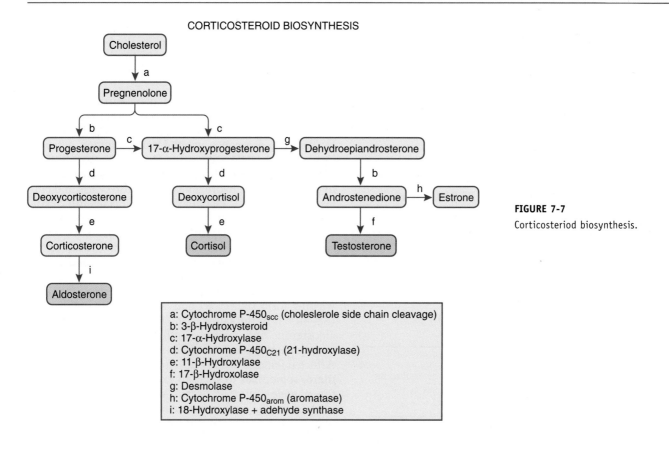

FIGURE 7-7

Corticosteriod biosynthesis.

CORTICOSTEROID BIOSYNTHESIS

a: Cytochrome P-450$_{scc}$ (choleslerole side chain cleavage)
b: 3-β-Hydroxysteroid
c: 17-α-Hydroxylase
d: Cytochrome P-450$_{C21}$ (21-hydroxylase)
e: 11-β-Hydroxylase
f: 17-β-Hydroxolase
g: Desmolase
h: Cytochrome P-450$_{arom}$ (aromatase)
i: 18-Hydroxylase + adehyde synthase

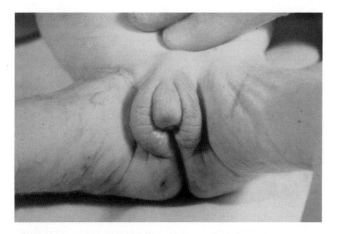

FIGURE 7-8

Ambiguous external genitalia of a genetically female patient with virilizing form of congenital adrenal hyperplasia 21-OHD.

CAH AND ASSOCIATED NODULES AND TUMORS

Patients with CAH may develop adrenocortical nodules and less frequently, may develop adrenocortical adenoma or carcinoma. Male patients appear to be at increased risk for testicular tumors (steroid type cells), which may be bilateral. Rarely, adrenal myelolipoma and bone sarcomas have been reported in association with CAH.

PATHOLOGIC FEATURES

Modern medical practice makes it rare to histologically examine adrenal glands of patients who have died of unrecognized or untreated CAH. With impaired cortisol secretion, adrenal cortical hyperplasia occurs as a result of increased and sustained levels of adrenocorticotropin hormone (ACTH) from the pituitary gland via the negative feedback system. The adrenal glands are enlarged with a convoluted, cerebriform surface (Figures 7-9 and 7-10). The glands may have a light brown color resulting from the sustained trophic effect of ACTH and conversion of the lipid-rich, pale-staining cortical cells to lipid-depleted compact eosinophilic cytoplasm (Figure 7-11).

ANCILLARY STUDIES

Molecular studies have elucidated the mutations responsible for the more common forms of the disorder. 21-Hydroxylase is a cytochrome P-450 enzyme and deficiency of this enzyme is caused by mutations in the *CYP21* gene, located on the short arm of chromosome 6, which encodes for the steroid 21-hydroxylase enzyme. Prenatal diagnosis is available. Mutations of the *CYP11B1* gene are believed to be related to CAH caused by 11-β-hydroxylase deficiency.

CONGENITAL ADRENAL HYPERPLASIA
PATHOLOGIC FEATURES

Gross Findings
▸ Enlarged adrenal glands bilaterally with cerebriform appearance; may be many times normal size
▸ Typically light brown
▸ Cholesterol desmolase deficiency characterized by yellow areas and diffuse nodularity

Microscopic Findings
▸ Hyperplastic cerebriform growth pattern
▸ Increased numbers of lipid-depleted cells with compact eosinophilic cytoplasm

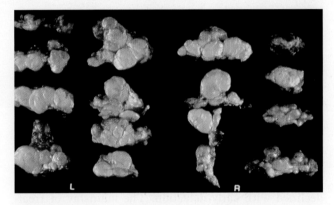

FIGURE 7-9
Left and right adrenals show a nodular, convoluted appearance in this example of CAH.

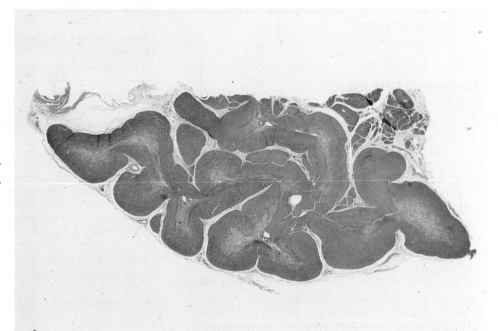

FIGURE 7-10
Highly convoluted and 'cerebriform' appearance of a CAH adrenal gland.

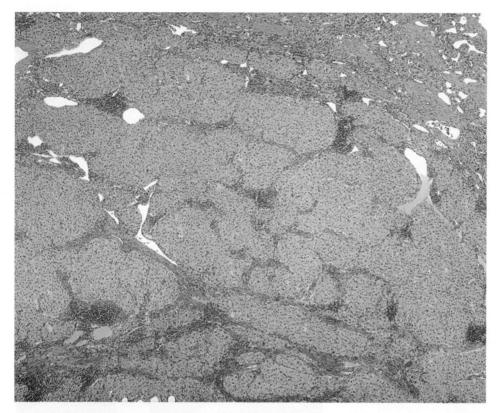

FIGURE 7-11
The cortical layer is composed of cells with compact, eosinophilic cytoplasm in this adrenal gland from a CAH patient.

PROGNOSIS AND THERAPY

Morbidity and mortality from salt wasting crisis has declined with early detection. The mainstay of treatment is replacement glucocorticoids and mineralocorticoids to suppress adrenal androgen secretion and to normalize electrolytes and plasma renin activity. Prenatal treatment of affected females with dexamethasone may help to prevent or minimize virilization of genitalia (dexamethasone crosses the placenta). New treatment approaches, such as gene therapy, are currently under investigation. Non-classic CAH does not always require treatment.

ADDISON'S DISEASE

Adrenocortical insufficiency, known as Addison's disease, is characterized by decreased levels of glucocorticoid production which eventually affects production of mineralocorticoids and sex steroids. Primary adrenal cortical insufficiency is caused by three broad etiologies: adrenal destruction, adrenal dysgenesis and impaired steroidogenesis. Secondary adrenal cortical insufficiency results from hypothalamic-pituitary impairment of the corticotropic axis, usually due to pituitary gland involvement by tumor. Adrenal destruction may result from infection (most often part of disseminated disease), adrenal hemorrhage, metastatic disease, adrenal amyloidosis, adrenoleukodystrophy and autoimmune adrenalitis (part of autoimmune polyglandular syndrome, APS). Adrenal dysgenesis may result from congenital adrenal hypoplasia (AHC), mutations of steroidogenic factor-1 (SF-1) and ACTH unresponsiveness (limited to glucocorticoid deficiency). Impaired steroidogenesis is seen in congenital adrenal hyperplasia (CAH), mitochondrial disorders, and Smith-Lemli-Opitz syndrome (SLOS), an enzyme deficiency in cholesterol metabolism. Tuberculosis used to be the most common cause of Addison's disease, but nowadays most cases are due to autoimmune etiologies and over 70% of patients have auto-adrenal steroid cell antibodies. Often times it is seen in association with other auto-immune disorders including thyroid disorders, diabetes mellitus, pernicious anemia, hypoparathyroidism, and ovarian failure or as part of polyglandular syndromes (type 1, 2 or 4).

CLINICAL FEATURES

Approximately 90% of the adrenal gland must be destroyed before clinical features of adrenocortical insufficiency are manifest. The signs and symptoms are protean and are non-specific, making it difficult to render a correct diagnosis. Symptoms, either acute or chronic, include anorexia, vomiting, diarrhea, weight loss (poor weight gain in a child), malaise, unexplained fatigue, salt craving, muscle weakness, arthralgia/myalgia, and dizziness. Clinical signs include postural

hypotension, dehydration, hyperpigmentation (only in primary adrenal insufficiency), fever, hyponatremia, hyperkalemia, elevated serum creatinine, anemia, and hypoglycemia. These signs and symptoms may occur in a variety of combinations and the 'classic triad' of hyperpigmentation, postural hypotension and hyponatremia is not often encountered. A concurrent viral illness is frequently the stress factor that leads to acute adrenal crisis. Specific drugs are known to inhibit cortisol biosynthesis (aminoglutethimide, etomidate, ketoconazole, methyrapone, suramin) which may lead to adrenal insufficiency.

PATHOLOGIC FEATURES

Pathologic features will depend on the cause of adrenal insufficiency. Infections, bleeding, metastatic neoplasms, and congenital causes all have unique pathologic features that are described elsewhere. The following pathologic features relate to autoimmune adrenalitis.

GROSS FINDINGS

The adrenal glands are markedly reduce in size and volume and are described as 'wafer-like'. It is often difficult to identify the glands at autopsy.

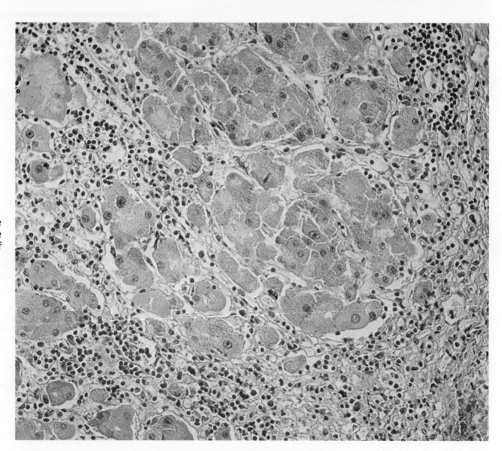

FIGURE 7-12
Eosinophilic cytoplasm in the adrenal cortical cells which are surrounded by an infiltrate of lymphocytes.

ADDISON'S DISEASE
PATHOLOGIC FEATURES

Gross Findings

▸ Thin and wafer-like, with loss of volume

Microscopic Findings

▸ Cortex is atrophic, thin and discontinuous with islands of cortical cells
▸ Cells have compact eosinophilic cytoplasm with mild nuclear pleomorphism
▸ Lymphocytic or plasma cell component may be present, especially if infectious etiology (organisms may be seen)

Pathologic Differential Diagnosis

▸ Non-specific adrenalitis

MICROSCOPIC FINDINGS

There is a nested, discontinuous cortical layer, the atrophic cortical nests surrounded by lymphocytes and plasma cells (Figure 7-12). The cells may be more eosinophilic with cytomegaly and nuclear atypia.

DIFFERENTIAL DIAGNOSIS

The pathologic differential diagnosis is limited to non-specific adrenalitis, in which the inflammatory cells are distributed around the perivascular regions and more haphazardly throughout the gland.

PROGNOSIS AND THERAPY

Advances in treatment (glucocorticoid and mineralo-corticoid replacement) have resulted in good patient outcomes, but delay in diagnosis may result in adrenal crisis, which often ends in death. There are no clear indications for androgen replacement.

INFECTIONS

Infections of the adrenal gland are usually part of systemic disease. Nearly any infection can occur in the adrenal glands, although some have a greater proclivity than others. Tuberculosis (TB) remains a common cause of infection of the adrenal gland in developing countries, causing approximately 70% of Addison's disease cases.

CLINICAL FEATURES

Signs and symptoms depend on the extent of adrenal gland involvement. If the infection is limited and does not destroy the majority of adrenal tissue, symptoms of adrenal insufficiency will be limited. However, if the infection destroys >90% of the adrenal tissue, adrenal insufficiency will occur. Clinical findings depend upon the organism. Bacterial infections tend to be more acute, occur in the setting of sepsis and have a high fever. Waterhouse-Friderichsen syndrome (WFS) results from bacterial sepsis/shock with sudden vascular collapse and disseminated intravascular coagulation with associated adrenal hemorrhage (Figure 7-13). This fulminant disorder is classically associated with meningococcal sepsis but can occur with other organisms such as *Streptococcus pneumoniae* and *Haemophilus*. Fungal and viral infections do not typically show acute symptoms but are discovered when working up a low-grade fever of unknown origin or adrenal cortical insufficiency. The most common fungal infection is histoplasmosis but others include blastomycosis, coccidiomycosis and cryptococcosis. Herpes simplex virus (HSV) and varicella-zoster (VZ) are among the viral organisms that may lead to adrenalitis. With AIDS, cytomegalovirus (CMV) adrenalitis has become more common. These patients are at particular risk for adrenal crisis during periods of severe illness, surgery or trauma. Disseminated CMV infection in the new-

---

INFECTIONS
DISEASE FACT SHEET

Definition

▸ Adrenal gland affected by infectious organisms, usually part of systemic disease

Incidence and Location

▸ Rare
▸ Infectious agents vary (TB in developing countries; CMV in AIDS)

Morbidity and Mortality

▸ Patient's overall health and type of infection affects outcome
▸ Without antimicrobial therapy morbidity and mortality is high
▸ Mortality rate from Waterhouse-Friderichsen syndrome (WFS) remains extremely high

Clinical Features

▸ Fever and general malaise
▸ Septic shock may develop
▸ Disseminated intravascular coagulation may lead to WFS
▸ Adrenal insufficiency may develop depending on extent of cortical destruction (>90% required)

Prognosis and Therapy

▸ Dependant on extent of involvement and timeliness of therapy
▸ Outcome of WFS remains poor
▸ Antimicrobial therapies based on infectious agent

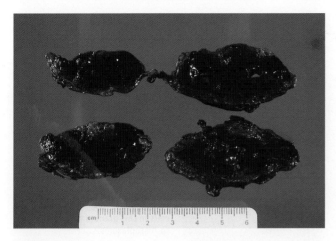

FIGURE 7-13
Bilateral adrenal gland hemorrhage as part of Waterhouse-Friderichsen syndrome (Courtesy of Dr JA Ohara).

MICROSCOPIC FINDINGS

TB of the adrenal gland is distinctly different from other organs; there is typically extensive caseating necrosis with only poorly formed granulomas. Epithelioid granulomas are usually not identified. Calcifications may also be seen. The poor granulomatous response is believe to be related to the relatively high concentration of corticosteroids dampening the inflammatory response. Similarly, the inflammatory process seen in mycotic infections is dominated by caseating necrosis with a blunted granulomatous response (Figure 7-14). The organisms are often seen aggregating within macrophages, identification based on their distinct yeast or fungal form (Figures 7-15 and 7-16). HSV and VZ show virtually identical histology with Cowdry type-A intranuclear inclusions in a background of necrosis with little or no inflammatory reaction (Figure 7-17). The pathognomonic large, eosinophilic intranuclear and basophilic cytoplasmic inclusions confirm the diagnosis of CMV adrenalitis (Figure 7-18).

ANCILLARY STUDIES

A battery of histochemical stains for microorganisms can be tailored to the agent suspected: Brown and Brenn or Brown and Hopps for bacteria in tissue sections; Ziehl-Neelsen for acid fast organisms; Gomori's methenamine silver (GMS) and Periodic acid Schiff (PAS) for fungi (Figure 7-16); and specific immunohistochemical studies for viruses (HSV, CMV).

DIFFERENTIAL DIAGNOSIS

The differential diagnosis will depend on the type of microorganism involved. Non-specific adrenalitis related to infarction and/or hemorrhage may suggest an underlying infection. Pseudocyst or hemorrhagic cyst may have an inflammatory component, mimicking an infectious etiology. If an infectious etiology is considered, it is wise to examine appropriate special stains. Rarely, cytologic atypia may mimic an adrenal cortical carcinoma or metastatic tumor.

PROGNOSIS AND THERAPY

Prognosis depends on the actual organism involved and the baseline health status of the patient. Immunocompromised patients have an increased risk of developing certain infections, with attendant higher morbidity and mortality. Typically, very young children, the elderly and those with immunocompromised status have a higher risk of poor outcomes. The earlier the infection is detected and the sooner therapy is started, the better the chance of good outcome without serious complications. Adrenal cortical insufficiency

born involves many organs, including the adrenal glands. Other infectious agents are individually case reported.

PATHOLOGIC FEATURES

GROSS FINDINGS

Adrenal glands involved by TB typically are enlarged and display caseating necrosis, occasionally with calcification. The adrenal glands in WFS are acutely congested and are partially or completely effaced by hemorrhage, but usually still normal size (Figure 7-13).

**INFECTIONS
PATHOLOGIC FEATURES**

Gross Findings
▸ Caseating necrosis in enlarged glands (tuberculosis)
▸ Acute congestion with hemorrhage (WFS)

Microscopic Findings
▸ Tuberculosis: extensive caseating necrosis with poorly formed granulomatous process (well-developed epithelioid granulomas not seen)
▸ Fungal infections: caseating necrosis with a blunted granulomatous response; organisms may aggregate in macrophages; specific fungi show unique characteristics
▸ HSV and VZ: Cowdry type-A intranuclear viral inclusions; extensive necrosis with little or no inflammatory reaction
▸ CMV infection: large eosinophilic intranuclear inclusions with peripheral halo; small basophilic cytoplasmic inclusions

Pathologic Differential Diagnosis
▸ Sarcoidosis, adrenal cortical carcinoma, lymphoma, metastatic carcinoma

---

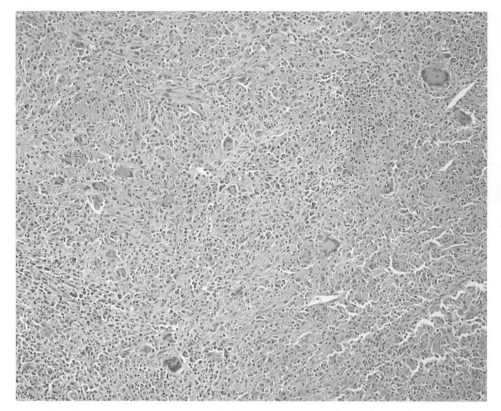

FIGURE 7-14

Epithelioid histiocytes and giant cells in this granulomatous response to histoplasmosis.

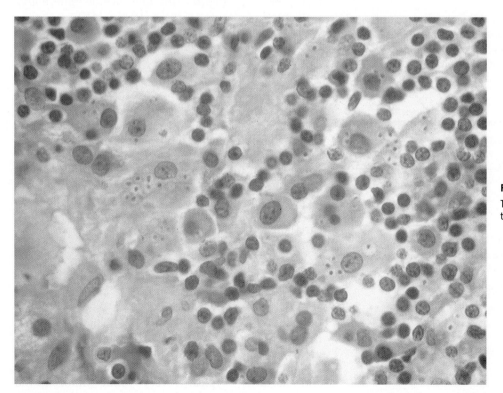

FIGURE 7-15

The cytoplasm of histiocytes contains Histoplasmosis organisms.

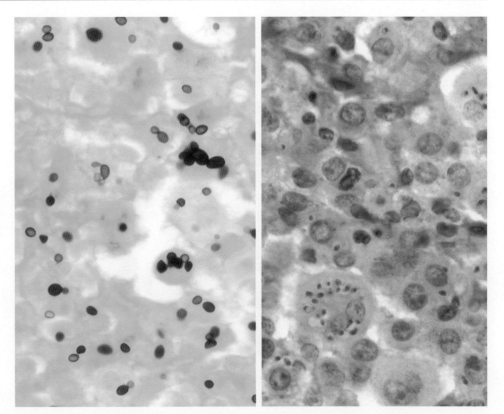

FIGURE 7-16

Left: A GMS impregnation stain highlights the *Histoplasma capsulatum* fungal organisms with black. Right: A PAS stain highlights the fungal organisms, such that the capsule is negatively stained, creating a small halo around the organism.

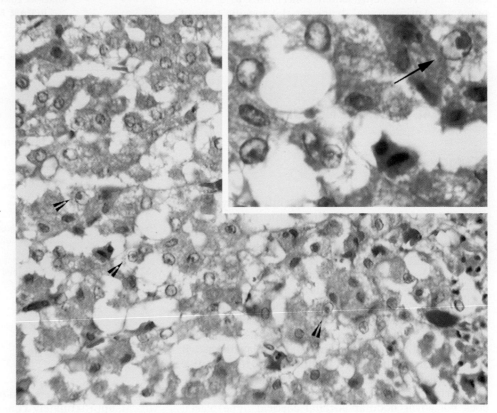

FIGURE 7-17

The HSV Cowdry type-A intranuclear inclusion is characteristic.

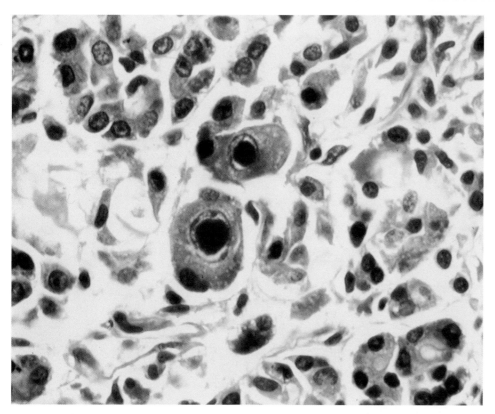

FIGURE 7-18
A large, eosinophilic intranuclear inclusion is characteristic for a CMV infection.

(Addison's disease) may develop depending on the extent of involvement, which contributes to a worse outcome. Antimicrobial drugs for the specific type of infection are available, generally controlling the infection.

ADRENAL CORTICAL NODULES

CLINICAL FEATURES

Adrenal cortical nodules are frequently discovered as an incidental finding on radiographic evaluation or during surgery for unrelated symptoms. Improvements in radiographic techniques have resulted in increased discovery, but perhaps not a true incidence increase. The incidence does increase with age, although seen over a wide age range. The nodules are nonfunctioning with no clinical, biochemical or histologic evidence of hyperfunction. Nodules are known to increase with chronic illnesses such as diabetes mellitus, hypertension and cardiovascular/peripheral vascular disease. It is hypothesized that these nodules are a regenerative hyperplasia resulting from localized ischemia and 'capsular arteriopathy' associated with hypertension. This does not cover nodular adrenal cortical hyperplasia, where hormone production results in a clinical presentation and specific biochemical alterations.

**ADRENAL CORTICAL NODULES
DISEASE FACT SHEET**

Definition
▸ Benign, nonfunctional nodules of adrenal cortical tissue

Incidence and Location
▸ Between 1.5% and 3%, although perhaps higher in elderly, hypertensive and diabetic patients

Gender, Race and Age Distribution
▸ Equal gender distribution
▸ Wide age range, although more frequent in elderly patients

Clinical Features
▸ No clinical symptoms
▸ Incidental discovery on radiographic studies or during surgery

Prognosis and Therapy
▸ Excellent; no treatment required

RADIOLOGIC FEATURES

While radiographic techniques highlight bilateral, multifocal, approximately 1 cm nodules, the studies may be insufficiently sensitive to detect the more common smaller nodules which comprise the disorder. Patho-

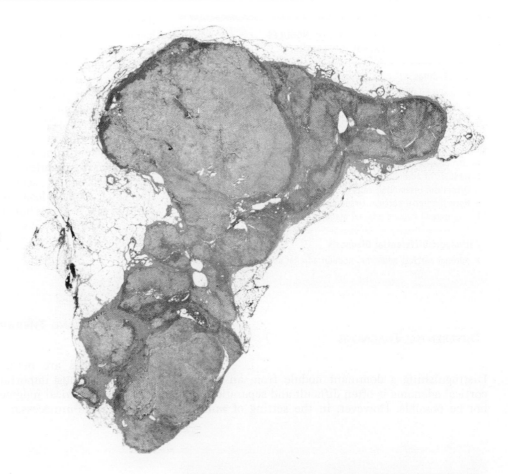

FIGURE 7-19
Macroscopic view of an adrenal gland with multiple cortical nodules.

logic examination is usually needed to define the extent and type of disease present.

PATHOLOGIC FEATURES

GROSS FINDINGS

The adrenal glands typically show multiple nodules of varying sizes, although one nodule may appear dominant or larger than the rest. In general, the nodules measure <1 cm (Figure 7-19), although larger nodules are seen (3 cm; Figure 7-20). Any asymptomatic, incidentally discovered nonfunctioning nodule >4 cm should be evaluated as an 'incidentaloma' of the adrenal.

MICROSCOPIC FINDINGS

The multiple nodules identified are circumscribed but typically unencapsulated, although the nodules may become confluent (Figure 7-21). The nodules may extend beyond the capsule of the gland into the periadrenal soft tissues. Cystic degeneration and/or calcification is rarely observed. The nodules are composed of adrenal cortical cells with abundant lipid-filled microvesiculated cytoplasm, occasionally admixed with eosinophilic cells. Lipomatous or myelolipomatous change may be seen.

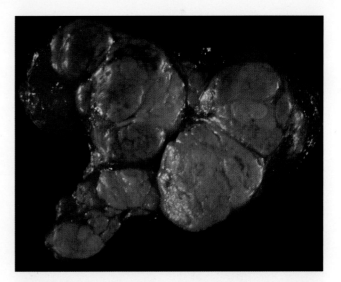

FIGURE 7-20
Macroscopic presentation of a gland affected by larger adrenal cortical nodules.

ANCILLARY STUDIES

Fine needle aspiration confirms adrenal cortical tissue, but it is unable to separate normal adrenal tissue from adenoma or nodule. It will, however, remove metastatic disease from clinical consideration.

ADRENAL CORTICAL NODULES
PATHOLOGIC FEATURES

Gross Findings

▶ Typically bilateral and multiple
▶ Variable size, with most <1 cm
▶ Single dominant nodule may be seen

Microscopic Findings

▶ Circumscribed and unencapsulated
▶ Nodules of adrenal cortical cells with abundant microvesiculated cytoplasm resembling cells of zona fasciculata
▶ Normal adrenal cortical tissue between nodules
▶ May extend beyond adrenal gland capsule

Pathologic Differential Diagnosis

▶ Adrenal cortical adenoma, nodular adrenal cortical hyperplasia

DIFFERENTIAL DIAGNOSIS

Distinguishing a dominant nodule from an adrenal cortical adenoma is often difficult and separation may not be possible. However, in the setting of multiple nodules, a non-functional dominant adrenal cortical lesion is probably best classified as a dominant nodule rather than a true neoplasm. Typically, nonfunctioning adenomas are unilateral and the remaining adrenal parenchyma is normal, without compensatory atrophy (as would be expected in a functional adenoma). Rarely, adenoma may be unencapsulated, 'blending almost imperceptibly' with the remaining parenchyma, making separation difficult. Adrenal hyperplasia of Cushing's syndrome gives a 'diffuse nodularity' rather than discrete nodules. No residual normal adrenal cortical tissue is seen. Likewise, hyperplasia of the zona glomerulosa produces a 'V-shaped' zone within the cortex, but is usually associated with clinical symptoms related to aldosterone production (Figure 7-22).

PROGNOSIS AND THERAPY

These nodules are benign and require no specific therapy. It is most important to recognize the nodularity and use clinical judgment and preoperative assessment to avoid unnecessary surgery.

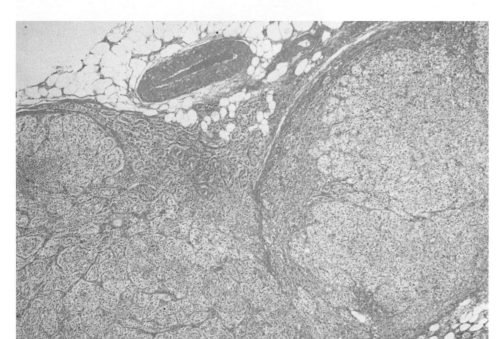

FIGURE 7-21
Unencapsulated nodules of adrenal cortical tissue.

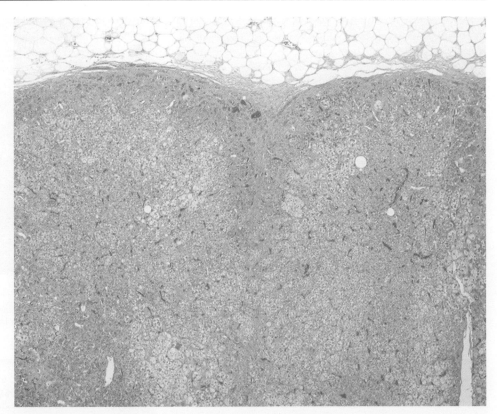

FIGURE 7-22
Zona glomerulosa hyperplasia is associated with increased aldosterone production.

ADRENAL GLAND CYSTS

Cysts of the adrenal gland are rare, separated into four categories: epithelial/retention, vascular/endothelial, parasitic and pseudocysts.

CLINICAL FEATURES

Adrenal cysts are usually discovered incidentally, although occasionally non-specific symptoms of abdominal pain and vomiting may result in their discovery. Rarely, cysts may be palpable. Adrenal cysts arise more commonly in women, and are most commonly discovered in the fifth and sixth decades, although all ages can be affected.

RADIOLOGIC FEATURES

Radiographs show an enlarged adrenal gland with cystic change within a dominant mass. Depending upon the cyst type, hemorrhage, fluid levels and/or degenerative changes (calcification, fibrosis) are seen (Figure 7-23). MRI has the best sensitivity but ultrasound and CT remain good diagnostic techniques. The typical adrenal pseudocyst is anechoic with a smooth cyst wall on ultrasound.

PATHOLOGIC FEATURES

PSEUDOCYSTS

Size usually varies between 2 and 10 cm, although they can be larger, often containing massive amounts of fluid (up to 12 liters). Pseudocyts are usually unilocular containing granulation tissue, brown-hemorrhagic fluid contents, and occasionally organizing blood clot with fibrosis (Figure 7-24). By definition, pseudocysts do not have an epithelial lining. Secondary degeneration of any of the other types of cysts may blur the distinction.

VASCULAR/ENDOTHELIAL CYSTS

These multilocular cysts are lined by flattened endothelial cells, and are related to hemangiomas and lymphangiomas (Figure 7-25), the latter called a 'serous cyst'. Cyst contents vary from hemorrhagic material to fibrin deposition and clear cyst fluid (Figure 7-26).

TRUE EPITHELIAL CYSTS

Epithelial cysts are usually small, incidental and typically filled with clear fluid. Believed to be developmental in origin or as a result of mesothelial inclusions, the

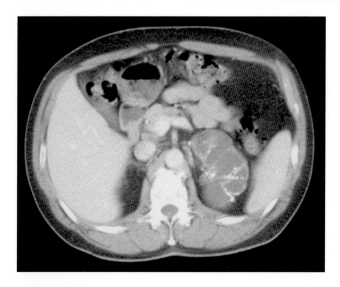

FIGURE 7-23
Computed tomography scan showing a multilocular adrenal gland cyst with fibrosis and calcifications.

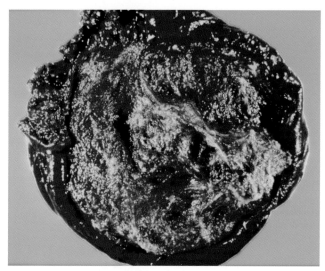

FIGURE 7-24
A pseudocyst contains granulation-type tissue with hemorrhage and clot. No lining was identified on microscopic examination.

ADRENAL GLAND CYSTS
DISEASE FACT SHEET

Definition
▸ Dominant cystic mass of adrenal gland which may be vascular (endothelial), epithelial/retention, parasitic, or pseudocyst

Incidence and Location
▸ Rare (<0.1% in autopsy series)

Gender, Race and Age Distribution
▸ Female > Male (3 : 1)
▸ Wide age distribution; most common in the fifth and sixth decades

Clinical Features
▸ Most are asymptomatic
▸ Symptoms non-specific and include abdominal pain, vomiting, and mass effect, depending on size

Prognosis and Therapy
▸ Good prognosis
▸ If symptomatic, >5 cm, or suspicion of malignancy, surgery is advocated

---

ADRENAL GLAND CYSTS
PATHOLOGIC FEATURES

Pathology Findings
▸ Cyst frequency: vascular/endothelial, 45%; pseudocyst, 39%; epithelial, 9%; parasitic, 7%
▸ Vascular/endothelial cysts: often multiloculated, with flattened endothelial cells and content ranging from hemorrhagic material and fibrin to clear fluid
▸ Pseudocysts: usually irregular contour, unilocular without an epithelial lining containing brown-hemorrhagic fluid; organizing blood clot, fibrosis and granulation tissue; variable size (2–10 cm), but may have massive fluid accumulation
▸ True epithelial cysts: usually small and incidental, often filled with clear fluid and lined by cuboidal or ciliated columnar epithelium
▸ Parasitic cysts: usually part of disseminated echinococcal infection; mature cyst has laminated chitinous membrane with inner nucleated germinal membrane and a central fluid filled cavity; daughter cysts have budding scolices within the germinal membrane

Immunohistochemical Features
▸ Vascular cysts: CD31, CD34, factor VIII-RAg
▸ Epithelial cysts: keratin

Pathologic Differential Diagnosis
▸ Cystic adrenal cortical neoplasms and pheochromocytoma

---

cyst lining shows cuboidal or ciliated columnar epithelium.

PARASITIC CYSTS

This rare cyst is usually part of disseminated echinococcal infection. The mature echinococcal cyst consists of a laminated chitinous membrane and inner nucleated germinal membrane and a central fluid filled cavity. Daughter cysts are formed in the germinal membrane where multiple scolices form by budding.

ANCILLARY STUDIES

Immunohistochemical stains may be helpful in identifying a cyst lining of either epithelial (keratin positive) or endothelial (CD34, CD31 positive) cells.

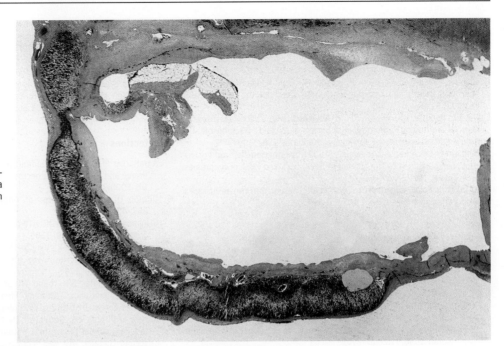

FIGURE 7-25
The adrenal cortical tissue is compressed to the periphery with a unilocular, endothelial lined cyst in this lymphangioma.

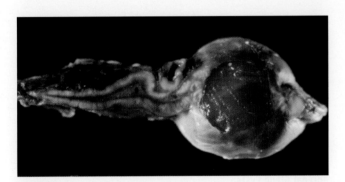

FIGURE 7-26
A simple lymphatic cyst contains clear fluid.

DIFFERENTIAL DIAGNOSIS

Adrenal cysts need to be differentiated from adrenal neoplasms with cystic change. In particular, adrenal cortical adenomas are well-known to undergo cystic degeneration with central hemorrhage and degeneration. Less frequently pheochromocytomas may show cystic degeneration and rarely, cystic change may be seen in adrenal cortical carcinomas.

PROGNOSIS AND THERAPY

Surgical excision is the treatment of choice under three scenarios: if symptomatic, if >5 cm, and if there is a suspicion of malignancy. When surgery is employed, an en block resection is recommended, even if performed laparoscopically.

SUGGESTED READING

Heterotopia and Accessory Adrenal Glands

Armin A, Castelli M. Congenital adrenal tissue in the lung with adrenal cytomegaly. Am J Clin Pathol 1984;82:225–228.

Chin I, Brody RI, Morales P, Black VH. Immunocytochemical characterization of intrarenal adrenal tissue. Urology 1994;44:429–432.

Czaplicki M, Bablok L, Kuzaka B. Heterotopic adrenal tissue. Int Urol Nephrol 1985;17:177–181.

Guschmann M, Vogel M, Urban M. Adrenal tissue in the placenta: a heterotopia caused by migration and embolism? Placenta 2000;21:427–431.

Lloyd RV, Douglas BR, Young WF Jr. Adrenal Gland. Endocrine Diseases. Atlas of Nontumor Pathology, First Series, Fascicle 1. Washington, DC: Armed Forces Institute of Pathology, 2002:171–258.

Medeiros LJ, Anasti J, Gardner KL, et al. Virilizing adrenal cortical neoplasm arising ectopically in the thorax. J Clin Endocrinol Metab 1992;75:1522–1525.

Okur H, Kucukaydin M, Kazez A, Kontas O. Ectopic adrenal tissue in the inguinal region in children. Pediatr Pathol Lab Med 1995;15:763–767.

Congenital Hypoplasia

Achermann JC, Silverman BL, Habiby RL, et al. Presymptomatic diagnosis of X-linked adrenal hypoplasia congenita by analysis of DAX1. J Pediatr 2000;137:878–881.

Lehmann SG, Lalli E, Sassone-Corsi P. X-linked adrenal hypoplasia congenita is caused by abnormal nuclear localization of the DAX-1 protein. Proc Natl Acad Sci USA 2002;99:8225–8230.

Lloyd RV, Douglas BR, Young WF Jr. Adrenal Gland. Endocrine Diseases. Atlas of Nontumor Pathology, First Series, Fascicle 1. Washington, DC: Armed Forces Institute of Pathology, 2002:171–258.

Peter M, Viemann M, Partsch CJ, et al. Congenital adrenal hypoplasia: clinical spectrum, experience with hormonal diagnosis, and report on new point mutations of the DAX-1 gene. J Clin Endocrinol Metab 1998;83:2666–2674.

Zaffanello M, Zamboni G, Tonin P, et al. Complex glycerol kinase deficient leads to psychomotor and body-growth failure. J Paediatr Child Health 2004;40:237–240.

Adrenal Cytomegaly

Aterman K., Kerenyi N, Lee M. Adrenal cytomegaly. Virchow Arch 1972;355:105–122.

DeBaun MR, Niemitz EL, Feinberg AP. Association of in vitro fertilization with Beckwith-Wiedemann syndrome and epigenetic alterations of LIT1 and H19. Am J Hum Genet 2003;72:156–160.

Favara BE, Steele A, Grant JH, Steele P. Adrenal cytomegaly: quantitative assessment by image analysis. Pediatr Pathol 1991;11:521–536.

Gosden R, Trasler J, Lucifero D, Faddy M. Rare congenital disorders, imprinted genes, and assisted reproductive technology. Lancet 2003; 361:1975–1977.

Lloyd RV, Douglas BR, Young WF Jr. Adrenal Gland. Endocrine Diseases. Atlas of Nontumor Pathology, First Series, Fascicle 1. Washington, DC: Armed Forces Institute of Pathology, 2002:171–258.

Oppenheimer EH. Adrenal cytomegaly: studies by light and electron microscopy. Comparison with the adrenal in Beckwith's and virilism syndromes. Arch Pathol 1970;90:57–64.

Yamashina M. Focal adrenocortical cytomegaly observed in two adult cases. Arch Pathol Lab Med 1986;110:1072–1075.

Congenital Adrenal Hyperplasia

Condom E, Villabona CM, Gómez JM, Carrera M. Adrenal myelolipoma in a woman with congenital 17-hydroxylase deficiency. Arch Pathol Lab Med 1985;109:1116–1118.

Duck SC. Malignancy associated with congenital adrenal hyperplasia. J Pediatr 1981;99:423–424.

Geley S, Kapelari K, Johrer K, et al. CYP11B1 mutations causing congenital adrenal hyperplasia due to 11 beta-hydroxylase deficiency. J Clin Endocrinol Metab 1996;81:2896–2901.

Lloyd RV, Douglas BR, Young WF Jr. Adrenal Gland. Endocrine Diseases. Atlas of Nontumor Pathology, First Series, Fascicle 1. Washington, DC: Armed Forces Institute of Pathology, 2002:171–258.

Merke D, Kabbani M. Congenital adrenal hyperplasia: epidemiology, management and practical drug treatment. Paediatr Drugs 2001;3:599–611.

Merke DP, Cutler GB Jr. New ideas for medical treatment of congenital adrenal hyperplasia. Endocrinol Metab Clin North Am 2001;30: 121–135.

New MI, Wilson RC. Steroid disorders in children: congenital adrenal hyperplasia and apparent mineralocorticoid excess. Proc Natl Acad Sci USA 1999;96:12790–12797.

Speiser PW, White PC. Congenital adrenal hyperplasia. N Engl J Med 2003;349:776–788.

White PC, Speiser PW. Congenital adrenal hyperplasia due to 21-hydroxylase deficiency. Endocr Rev 2000;21:245–291.

Winters JL, Chapman PH, Powell DE, et al. Female pseudohermaphroditism due to congenital adrenal hyperplasia complicated by adenocarcinoma of the prostate and clear cell carcinoma of the endometrium. Am J Clin Pathol 1996;106:660–664.

Addison's Disease

Alevritis EM, Sarubbi FA, Jordan RM, Peiris AN. Infectious causes of adrenal insufficiency. South Med J 2003;96:888–890.

Arlt W, Allolio B. Adrenal insufficiency. Lancet 2003;361:1881–1893.

Barker JM, Ide A, Hostetler C, et al. Endocrine and immunogenetic testing in individuals with type 1 diabetes and 21-hydroxylase autoantibodies: Addison's Disease in a high risk population. Clin Endocrinol Metab 2005;90:128–134.

Brosnan CM, Gowing NF. Addison's disease. Br Med J 1996;312:1085–1087.

Falorni A, Laureti S, De Bellis A, et al. Italian addison network study: update of diagnostic criteria for the etiological classification of primary adrenal insufficiency. J Clin Endocrinol Metab 2004;89:1598–1604.

Lloyd RV, Douglas BR, Young WF Jr. Adrenal Gland. Endocrine Diseases. Atlas of Nontumor Pathology, First Series, Fascicle 1. Washington, DC: Armed Forces Institute of Pathology, 2002:171–258.

Lovas K, Husebye ES. Replacement therapy in Addison's disease. Expert Opin Pharmacother 2003;4:2145–2149.

Mantzios G, Tsirigotis P, Veliou F, et al. Primary adrenal lymphoma presenting as Addison's disease: case report and review of the literature. Ann Hematol 2004;83:460–463.

Simm P, McDonnell C, Zacharin M. Primary adrenal insufficiency in childhood and adolescence: advances in diagnosis and management. J Paediatr Child Health 2004;40:596–599.

Soderbergh A, Myhre AG, Ekwall O, et al. Prevalence and clinical associations of 10 defined autoantibodies in autoimmune polyendocrine syndrome type I. J Clin Endocrinol Metab 2004;89:557–562.

Ten S, New M, Maclaren N. Clinical review 130: Addison's disease 2001. J Clin Endocrinol Metab 2001;86:2909–2922.

Infections

Agraharkar M, Fahlen M, Siddiqui M, et al. Waterhouse-Friderichsen syndrome and bilateral renal necrosis in meningococcal sepsis. Am J Kidney Dis 2000;36:396–400.

Dunlop D. Eighty-six cases of Addison's disease. Br Med J. 1963;12: 887–896.

Grinspoon SK, Bilezikian JP. HIV disease and the endocrine system. N Engl J Med 1992;327:1360–1365.

Karakousis PC, Page KR, Varello MA at al. Waterhouse-Friderichsen syndrome after infection with group A streptococcus. Mayo Clin Proc 2001;76:1167–1170.

Lloyd RV, Douglas BR, Young WF Jr. Adrenal Gland. Endocrine Diseases. Atlas of Nontumor Pathology, First Series, Fascicle 1. Washington, DC: Armed Forces Institute of Pathology, 2002:171–258.

Razzaq F, Dunbar EM, Bonington A. The development of cytomegalovirus-induced adrenal failure in a patient with AIDS while receiving corticosteroid therapy. HIV Med. 2002;3:212–214.

Rotterdam H, Dembitzer F. The adrenal glands in AIDS. Endocr Pathol 1993;4:4–14.

Adrenal Cortical Nodules

Cohen RB. Observations on cortical nodules in human adrenal glands. Cancer 1966;19:552–556.

Copeland PM. The incidentally discovered adrenal mass. Ann Surg 1984; 199:116–122.

Dobbie JW. Adrenocortical nodular hyperplasia: the aging adrenal. J Pathol 1969;99:1–18.

Mansmann G, Lau J, Balk E, et al. The clinically inapparent adrenal mass: update in diagnosis and management. Endocr Rev 2004;25:309–340.

Neville AM. The nodular adrenal. Invest Cell Pathol 1978;1:99–111.

Adrenal Gland Cysts

Akcay MN, Akcay G, Balik AA, Boyuk A. Hydatid cysts of the adrenal gland: review of nine patients. World J Surg 2004;28:97–99.

Erickson LA, Lloyd RV, Hartman R, Thompson G. Cystic adrenal neoplasms. Cancer 2004;101:1537–1544.

Gaffey MJ, Mills SE, Fechner RE, et al. Vascular adrenal cysts. A clinicopathologic and immunohistochemical study of endothelial and hemorrhagic (pseudocystic) variants. Am J Surg Pathol 1989;13:740–747.

Gaffey MJ, Mills SE, Medeiros LJ, et al. Unusual variants of adrenal pseudocysts with intracystic fat, myelolipomatous metaplasia, and metastatic carcinoma. Am J Clin Pathol 1990;94:706–713.

Groben PA, Roberson JB, Anger SR, et al. Immunohistochemical evidence for the vascular origin of primary adrenal pseudocysts. Arch Pathol Lab Med 1986;110:121–123.

Jennings TA, Ng B, Boguniewicz A, et al. Adrenal pseudocysts: Evidence of their posthemorrhagic nature. Endocr Pathol 1998;9:353–361.

Lal TG, Kaulback KR, Bombonati A, et al. Surgical management of adrenal cysts. Am Surg 2003;69:812–814.

Lloyd RV, Douglas BR, Young WF Jr. Adrenal Gland. Endocrine Diseases. Atlas of Nontumor Pathology, First Series, Fascicle 1. Washington, DC: Armed Forces Institute of Pathology, 2002:171–258.

Lockhart ME, Smith JK, Kenney PJ. Imaging of adrenal masses. Eur J Radiol 2002;41:95–112.

Newhouse JH, Heffess CS, Wagner BJ. Large degenerated adrenal adenomas: Radiologic-Pathologic correlation. Radiology 1999;210:385–391.

8 Benign Neoplasms of the Adrenal Gland

Lester DR Thompson • Jacqueline A Wieneke

ADRENAL CORTICAL ADENOMA

Adrenal cortical adenoma (ACA) is a benign neoplastic proliferation of adrenal cortical tissue that may be functionally active (hormone producing) or may be non-functional. The vast majority are solitary, unilateral masses.

**ADRENAL CORTICAL ADENOMA
DISEASE FACT SHEET**

Definition
▸ Benign neoplastic proliferation of adrenal cortical tissue

Incidence and Location
▸ Incidence ranges from 1–5 % of patients

Morbidity and Mortality
▸ Morbidity related to endocrine hyperfunction (hypertension, Cushing symptoms, and virilization)
▸ Mortality is low unless untreated

Gender, Race and Age Distribution
▸ Equal gender distribution
▸ Peak age is fourth and fifth decades

Clinical Features
▸ Depends on hormone secretion:
  – Aldosterone producing tumors (75 % of primary hyperaldosteronism) cause Conn syndrome with hypertension
  – 15 % of Cushing syndrome caused by a cortisol producing adenoma (more common in children): truncal obesity, hirsutism, abdominal striae, glucose intolerance, osteoporosis, weakness and fatigue, amenorrhea, hypertension
  – Pure virilizing and feminizing ACAs are rare: virilizing tumors in females cause male hair pattern with facial hair development; feminizing tumors in males cause gynecomastia, decreased libido, feminized hair pattern and testicular atrophy

Radiographic Features
▸ CT and MRI give size, location and possible functional status
▸ T2 weighted MRI out of phase studies show lipid content

Prognosis and Therapy
▸ Excellent prognosis once surgically excised
▸ Supportive hormone replacement may be necessary due to suppression of the contralateral adrenal gland

---

CLINICAL FEATURES

The prevalence of ACAs ranges from 1–5 % of patients, many discovered incidentally during radiographic imaging for other disorders. These 'incidentalomas' usually refer to cortical not medullary tumors. Incidentalomas are uncommon in the young, but increase as patients age. There is no gender predilection. For the most part, these incidentalomas are non-functioning (about 80 % of cases). Furthermore, while hormones may be secreted, it may not result in clinical symptoms. Tumor size plays a role in the management of these lesions, with most physicians surgically excising lesions >6 cm, while radiographically or biochemically monitoring lesions <4 cm. It has been suggested that tumors that remain stable on two imaging studies at least six months apart and do not exhibit hormonal hypersecretion over four years, may not warrant further follow-up.

When symptomatic, the most common endocrine abnormality is primary hyperaldosteronism followed by Cushing syndrome, while virilizing and feminizing tumors are rare. Most patients present with either pure hyperaldosteronism (Conn syndrome) or hypercortisolism (Cushing syndrome); mixed endocrine syndromes may occur and increase the likelihood of malignancy. When tumors are non-functional, abdominal pain or abdominal mass is a common presentation. Primary hyperaldosteronism is most frequently caused by aldosterone secreting ACA (75 % of cases), perhaps detected more frequently with the use of the aldosterone/plasma renin activity ratio (ARR) as a screening test. An aldosterone secreting adenoma represents one of the surgically curable causes of hypertension (but represents only 2 % of all hypertensive patients). Only about 15 % of Cushing syndrome are caused by cortisol secreting ACA, the vast majority caused by pituitary adenomas or ectopic ACTH production. Virilizing and feminizing tumors are much less common, usually part of a mixed endocrine syndrome, but rarely pure virilizing or feminizing tumors are encountered. In adults, a virilizing or feminizing adrenal cortical neoplasm suggests malignancy.

RADIOLOGIC FEATURES

Computed tomography (CT) and magnetic resonance imaging (MRI) allow for highly accurate determination of the size, localization and possible functional status of ACA. MRI has the added advantage of categorizing the lesions based on signal intensity of T2 weighted images. Non-hyperfunctioning adenomas have low signal intensity relative to pheochromocytomas (which display high signal intensity), while the presence of intracellular lipid causes ACA to appear dark on 'out of phase' MRI imaging studies (Figures 8-1 and 8-2).

PATHOLOGIC FEATURES

GROSS FINDINGS

ACAs are characteristically unilateral, solitary masses. They are usually small, weighing less than 100 g and

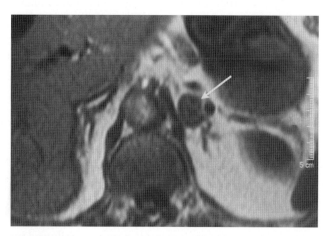

FIGURE 8-1
A T2 weighted MRI of an adrenal cortical adenoma, in phase.

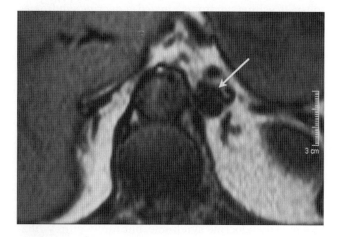

FIGURE 8-2
A T2 weighted MRI of an adrenal cortical adenoma, out of phase, shows a much darker appearance.

ADRENAL CORTICAL ADENOMA PATHOLOGIC FEATURES

Gross Findings

▸ Vast majority are unilateral and solitary masses
▸ Average 2 cm and weigh less than 100 g
▸ Well circumscribed with a yellow-brown cut surface
▸ Secondary changes may be present
▸ Residual adrenal cortex may be nodular (aldosterone secreting tumors) or atrophic (cortisol tumors)

Microscopic Findings

▸ Usually unencapsulated with blending into the surrounding cortex
▸ Mixture of growth patterns may be seen including nests, cords, solid growth
▸ Dominant cell type has a lipid-filled microvesiculated cytoplasm resembling cells of the zona fasciculata
▸ Occasionally may have cells interspersed with more compact, dense eosinophilic cytoplasm
▸ Pleomorphism may be seen
▸ Mitotic figures are infrequent; no atypical forms
▸ Degenerative changes may be present (fibrosis, calcification, hemosiderin, cystic change, re-canalization of thrombus)
▸ Myelolipomatous metaplasia may be present
▸ Spironolactone bodies may be present in patients treated with spironolactate, an aldosterone antagonist medication

Immunohistochemical Results

▸ Inhibin, melan-A (clone A103) and vimentin positive

Fine Needle Aspiration

▸ A hypercellular smear composed of small, round and regular naked nuclei in a background of disrupted, granular to bubbly cytoplasm; occasional lipid-containing cells are noted
▸ A hypocellular pattern is composed of intact cells with bubbly cytoplasm
▸ Nuclei are small, nucleoli are inconspicuous
▸ Necrosis and mitotic figures are absent

Pathologic Differential Diagnosis

▸ Dominant nodule of adrenal cortical hyperplasia, non-functional adrenal cortical nodules, adrenal cortical carcinoma, renal cell carcinoma, other metastatic clear cell tumors

---

measuring less than 4 cm in size, with an average size of 2 cm. They typically are well circumscribed but not always encapsulated. ACAs are often yellow-brown, and depending on hormone production, there may be an atrophic uninvolved rim of adrenal cortex (Figure 8-3). A 'black adenoma' is highly pigmented, most commonly associated with Cushing syndrome (Figure 8-4). Secondary changes such as hemorrhage, fibrosis, cyst formation, and calcification may be present (Figure 8-5).

MICROSCOPIC FINDINGS

If encapsulated, the tumor capsule is thinner and less well developed than is seen in malignant adrenal cortical neoplasms and often times the ACA blends with the surrounding residual adrenal cortical tissue (Figures 8-6

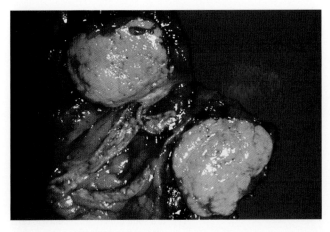

FIGURE 8-3

A bright yellow adrenal cortical adenoma shows a small portion of uninvolved parenchyma.

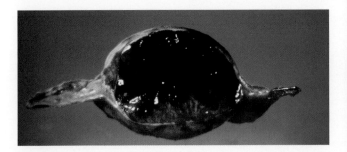

FIGURE 8-4

This black adenoma was dark on cross section and associated with Cushing syndrome clinically.

and Figure 8-7). In cases of adrenal cortical adenoma with hyperaldosteronism, there may be some nodularity in the residual adrenal cortex (Figure 8-8).

Typical ACAs are composed predominantly of bland appearing, well differentiated adrenal cortical cells with a prominent lipid-filled, microvesiculated cytoplasm similar to cells of the zona fasciculata (Figure 8-9). There is often a nested or cord-like growth of the neoplastic cells (Figure 8-10). The lipid-filled component is often interspersed by cells with a more compact, dense eosinophilic cytoplasm, resembling cells of the zona reticularis (Figure 8-11). Nuclei are usually round to oval, although occasionally nuclear pleomorphism may

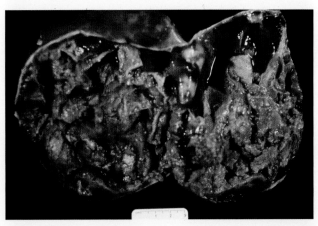

FIGURE 8-5

Extensive degenerative changes are noted within this adrenal cortical adenoma.

FIGURE 8-6

An adrenal cortical adenoma composed of compact eosinophilic cells blends with the surrounding cortex and is only circumscribed rather than encapsulated.

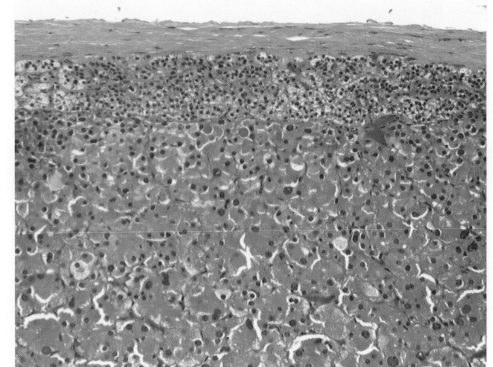

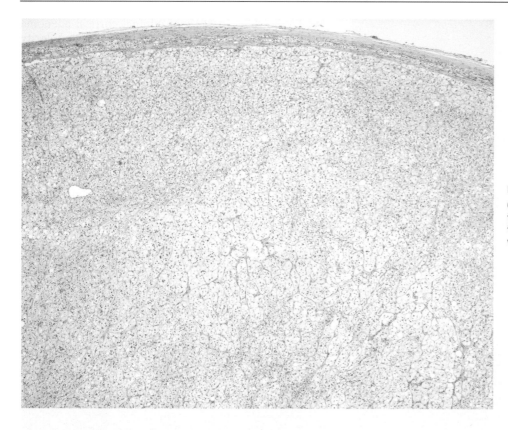

FIGURE 8-7

Compressed adrenal cortical tissue is noted at the periphery. The tumor is a solid growth of neoplastic cells with pale cytoplasm.

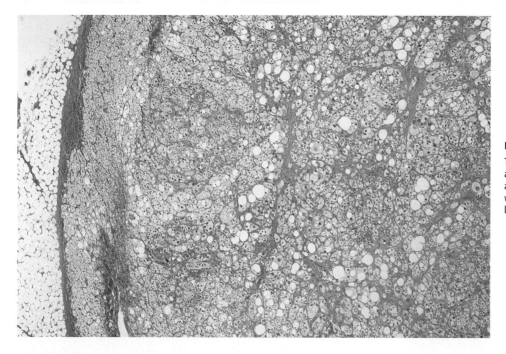

FIGURE 8-8

The far left shows a slightly nodular adrenal cortex, a finding common in aldosterone producing adenomas, while the tumor mass shows much larger cells.

be quite remarkable (Figure 8-12). Intracytoplasmic eosinophilic globules may also be present in adenomas. Mitotic activity is inconspicuous and atypical mitotic figures are not seen. It is not uncommon to have degenerative changes within an adenoma, including hemorrhage, fibrosis, cyst formation and calcifications.

Sometimes clot organization can be misinterpreted to represent a vascular neoplasm (Figure 8-13). However, the presence of typical adrenal cortical adenoma cells is usually noted at the periphery or in areas of viability (Figure 8-14). Eosinophilic, whorled or lamellated intracytoplasmic inclusions surrounded by a clear halo are

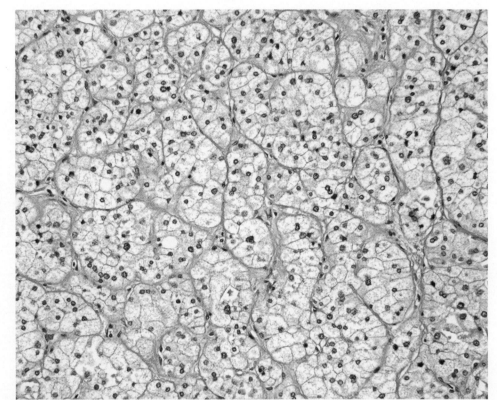

FIGURE 8-9

An adrenal cortical adenoma showing the characteristic microvesiculated cytoplasm mimicking the adrenal zona fasciculata, with the cells arranged in a cord-like pattern.

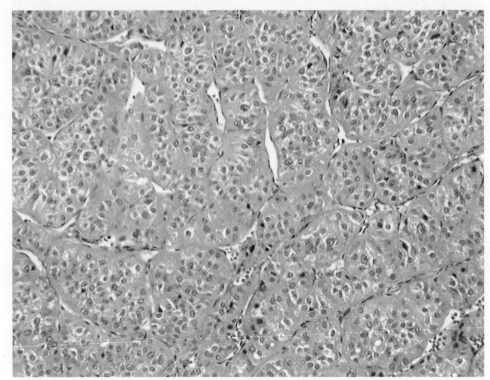

FIGURE 8-10

This cord-like to trabecular pattern of growth is comprised of cells with more compact cytoplasm.

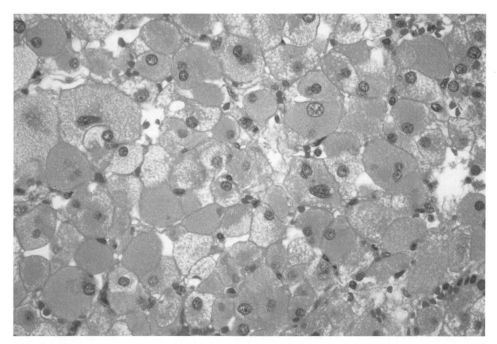

FIGURE 8-11
Compact cells with eosinophilic cytoplasm are seen interspersed with cells with microvesciculated cytoplasm.

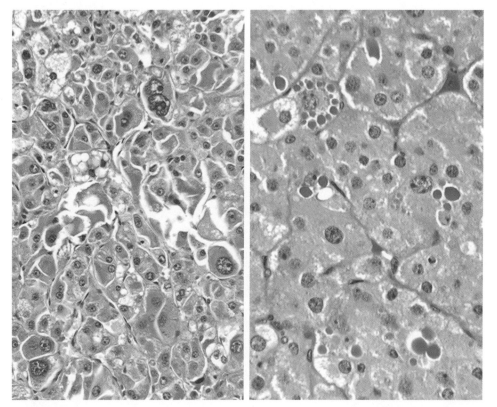

FIGURE 8-12
Left: Compact cells with rare lipid rich cells and remarkably atypical cells blend in this adrenal cortical adenoma. Right: Intracytoplasmic eosinophilic globules can be seen in adrenal cortical adenoma.

referred to as spironolactone bodies and may be found in adenomas from patients with hyperaldosteronism who have been treated with spironolactone (Figure 8-15), although they are more easily identified in the non-neoplastic zona glomerulosa cells (Figure 8-16). They

are believed to be tightly packed tubules of endoplasmic reticulum. Rarely, ACAs may show myelolipomatous metaplasia or myxoid degeneration (Figure 8-17). Black adenomas have a similar histologic appearance to other ACAs with the exception that there is a conspicuous

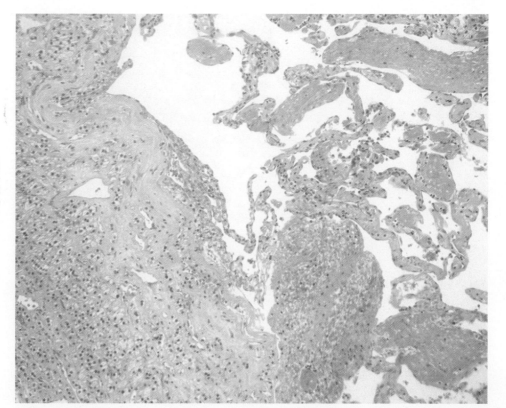

FIGURE 8-13

An adrenal cortical adenoma with degenerative changes, with vascular endothelial hyperplasia noted within an organizing clot. Note the neoplastic cells to the left.

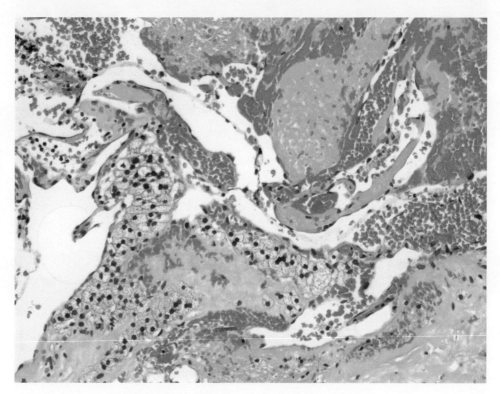

FIGURE 8-14

Small collections of adrenal cortical cells within the degenerated and organizing regions confirm that the adenoma has undergone degenerative changes, rather than representing a vascular neoplasm within the adrenal gland.

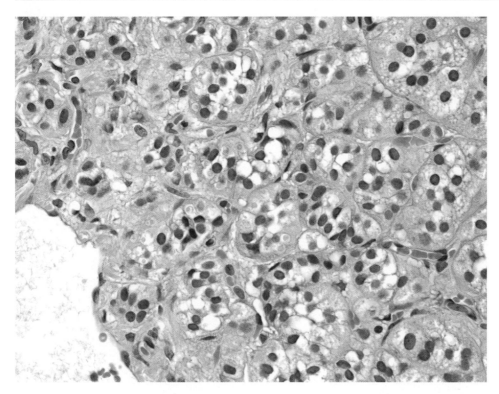

FIGURE 8-15

Adrenocortical adenoma demonstrating numerous spironolactone bodies. These small esosinophilic concentric bodies are noted in the cytoplasm, frequently surrounded by a slight halo.

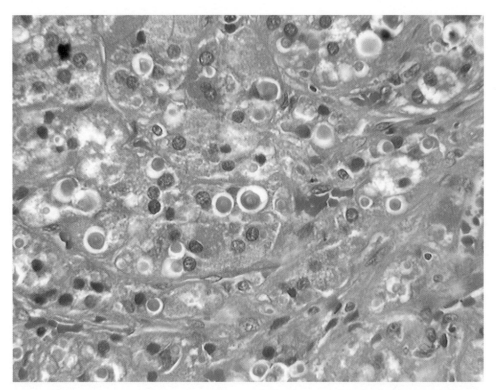

FIGURE 8-16

Numerous spironolactone bodies, concentrically laminated concretions, are frequently found in the zona glomerulosa of aldosterone producing tumors when patients have been treated with spironolactone (aldosterone agonist)

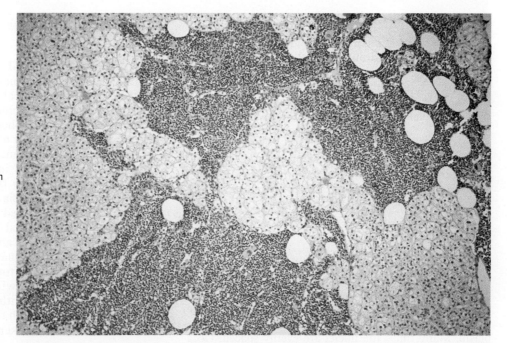

FIGURE 8-17

An adrenal cortical adenoma with myelolipomatous metaplasia.

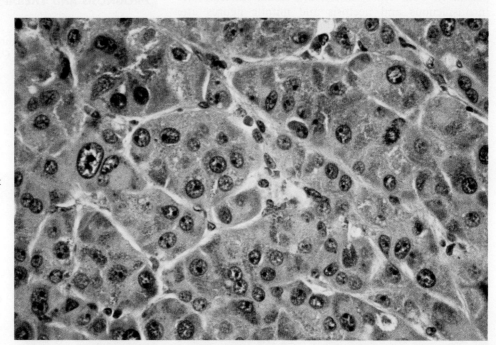

FIGURE 8-18

A black adenoma with abundant granular intracytoplasmic pigment.

brown or golden brown granular cytoplasmic pigment with staining characteristic similar to lipofuscin (Figure 8-18). Rarely, ACAs are composed predominantly of oncocytic cells with abundant finely granular eosinophilic cytoplasm, referred to as adrenal cortical oncocytoma.

ANCILLARY STUDIES

ULTRASTRUCTURAL FEATURES

Electron microscopy demonstrates abundant mitochondria in the cytoplasm of neoplasms with oncocytic differentiation, while smooth endoplasmic reticulum is common.

IMMUNOHISTOCHEMICAL RESULTS

Immunohistochemistry is seldom necessary to prove the diagnosis of an adrenal cortical adenoma, but sometimes on scant core needle biopsy specimens, antibodies against the alpha inhibin subunit or melan-A protein (A103) may help to confirm adrenal cortical tissue. However, positive reactivity with inhibin with cytoplasmic granular staining is focal to absent in clear cells, and doesn't separate between cortical lesions (Figure 8-19). Immunoreactivity with melan-A (clone A-103) and calretinin in adrenal cortical neoplasms has been reported as strong and diffuse with granular cytoplasmic staining, but further analysis is necessary before these markers become clinically valuable.

FINE NEEDLE ASPIRATION

Two different patterns are usually present: a hypercellular and a hypocellular one. The hypercellular one is composed of small, round and regular naked nuclei in a background of disrupted, granular to bubbly cytoplasm. Many times the nuclei are evenly spaced. Occasional lipid-containing cells are noted. The hypocellular pattern is composed of intact cells with bubbly cytoplasm. In both types, nuclei are small, nucleoli are inconspicuous and necrosis and mitotic figures are absent. Separation from other adrenal cortical neoplasms, hepatocytes, and other small cell tumors may be difficult on FNA alone.

DIFFERENTIAL DIAGNOSIS

The pathologic differential diagnosis of ACA includes a dominant nodule of adrenal cortical hyperplasia, nonfunctioning adrenocortical nodules, adrenal cortical carcinoma, renal cell carcinoma, other metastatic clear cell tumors and rarely pheochromocytoma with lipid degeneration. Assessment of the residual adrenal cortical tissue as well as the contralateral gland (radiographically or histologically) is important in distinguishing adrenal cortical adenoma from a dominant nodule of adrenal cortical hyperplasia or non-functioning adrenocortical nodules. Increased cellularity, diffuse or trabecular growth, increased mitotic activity, including atypical forms, necrosis, and invasion are features of carcinoma. Metastatic renal cell carcinoma (RCC) or direct extension of RCC from the kidney can present a dilemma. However, PAS will highlight the presence of glycogen in a RCC, with pertinent immunohistochemistry able to help with the separation (EMA, CD10, renal cell carcinoma marker, melan-A, inhibin).

PROGNOSIS AND THERAPY

Prognosis is excellent. There is a risk of adrenocortical insufficiency in cases of Cushing syndrome once the

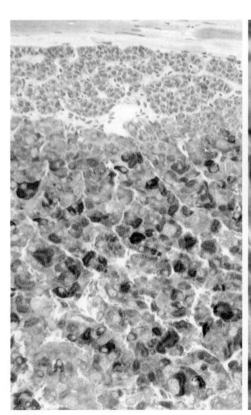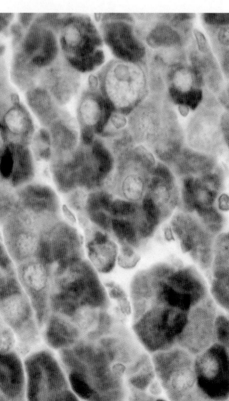

FIGURE 8-19

Left: Inhibin is reactive in adrenal cortical tissue, more strongly in adenomas which are of an eosinophilic nature. Right: Granular, heavy, cytoplasmic reaction with inhibin is noted.

hyperfunctioning mass has been resected due to long-standing suppression of the contralateral adrenal gland. Supportive administration of glucocorticoids and mineralocorticoids may be necessary for an extended period of time. Surgery is the treatment of choice, whether laparoscopic or by open technique.

PHEOCHROMOCYTOMA

The designation of pheochromocytoma (adrenal medullary paraganglioma) refers to catecholamine secreting tumors arising from the chromaffin cells of adrenal medullary tissue, also referred to as paragangliomas when they arise from sympathetic paraganglia. The majority of pheochromocytomas have a benign clinical course but can have a malignant potential. A 10% rule

---

PHEOCHROMOCYTOMA
DISEASE FACT SHEET

Definition
▸ Catecholamine secreting tumor arising from the chromaffin tissue of the adrenal medulla

Incidence and Location
▸ Rare, with 8/million population
▸ Adrenal medulla, but other sympathetic ganglia may be affected by paraganglioma

Morbidity and Mortality
▸ Morbidity related to associated clinical findings, in particular, hypertension, headaches and diaphoresis

Gender, Race and Age Distribution
▸ Equal gender distribution
▸ Peak age, fifth decade, although younger in syndrome associated patients (second decade)

Clinical Features
▸ '10 % tumor': 10 % bilateral, 10 % extraadrenal, 10 % malignant, 10 % familial, and 10 % in children
▸ Most are sporadic (90 %), but familial syndromes include MEN2A or 2B, von Recklinghausen disease, von Hippel-Lindau disease
▸ Symptoms are determined by excess catecholamines and include hypertension, palpitations, headaches, diaphoresis, flushing, anxiety, nausea, constipation, pain, epistaxis
▸ May have a palpable abdominal mass
▸ Elevated urine and/or serum catecholamines, norepinephrine, epinephrine, metanephrine, dopamine, VMA

Prognosis and Therapy
▸ Excellent prognosis, although some may have aggressive biologic behavior
▸ Clinical and biochemical follow-up suggested, in spite of histologic features
▸ Surgery with pre- and intraoperative hypertension management
▸ Intraoperative evaluation for multicentric disease

---

of thumb can be applied to this tumor: 10% bilateral, 10% extraadrenal, 10% malignant, 10% in childhood, and 10% familial.

CLINICAL FEATURES

Pheochromocytomas are rare tumors with an estimated incidence of 8/1 000 000 population. Most pheochromocytomas (90%) are sporadic and about 10% are familial, whether part of a specific syndrome or arising in a familial setting. Syndromes include multiple endocrine neoplasia (MEN2A or 2B), von Recklinghausen disease and von Hippel-Lindau disease, among others. In a sporadic setting, >95% of cases are solitary, unilateral lesions, while 5% are bilateral. Within familial patients, >50% are bilateral and/or multicentric. The peak age in sporadic cases is the fifth decade, while familial cases tend to be diagnosed within the first two decades of life. Pediatric patients account for about 10% of tumors, where there is also an increased incidence of bilateral and multicentric disease. There is no gender predilection.

Symptoms are referable to excess catecholamine production and include episodic, sustained, labile, and/or paroxysmal (erratic) hypertension, frequently induced by postural changes, palpitations, headaches, diaphoresis, flushing, anxiety, nausea, epistaxis, constipation, and pain. The classic diagnostic triad is paroxysmal hypertension, headaches, and diaphoresis. Tumor hormone production may give differences in the type of hypertension: norepinephrine is more frequently associated with sustained hypertension while epinephrine along with norepinephrine is associated with episodic hypertension. Pure epinephrine secreting tumors may be associated with hypotension. Occasionally, a palpable abdominal mass may be the presenting symptom. Laboratory investigation is vital to the diagnostic work-up of pheochromocytoma and includes remarkably elevated levels of serum and/or urine catecholamines, norepinephrine, epinephrine, metanephrine, dopamine, vanillylmandelic acid (VMA), or other metabolites.

RADIOLOGIC FEATURES

Preoperative localization of pheochromocytoma is possible with a combination of techniques, including high resolution CT, MRI and nuclear medicine studies. Benign lesions are characteristically homogeneous, fairly well-circumscribed masses. Cystic degeneration, calcification, hemorrhage and necrosis lead to a non-homogeneous appearance, especially on contrast enhanced imaging. With MRI T2 weighted images, pheochromocytomas typically show high signal intensity and appear bright on imaging, sometimes referred to as the 'light-bulb' sign (Figures 8-20 and 8-21). The use of the radiopharmaceutical and guanethidine analog ^{131}I-meta-iodobenzylguanidine (MIBG) for scintigraphy

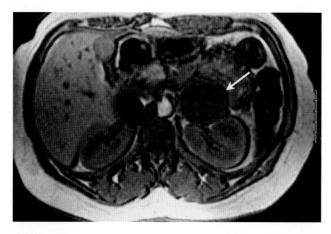

FIGURE 8-20
A T1 weighted MRI demonstrates an intermediate signal mass in the adrenal gland.

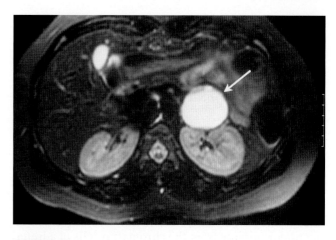

FIGURE 8-21
A T2 weighted MRI shows a high signal intensity, bright mass, giving the 'light-bulb' designation.

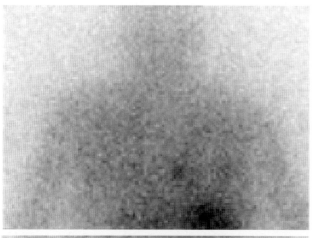

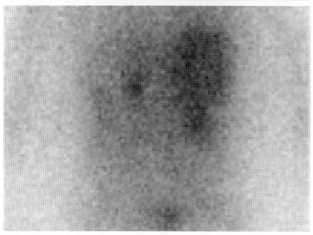

FIGURE 8-22
This MIBG scintigraphy shows increased uptake in the right adrenal gland and also in the chest in this syndromic associated patient who had two separate tumors: a pheochromocytoma and a paraganglioma.

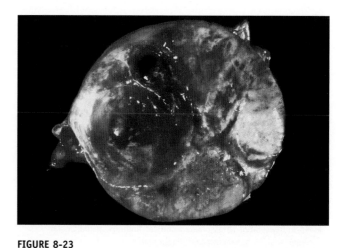

FIGURE 8-23
Cross section through a pheochromocytoma shows a small remnant of adrenal cortex with the tumor mass demonstrating extensive degenerative changes including cyst formation and hemorrhage.

shows a remarkable affinity for adrenal medullary tissue (Figure 8-22), but does not separate between different neuroendocrine tumors types. Angiography reveals a vascular tumor mass in the adrenal gland, but is seldom employed.

PATHOLOGIC FEATURES

GROSS FINDINGS

Pheochromocytomas are typically well-circumscribed and spherical or oval in shape. Tumors weigh between 12 g and 650 g (mean, 200 g) and measure 1–18 cm in greatest size (mean, 6 cm). On cut section, the tumors are usually firm with a glistening gray-white surface. Some tumors exhibit degenerative changes such as congestion, hemorrhage, necrosis and even cystic change (Figure 8-23). Although they may appear encapsulated,

Gross Findings

▸ Sporadic pheochromocytomas are usually unilateral masses
▸ Familial tumors tend to be bilateral, multicentric and/or extraadrenal
▸ Typically well-circumscribed and spherical or oval
▸ Most lack a well-developed fibrous capsule
▸ Average size 6 cm and 200 g
▸ Cut section is usually firm, glistening, gray-white with some tumors showing degenerative changes

Microscopic Findings

▸ Zellballen, alveolar, nested, trabecular, solid or diffuse patterns of growth, one of which predominates
▸ 'Balls' of cells are surrounded by a rich vascular sustentacular supporting framework
▸ Polygonal cells with granular, basophilic cytoplasm
▸ Nuclei have stippled ('salt-and-pepper') chromatin pattern, with occasionally pleomorphic nuclei noted
▸ PAS positive globules and intranuclear cytoplasmic inclusions may be seen
▸ Mitotic activity is scarce
▸ Degenerative changes are seen, along with rare cases showing amyloid or melanin

Ultrastructural Features

▸ Dense core neurosecretory granules
▸ Norepinephrine granules have large, eccentric, electron-lucent halos between the dense core and the membrane
▸ Epinephrine granules are smaller and more uniform

Immunohistochemical Results

▸ Pheochromocytes are chromogranin and synaptophysin positive
▸ Sustentacular cells are S-100 protein positive
▸ Other neuroendocrine markers or neuropeptides may be positive

Fine Needle Aspiration

▸ Hypercellular smears
▸ Single, small groups or 'pseudorosettes'
▸ Three cell types: small to moderate-size *polygonal* shaped with delicate, granular cytoplasm; *spindle* cells with ample cytoplasm and elongated nuclei; and *large, 'strap-like'* cells with large, eccentric nuclei and prominent nucleoli

Molecular Analysis

▸ Ret proto-oncogene, VHL tumor suppressor gene, succinate dehydrogenase subunit D and subunit B genes

Pathologic Differential Diagnosis

▸ Adrenal cortical adenoma, adrenal cortical carcinoma, malignant pheochromocytoma, metastatic neuroendocrine neoplasms, alveolar soft parts sarcoma, mixed medullary neoplasms

close inspection shows a 'pseudocapsule'. The adrenal cortex may be atrophic, or may show paradoxical hyperplasia in response to the hypertension.

MICROSCOPIC FINDINGS

Various architectural patterns may be present but often one pattern predominates. 'Zellballen' (alveolar or nested; Figure 8-24) and trabecular patterns are seen most commonly. Solid, diffuse, and spindle cell patterns are rare, and are not dominant. The 'balls' of cells are supported by a rich vascular plexus and a delicate, dendritic to spindle cell sustentacular meshwork (Figure 8-25). The sustentacular supporting cells are difficult to absolutely identify on light microscopy. The pheochromocytes are polygonal and may have sharply defined cell borders or may interdigitate with indistinct borders (Figure 8-26). The cytoplasm of the neoplastic cells varies from eosinophilic to basophilic and typically has a finely granular character (Figure 8-27). Nuclei are round to oval in shape with a stippled 'salt-and-pepper' chromatin pattern. The cytoplasm may be vacuolated in some cases and may also display PAS-positive globules (Figure 8-28). Pleomorphism may be present and bizarre hyperchromatic nuclei, often with intranuclear cytoplasmic inclusions are not uncommon (Figure 8-28). Mitotic activity is sparse, and usually <3/10 HPFs. Degenerative changes such as fibrosis, hemorrhage, hemosiderin deposition and cystic change can also be seen, while stromal amyloid and melanin is occasionally identified (Figure 8-29).

ANCILLARY STUDIES

ULTRASTRUCTURAL FEATURES

The diagnostic hallmark are dense core neurosecretory granules that range in size from 150–250 nm. Norepinephrine granules are separated from epinephrine granules by a large, eccentric, electron-lucent zone or 'halo' between the dense core and the granule membrane. The granules may vary in size, shape, distribution and density. Epinephrine granules tend to be more uniform. Both epinephrine and norepinephrine granules may be seen in the same tumor.

IMMUNOHISTOCHEMICAL RESULTS

Pheochromocytes are characteristically chromogranin and synaptophysin positive while the supporting sustentacular cell population is highlighted with antibodies to S-100 protein (Figures 8-30 and 8-31). Many different patterns of growth and size of nests will be accentuated by the S-100 protein (Figure 8-32) Occasionally, S-100 protein may non-specifically cross react with the cytoplasm of the pheochromocytes. While unnecessary for the diagnosis, pheochromocytes express a broad range of neuroendocrine markers and neuropeptides, including leu- and met-enkephalins, serotonin, somatostatin, vasoactive intestinal peptide, ACTH, calcitonin, CD56 and NSE (Figure 8-33)

FINE NEEDLE ASPIRATION

Smears are usually hypercellular with cells arranged singly or in small groups, often creating a 'pseudorosette' (Figure 8-34). Cells are small to moderate-sized, and polygonal shaped with delicate, granular cytoplasm;

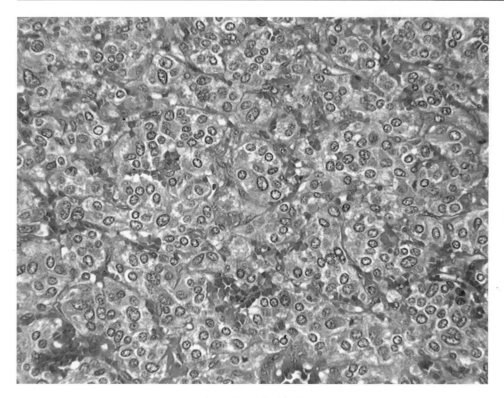

FIGURE 8-24

Zellballen architecture with a rich vascular, sustentacular framework in this pheochromocytoma.

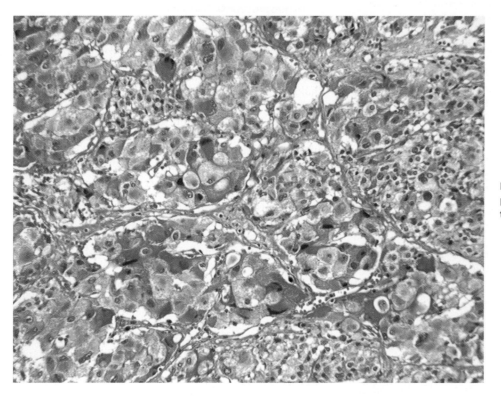

FIGURE 8-25

Nests of variable size are present in this pheochromocytoma.

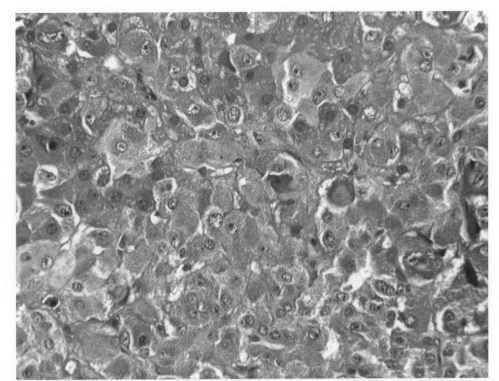

FIGURE 8-26

A syncytial architecture of cells with prominently granular basophilic cytoplasm can be seen in pheochromocytoma.

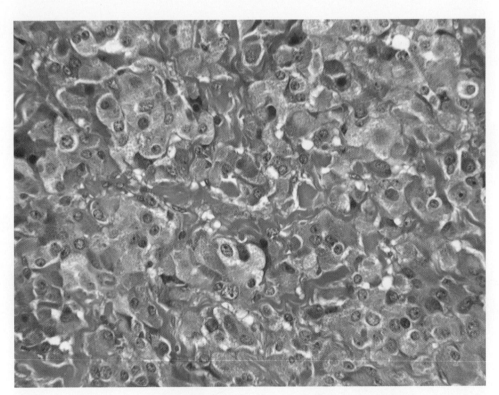

FIGURE 8-27

Heavily basophilic granular cytoplasm surrounding round to oval nuclei with stippled chromatin. Fibrous connective tissue may sometimes meander through the neoplam.

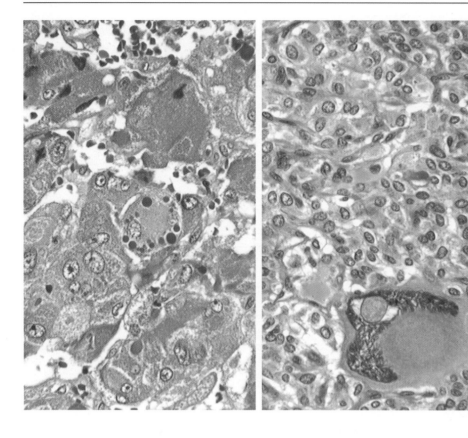

FIGURE 8-28
Left: Intracytoplasmic, eosinophilic globules may be seen. Right: Focal, bizarre nuclei with intranuclear cytoplasmic inclusion within this benign pheochromocytoma.

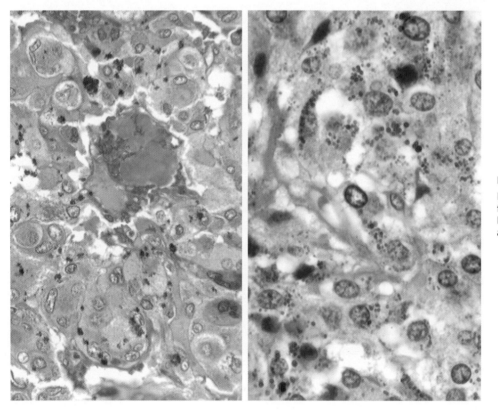

FIGURE 8-29
Left: Amyloid can sometimes be found within a pheochromocytoma. Right: Melanin pigment is occasionally identified.

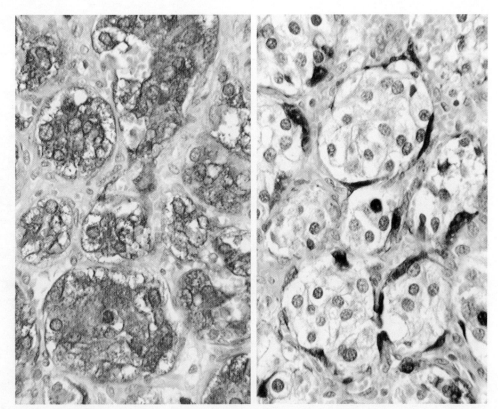

FIGURE 8-30

Left: The pheochromocytes react strongly and diffusely with chromogranin. Right: The sustentacular cells are highlighted by S-100 protein immunoreactivity.

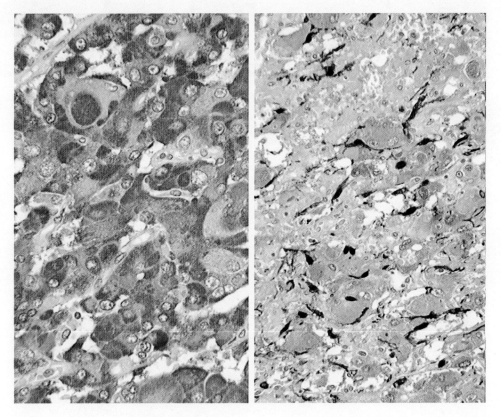

FIGURE 8-31

Left: The pheochromocytes react strongly and diffusely with chromogranin. Right: The sustentacular cells are highlighted by S-100 protein, but the staining is discontinuous in this example.

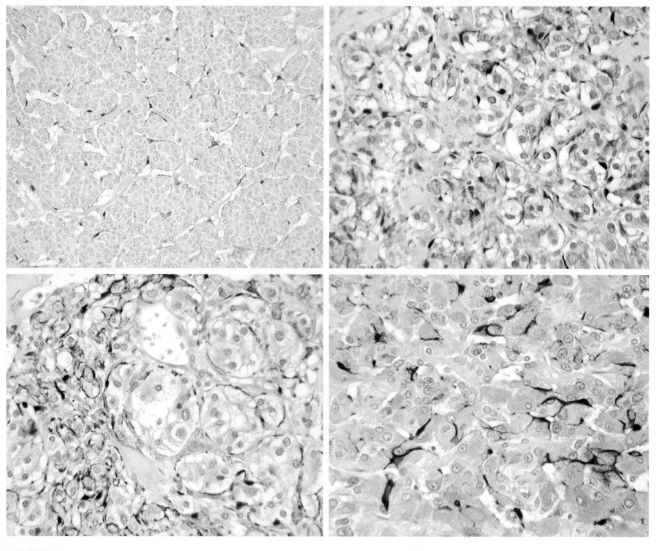

FIGURE 8-32
The variety of S-100 protein reaction patterns displayed in this selection demonstrates small nests, larger nests, individual cell staining and more discontinous staining.

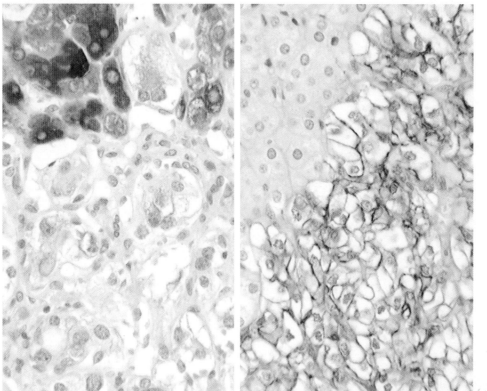

FIGURE 8-33
Left: Inhibin will react with the cortical cells but not the cells of a pheochromocytoma. Right: CD56 is one of the neuroendocrine type markers which is positive in pheochromocytoma. Note the nonreactive adrenal cortex in the upper left.

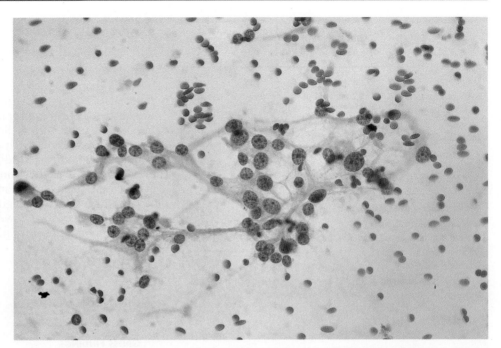

FIGURE 8-34

A fine needle aspiration shows small cells with delicate, feathered cytoplasm surrounding nuclei with coarse, 'salt-and-pepper' nuclear chromatin distribution. Fibrovascular channels and blood is noted in the background.

spindle cells with ample cytoplasm and elongated nuclei; and large, 'strap-like' cells with large, eccentric nuclei with prominent nucleoli. All three cell types are interspersed throughout the smear, requiring complete examination of the aspirated material.

GENETIC STUDIES

Familial pheochromocytoma may arise without associated disease but is usually seen in the setting of MEN2A or 2B, von Recklinghausen disease and von Hippel-Lindau disease. A group of susceptibility genes has been identified and includes the *RET* proto-oncogene (associated with MEN2), the tumor suppressor gene VHL (associated with von Hippel-Lindau disease) and the newly identified genes for succinate dehydrogenase subunit D (SDHD) and succinate dehydrogenase subunit B (SDHB), which predispose to pheochromocytoma and glomus tumor.

DIFFERENTIAL DIAGNOSIS

The differential diagnosis includes adrenal cortical adenoma, adrenal cortical carcinoma, malignant pheochromocytoma, and mixed medullary neoplasms. Usually, the basophilic, granular cytoplasm, the zellballen architecture, and the immunohistochemistry profile allows for separation. However, it may be more difficult, especially on core needle biopsy specimens. Granular neoplasms often display diffusion artifact or 'background' staining with immunohistochemical techniques, requiring caution in over interpreting these results. Neoplasms may metastasize to the adrenal gland and include renal cell carcinoma, alveolar

soft parts sarcoma, and metastatic neuroendocrine carcinoma, all of which require additional clinical and radiographic information to make the appropriate separation.

PROGNOSIS AND THERAPY

Pheochromocytoma usually portends an excellent overall prognosis. However, pheochromocytomas are known to be capricious, occasionally demonstrating a malignant behavior years after the original resection. A constellation of histologic features may help to predict which tumors may portend an aggressive biologic behavior, but close clinical and biochemical follow-up is still recommended in all cases. The treatment of choice is surgical resection, with aggressive preoperative antihypertensive management to avert a hypertensive crisis intraoperatively. Intraoperative evaluation for multicentric disease should be performed.

GANGLIONEUROMA

Ganglioneuroma (GN) represents the benign end of the spectrum of ganglioneuroma, ganglioneuroblastoma (GNB) and neuroblastoma (NB), referred to collectively as neuroblastic tumors (NTs). NTs are embryonal tumors of the sympathetic nervous system and derive from neural crest tissue. They arise in the adrenal medulla, paravertebral sympathetic ganglia and sympathetic paraganglia, such as the Organ of Zuckerkandl. GN is a mature benign neoplasm and

GANGLIONEUROMA
DISEASE FACT SHEET

Definition

▶ Benign neuroblastic tumor composed of mature ganglion cells and Schwannian stroma

Incidence and Location

▶ Rare tumor within the neuroblastic tumor group
▶ Most arise in the posterior mediastinum, with adrenal tumors comprising about 20 % of all tumors

Gender, Race and Age Distribution

▶ Equal gender distribution
▶ Mean age for adrenal tumors is third to fifth decades

Clinical Features

▶ Tumors grow slowly, resulting in large tumors at time of discovery
▶ Symptoms, if present, are related to mass effect, and include cough, dyspnea, abdominal pain, emesis, fever, weight loss, and constipation
▶ Rarely, functional symptoms develop (hypertension, virilization)

Radiographic Features

▶ Well-defined, homogenous masses
▶ CT shows low attenuation, with contrast induced enhancement
▶ MRI shows a heterogeneous high signal intensity on T2 weighted images
▶ Calcifications are common

Prognosis and Therapy

▶ Outcome is generally excellent with only rare cases of malignant transformation
▶ Immature ganglion cells do not change prognosis
▶ Surgery is the treatment of choice

is composed of mature Schwannian stroma and ganglion cells. It may arise de novo or evolve from a differentiating/maturing neuroblastoma or ganglioneuroblastoma.

CLINICAL FEATURES

GNs are rare in the adrenal gland, with most presenting in the posterior mediastinum. While most GNs occur within the first three decades, adrenal GNs occur more commonly in the third to fifth decades, typically in much older patients than neuroblastomas and ganglioneuroblastomas (median age: 7 years). There is no well documented gender preference. Due to slow growth, the tumors may be large by the time they are incidentally discovered; less commonly, symptoms are related to mass effect and include cough, dyspnea, abdominal pain, emesis, fever, weight loss, and constipation. Rarely, patients may have functional symptoms (hypertension, virilization).

RADIOLOGIC FEATURES

Despite the fact that GNs tend to be homogeneous, they have similar imaging characteristics to GNB and NB; thus, they cannot be distinguished by imaging evaluation alone. Ultrasound typically shows a homogeneous, hypoechoic mass with well-defined borders. CT demonstrates a mass lesion, with a homogeneous, low attenuation, while contrast studies show slight to moderate enhancement. Calcifications are present in up to 60 % of cases. MRI imaging demonstrates low signal intensity on T1-weighted imaging and heterogeneous high signal intensity on T2 weighted imaging. ^{123}I-MIBG uptake may be present, failing to separate among NB, GNB and GN.

PATHOLOGIC FEATURES

GROSS FINDINGS

GNs typically are well-circumscribed tumors with a firm, rubbery, gray-white to tan-yellow cut surface (Figure 8-35). There may be a whorled or trabecular appearance reminiscent of leiomyoma. They may appear

GANGLIONEUROMA
PATHOLOGIC FEATURES

Gross Findings

▶ Mean size, 8 cm (range up to 18 cm)
▶ Well-circumscribed, firm, rubbery, gray white to tan-yellow tumors
▶ Hemorrhage or cystic change may be seen in larger tumors, but requires careful sampling to exclude neuroblastomatous foci

Microscopic Findings

▶ Mixture of mature Schwannian stromal component and interspersed ganglion cells
▶ Ganglion cells are polygonal with eccentrically placed nuclei and prominent nucleoli with cytoplasm showing Nissl substance and/or neuromelanin pigment
▶ Dysmorphic and immature ganglion cells may be observed
▶ Distribution and density of ganglion cells is variable
▶ Proliferating Schwann cells with spindled nuclei and variable amount of collagen fibers
▶ Fat and lymphocytes may be seen

Immunohistochemical Results

▶ Schwannian component is S-100 protein positive
▶ Ganglion cells are NFP, synaptophysin, chromogranin, NSE, and sometimes S-100 protein positive
▶ Vimentin is usually positive; keratin negative
▶ Lymphocytes will be CD45RB, CD43 positive

Pathologic Differential Diagnosis

▶ Ganglioneuroblastoma, neurofibroma, schwannoma

encapsulated but on close inspection a true capsule is infrequent. The average size is 8 cm (range up to 18 cm), with thoracic lesions usually larger than adrenal tumors. Hemorrhage and cystic change may be seen, especially in large tumors, requiring careful sampling to exclude neuroblastic foci.

MICROSCOPIC FINDINGS

Microscopically, the tumor is composed of a mature Schwannian stromal component with individual or groups of ganglion cells randomly interspersed throughout the stroma (Figures 8-36 and 8-37). Most ganglion cells are mature, with eccentrically placed nuclei and prominent nucleoli, although immature forms may be seen. The ganglion cell cytoplasm often contains Nissl substance and/or granular tan to brown 'neuromelanin' pigment (Figure 8-38). The distribution and density of the ganglion cells varies considerably within a tumor. The Schwannian stromal component consists of proliferating Schwann cells with spindled nuclei and variable amounts of collagen fibers. Mature fat may be incorporated into the neoplasm at the advancing edge. Aggregates of lymphocytes may need to be separated from neuroblastic elements with immunohistochemical evaluation. When dysmorphic or immature ganglion cells are dominant, the tumors are called immature GNs.

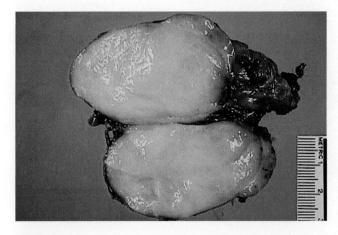

FIGURE 8-35
A macroscopic ganglioneuroma shows a firm, rubbery, tan-yellow cut surface with a somewhat whorled appearance.

ANCILLARY STUDIES

ULTRASTRUCTURAL FEATURES

Axons are seen containing neurofilaments, almost invariably accompanied by microtubules. Scattered neurosecretory granules are also present.

IMMUNOHISTOCHEMICAL RESULTS

The Schwannian component demonstrates strong S-100 reactivity, while the ganglion cells express neural

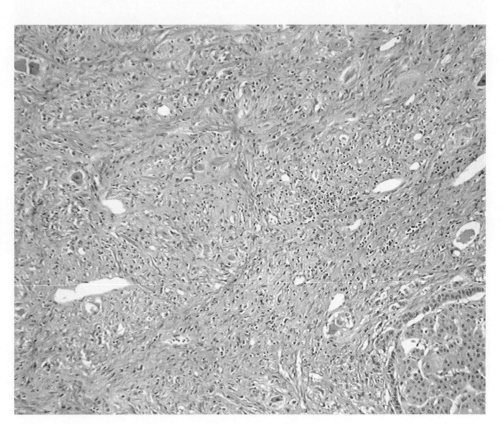

FIGURE 8-36
Mature Schwannian stroma contains large ganglion cells dotted throughout the tumor. A portion of benign adrenal cortex is noted in the lower right corner.

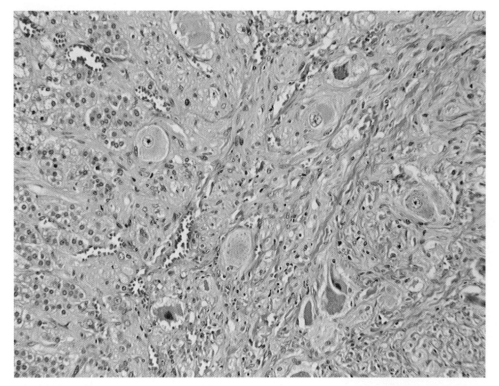

FIGURE 8-37

An adrenal ganglioneuroma showing the characteristic ganglion cells separated by the background neural component. Pigment is seen within the ganglion cells. Benign adrenal cortical tissue is seen in the left.

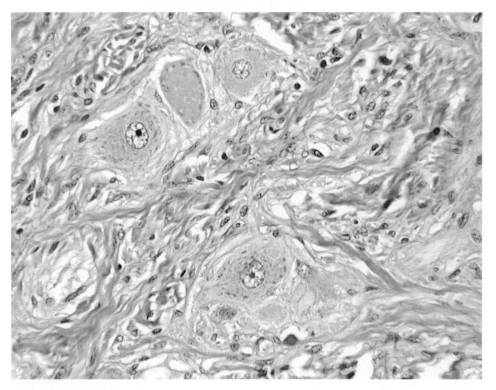

FIGURE 8-38

Large ganglion cells have eccentric nuclei with prominent nucleoli. Neuromelanin and Nissl substance is seen in the cytoplasm of the ganglion cells.

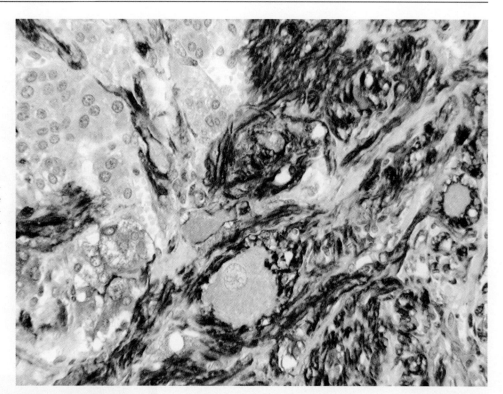

FIGURE 8-39
The adrenal cortical cells are non-reactive with S-100 protein, while the background Schwannian material is strongly reactive. The ganglion cell is also non-reactive.

markers such as neurofilament protein, synaptophysin, chromogranin, neuron specific enolase and occasionally S-100 protein (Figure 8-39). Vimentin is also typically positive. Lymphocytes will be CD45RB and CD43 positive.

MOLECULAR TECHNIQUES

In contrast to many NBs and GNBs, abnormalities of chromosome 1 and/or amplification of *MYCN* gene are not present.

DIFFERENTIAL DIAGNOSIS

The differential diagnosis includes ganglioneuroblastoma (GNB), neurofibroma, and neurilemmoma (schwannoma). Tumors may have an obvious neuroblastomatous component making the diagnosis of GNB straightforward. However, occasionally the neuroblastomatous component is sparse and careful examination with serial sectioning is necessary to identify it. Therefore, all GN should be closely examined macroscopically to identify areas of hemorrhage or discoloration that might contain neuroblastomatous elements. The density and distribution of ganglion cells in GN varies considerably and may be quite sparse. In this case, neurofibroma and schwannoma come into the differential diagnosis. Once again, thorough sampling should identify the ganglion cells.

PROGNOSIS AND THERAPY

Outcome, in general, is excellent following resection of the tumor. Rare cases of malignant transformation (fibrosarcoma, malignant peripheral nerve sheath tumor) have been reported. Immature ganglion cells do not influence the biologic behavior. Surgical resection is the treatment of choice, including laparoscopic techniques.

MYELOLIPOMA

Myelolipoma is a tumor-like lesion composed of mature adipose tissue and mature hematopoietic elements in various proportions. This lesion accounts for approximately 3% of primary adrenal gland neoplasms. The histogenesis is unknown, but may result from metaplastic alterations of adrenal cortical or stromal cells, bone marrow emboli, or embryonic rests of bone marrow in the adrenal gland.

CLINICAL FEATURES

Most patients are asymptomatic and the lesion is discovered incidentally on examination for other reasons.

MYELOLIPOMA
DISEASE FACT SHEET

Definition
▶ Benign tumor-like lesion composed of mature adipose tissue and hematopoietic elements in various proportions

Incidence and Location
▶ Approximately 3% of primary adrenal gland neoplasms
▶ Adrenal is most common location, but other sites include mediastinum, liver and gastrointestinal tract

Morbidity and Mortality
▶ Risk of rupture and hemorrhage in large tumors

Gender, Race and Age Distribution
▶ Equal gender distribution
▶ Fifth to seventh decades

Clinical Features
▶ Most are asymptomatic, discovered incidentally
▶ When symptomatic, symptoms relate to a mass effect: abdominal or flank pain, hematuria, palpable mass, hypertension, retroperitoneal hemorrhage
▶ Can be seen as a metaplastic process in other adrenal gland disorders

Radiographic Findings
▶ Unilateral, solitary mass with a density identical to fat
▶ T1 weighted MRI shows high signal intensity
▶ If fat is scarce or there is hemorrhage, infarction or calcification, radiographic features are obscured

Prognosis and Therapy
▶ Complete surgical excision prevents recurrence
▶ Small, clinically silent lesions can be observed

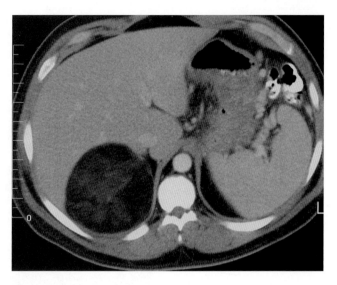

FIGURE 8-40
A myelolipoma of the right adrenal demonstrating an identical density to the subcutaneous fat.

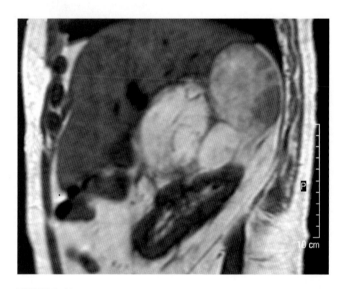

FIGURE 8-41
A heterogeneous signal on T1 weighted MRI scan, with a signal intensity identical to fat.

PATHOLOGIC FEATURES

GROSS FINDINGS

Adrenal myelolipomas vary considerably in size, ranging from incidentally discovered lesions radiographically to clinically palpable (up to 34 cm). Tumors are usually well-circumscribed but unencapsulated, blending with the uninvolved cortical tissue. The cut surface is variegated, ranging from pale yellow to deep red or red brown depending on the proportions of fat and hematopoietic elements (Figure 8-42). Areas of hemorrhage and infarction are more frequent in large lesions.

When symptoms are reported, they relate to mass effect and include abdominal or flank pain, hematuria, a palpable mass, hypertension or rarely retroperitoneal hemorrhage. Most tumors are discovered during the fifth to seventh decades without a gender predilection. Occasionally myelolipomas are seen in association with other adrenal lesions, giving support to the metaplastic hypothesis. Rarely, endocrine dysfunction has been reported.

RADIOLOGIC FEATURES

The vase majority of tumors are unilateral and solitary. CT and MRI demonstrate areas of obvious fat with a well-circumscribed adrenal mass lesion (Figure 8-40). T1-weighted images on MRI show high signal intensity due to fat content (Figure 8-41), however lesions with scarce fat, hemorrhage, infarction or calcifications may not be able to be distinguished from other adrenal tumors.

MYELOLIPOMA
PATHOLOGIC FEATURES

Gross Findings

▸ Size is variable, up to 34 cm
▸ Usually well-circumscribed, unencapsulated masses
▸ Cut surface is variegated, pale-yellow to red-brown depending on proportion of fat and hematopoietic elements
▸ Hemorrhage and infarction are more common in large lesions

Microscopic Findings

▸ Admixture of mature adipose tissue and hematopoietic elements
▸ Full trilineage maturation of myeloid, erythroid and megakaryocytic lines
▸ Osseous metaplasia, hemorrhage, and fibrosis may be seen

Fine Needle Aspiration

▸ Smears contain mature fat and mature and immature hematopoietic elements

Pathologic Differential Diagnosis

▸ Separation of *tumor mass* from myelolipomatous foci in other adrenal gland lesions, accidental bone marrow FNA

MICROSCOPIC FINDINGS

Tumors are a mixture of mature adipose tissue and hematopoietic elements resembling bone marrow (Figure 8-43). Full trilineage maturation is present with the hematopoietic component, including myeloid, ery-

throid and megakaryocytic lines (Figure 8-44). Osseous metaplasia, hemorrhage, and fibrosis may be seen.

ANCILLARY STUDIES

The smears are composed of mature fat, and mature and immature hematopoietic elements, including erythroid, myeloid, and megakaryocytic. Occasionally, on non-radiographically guided samples, it is important to make sure that bone marrow has not inadvertently been sampled.

DIFFERENTIAL DIAGNOSIS

Myelolipoma is a distinctive lesion, unlikely to be confused with other tumors. The main difficulty is separating myelolipomatous foci within other adrenal lesions versus a discrete mass lesion. This distinction at times is arbitrary. In general, if there is no other adrenal pathology, myelolipoma is warranted.

PROGNOSIS AND THERAPY

Myelolipoma is a benign process and does not recur following complete surgical resection. Large lesions carry the risk of rupture and hemorrhage. Therefore, while clinically small lesions may be observed, larger lesions are usually excised.

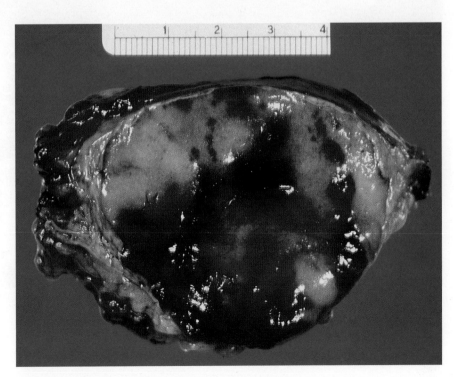

FIGURE 8-42

The adrenal gland shows a large well-demarcated mass composed of yellow adipose tissue and red bone marrow elements. A rim of residual adrenal cortical tissue is noted on the top and left of the specimen.

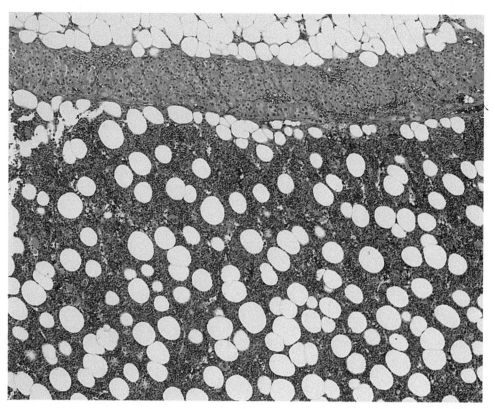

FIGURE 8-43
Low power shows the adipose component of this myelolipoma. Adrenal cortical tissue is present at the top of the illustration.

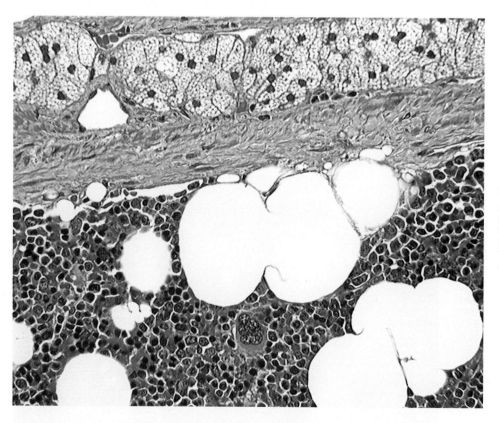

FIGURE 8-44
A mixture of mature adipose tissue and bone marrow elements including erythroid, myeloid and megakaryocytes are present in the tumor. There is compression of the adjacent adrenal cortex.

COMPOSITE TUMOR

Composite tumors of the adrenal gland are rare neoplasms, usually considered as medullary lesions, although rare reports of mixed medullary and cortical tumors are documented (Figures 8-45 and 8-46). Tumors typically combine features of pheochromocytoma with neuroblastoma, ganglioneuroblastoma or ganglioneuroma. Ganglioneuroma is the most frequently encountered component (80%) followed by ganglioneuroblastoma (20%).

CLINICAL FEATURES

Composite tumors are uncommon, comprising <3% of all adrenal gland neoplasms. They arise in adults (mean, 50 years) without a gender predilection. Occasionally cases may be associated with von Recklinghausen disease and MEN2A. Symptoms are uncommon, but may relate to mass effect or be associated with catecholamine hypersecretion similar to pheochromocytoma. Other hormones may be produced. These tumors are not uniformly benign and may go on to aggressive biologic behavior with metastases.

**COMPOSITE TUMOR
DISEASE FACT SHEET**

Definition
▸ Mixed adrenal tumor composed of pheochromocytoma and ganglioneuroma, ganglioneuroblastoma or neuroblastoma

Incidence and Location
▸ <3% of adrenal gland neoplasms
▸ >90% occur in the adrenal gland

Morbidity and Mortality
▸ Depends on tumor components present

Gender, Race and Age Distribution
▸ Equal gender distribution
▸ Mean, 50 years

Clinical Features
▸ Most are asymptomatic
▸ If symptomatic, usually a mass effect
▸ Rarely may have catecholamine hypersecretion
▸ Occasionally associated with familial syndromes

Prognosis and Therapy
▸ Prognosis is considered good following complete surgical resection, although biologic aggressiveness may occasionally develop
▸ Metastasis may develop via hematogenous or lymphatic routes
▸ Continued follow-up is required
▸ Surgical excision is treatment of choice

PATHOLOGIC FEATURES

GROSS FINDINGS

Tumors are usually well circumscribed, measuring up to 15 cm. The cut surface varies depending on the proportion of various tumor elements, ranging from gray-white to tan to purple with areas of hemorrhage. Areas which contain neuroblastomatous elements are soft and may be necrotic. Typically, the composite nature of the tumor is not discovered until histologic examination is performed.

MICROSCOPIC FINDINGS

Histologically, composite tumors have a mixture of growth patterns. There is an identifiable pheochromocytoma component with an organoid/trabecular growth pattern and characteristic cells with basophilic to eosinophilic granular cytoplasm (Figure 8-47). The pheochromocytoma component is usually the predominant component. The additional component shows areas of ganglioneuroma, ganglioneuroblastoma or neuroblastoma. The two components are intimately admixed distinguishing it from a collision tumor of two separate

---

**COMPOSITE TUMOR
PATHOLOGIC FEATURES**

Gross Findings
▸ Well circumscribed, up to 15 cm
▸ Cut surface varies depending on the proportion of various tumor elements; gray white to tan to purple, with areas of hemorrhage
▸ Areas of neuroblastomatous elements are soft and may be necrotic

Microscopic Findings
▸ Mixture of growth patterns, characteristic histology for each component
▸ Pheochromocytoma is almost always present and the predominant component
▸ Ganglioneuroma, ganglioneuroblastoma, neuroblastoma components juxtaposed with pheochromocytoma
▸ Ganglion cells have abundant pink granular cytoplasm with distinct borders and eccentrically placed round nuclei
▸ Primitive small cell component is part of neuroblastomatous cells (must be separated from lymphocytes)
▸ If metastases develop, ganglioneuroblastomatous foci are more frequently identified

Immunohistochemical Results
▸ Pheochromocytoma component has strong and diffuse reactivity with chromogranin and synaptophysin, while S-100 protein highlight sustentacular cells
▸ Ganglioneuroma is highlighted with S-100 protein; NFP highlights axon-like processes

Pathologic Differential Diagnosis
▸ Pheochromocytoma, ganglioneuroma, ganglioneuroblastoma, neuroblastoma

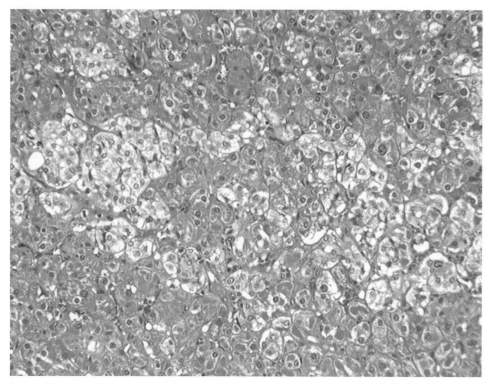

FIGURE 8-45
A mixed medullary and cortical neoplasm in which there is blending of cortical and medullary cells.

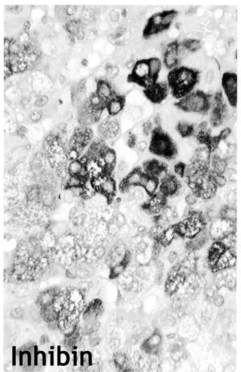

Inhibin

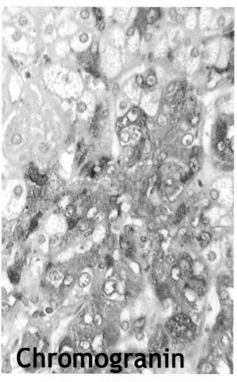

Chromogranin

FIGURE 8-46
The the overall interposition of the cellular components with inhibin (cortex) and chromogranin (medullary) positive cells in this mixed medullary and cortical neoplasm.

origins. Neuronal or ganglionic cell features are present often in a loose fibrillar matrix resembling neuropil (Figure 8-48). Ganglion cells have abundant pink granular cytoplasm with distinct borders and eccentrically placed round nuclei (Figure 8-49); Nissl substance may be seen. In the setting of a ganglioneuroblastoma or neuroblastoma component, a more primitive small cell component is seen. The transition between the two components may be abrupt or there may be blending.

ANCILLARY STUDIES

Immunohistochemical reactions of the individual tumor components are similar to their pure tumor counterparts. The pheochromocytoma component stains strongly and diffusely with chromogranin and the sustentacular cell component is highlighted with S-100 protein (Figure 8-50). Specifically for ganglioneuroma,

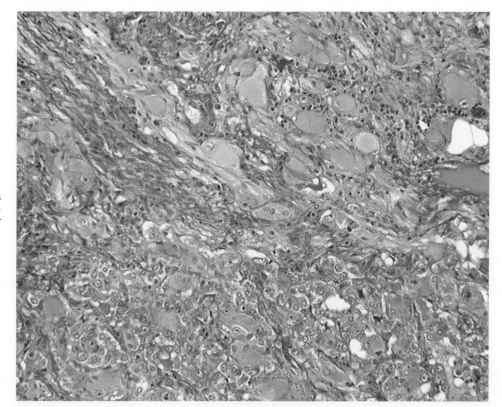

FIGURE 8-47

A pheochromocytoma component is noted in the lower left, while a ganglioneuroma is noted in the upper right.

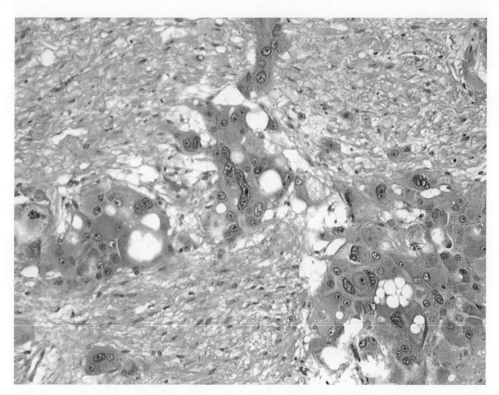

FIGURE 8-48

The loose fibrillar matrix of the ganglioneuroma component is seen in sharp contrast to the nests of pheochromocytes.

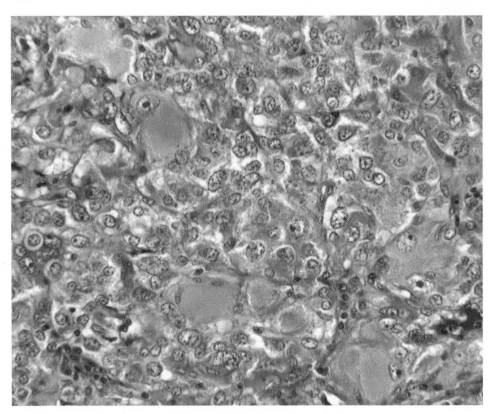

FIGURE 8-49
A number of ganglion cells are noted within a background of pheochromocytoma.

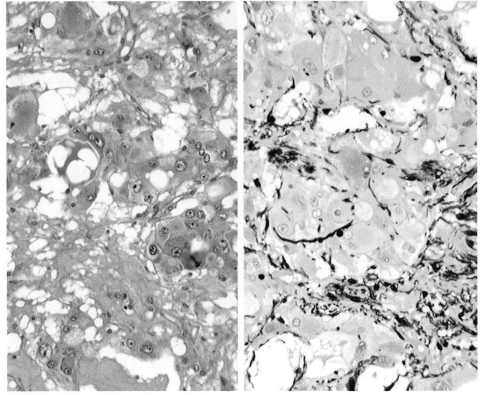

FIGURE 8-50
Left: A ganglioneuroma and pheochromocytoma intersect with one another. Right: An S-100 protein highlights both the ganglioneuroma component and the sustentacular cells of the pheochromocytoma.

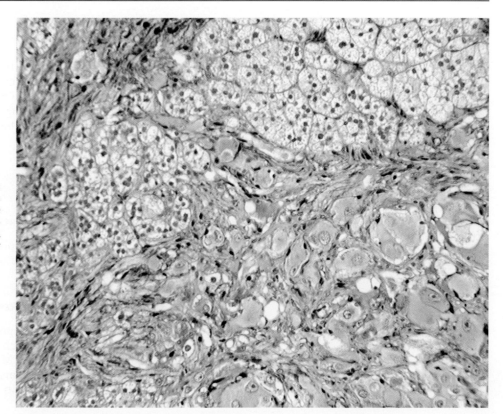

FIGURE 8-51

An S-100 protein immunoreaction accentuates the ganglioneuroma component as well as showing the zellballen architecture of the pheochromocytoma. Unstained adrenal cortical cells are noted in the upper right.

S-100 protein is easily identified in the Schwannian areas (Figure 8-51). Neurofilament protein aids in identifying axon-like processes.

DIFFERENTIAL DIAGNOSIS

The differential usually lies with confirming two separate neoplasms rather than a single lesion. Pattern of growth, cellular components, and immunohistochemistry usually allow separation.

PROGNOSIS AND THERAPY

Histological appearance does not necessarily correlate with biologic outcome, as occasional malignant behavior is noted. Malignant composite pheochromocytomas metastasize via hematogenous or lymphatic routes and spread has been reported to liver, lung, bone and lymph nodes. Seeding of the omentum and diaphragm may also occur. The metastatic deposits usually have the characteristics of ganglioneuroblastoma, while only rarely are the deposits of pheochromocytoma. Complete surgical excision is the goal.

ADENOMATOID TUMOR

CLINICAL FEATURES

Adenomatoid tumor is a rare benign tumor of mesothelial origin arising in the adrenal gland. Patients are typically asymptomatic and the tumors are discovered incidentally as part of a workup for other reasons. Patients rarely report painless hematuria. Middle aged (mean, 42 years) men are affected much more commonly than women (10:1). Radiographic findings are non-specific with a solid enhancing mass with cystic components.

PATHOLOGIC FEATURES

GROSS FINDINGS

The tumors are solitary and well circumscribed masses, lacking a distinct capsule. The tumors range from 0.5–11 cm (mean, 4 cm). The cut surface is firm, smooth and white, typically without hemorrhage. Cystic change may be present.

ADENOMATOID TUMOR
DISEASE FACT SHEET

Definition
▸ Benign neoplasm of mesothelial origin

Incidence and Location
▸ Rare
▸ More common in the genital tract than adrenal gland

Gender, Race and Age Distribution
▸ Male >>> Female (10:1)
▸ Mean, 42 years

Clinical Features
▸ Usually asymptomatic, discovered incidentally on radiographic, surgical or autopsy examination
▸ Rarely may have painless hematuria

Prognosis and Therapy
▸ Benign and will not recur if completely excised
▸ Small asymptomatic tumors can be radiographically followed
▸ Surgery

MICROSCOPIC FINDINGS

Histologically, the tumors are well circumscribed, exhibiting anastomosing, variably sized tubules or gland-like spaces lined by epithelioid cells. Extension into adrenal gland and periadrenal adipose tissue is frequently noted (Figure 8-52). The cells may be arranged as papillary, solid or cystic structures. The nests and cords of epithelioid cells are often flattened, containing round, uniform nuclei, with intracytoplasmic vacuoles reminiscent of signet ring cells, although lacking mucin. The epithelioid cells may be plump with a characteristic single, small 'dot-like' nucleolus. Often there is a background stromal component composed of fibroblastic cells and collagen. A lymphoid component, sometimes arranged in germinal centers, can be seen.

ANCILLARY STUDIES

ULTRASTRUCTURAL FEATURES

The long, 'bushy' cytoplasmic microvilli characteristic of mesothelial cells are seen on electron microscopic examination.

IMMUNOHISTOCHEMICAL RESULTS

The immunostaining profile is fairly characteristic and includes positive reactions with cytokeratin (AE1/AE3, CAM 5.2, CK7), EMA, calretinin and vimentin (Figure 8-53). The cells are negative for CD31, CD34, CK20, CEA, chromogranin and inhibin.

DIFFERENTIAL DIAGNOSIS

Adenomatoid nodules have fairly distinctive histological appearance, but metastatic adenocarcinoma (signet-

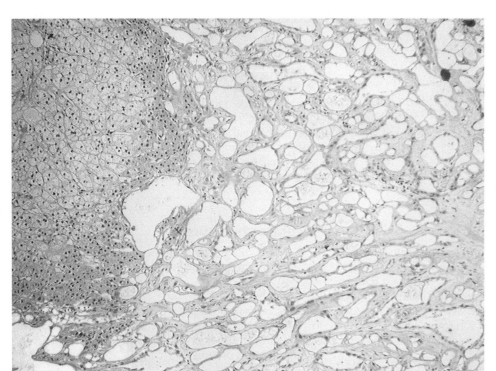

FIGURE 8-52

Mesothelial inclusions within the adrenal gland create a glandular or pseudo-glandular growth. Adrenal cortex is noted on the left.

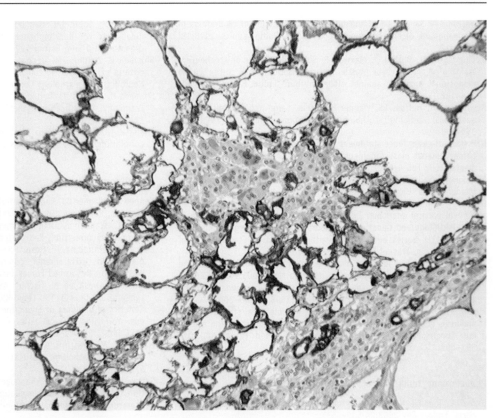

FIGURE 8-53
The mesothelial proliferation of this adenomatoid tumor is highlighted with keratin, while the adrenal tissue is not-reactive. Calretinin gives a similar reaction.

ADENOMATOID TUMOR PATHOLOGIC FEATURES

Gross Findings

▸ Well circumscribed, lacking a capsule
▸ Mean, 4 cm (range, 0.5–11 cm)
▸ Firm, smooth, white, usually without hemorrhage
▸ Cystic change may be seen

Microscopic Findings

▸ Circumscribed, but blends with adrenal cortical tissue
▸ Anastomosing, variably sized tubules or gland-like (sieve-like) spaces
▸ Epithelioid cells arranged in papillary, solid or cystic structures
▸ Foci of dystrophic calcifications, fibroblastic cells and lymphoid elements may be seen

Immunohistochemical Results

▸ Positive reactivity for keratin (AE1/AE3, CAM 5.2, CK7), calretinin, EMA, vimentin
▸ Negative for CD31, CD34, CK20, CEA, chromogranin, inhibin

Pathologic Differential Diagnosis

▸ Metastatic adenocarcinoma (signet ring type) angiosarcoma, mesothelioma, adrenal cysts, cystic adrenal cortical neoplasms

---

ring type specifically), angiosarcoma, mesothelioma, adrenal cysts, and cystic adrenal cortical adenoma are included in the differential diagnosis depending on the pattern of growth. Morphologic, immunohistochemical and ultrastructural features will separate these lesions. Interestingly, true 'epithelial' cysts of the adrenal gland are thought to arise from mesothelial inclusions, similar to adenomatoid tumor.

PROGNOSIS AND THERAPY

Adenomatoid tumors are benign lesions and do not recur if completely excised. Occasionally, small, asymptomatic tumors can be radiographically observed.

SUGGESTED READING

Adrenal Cortical Adenoma

Brunaud L, Duh QY. Aldosteronoma. Curr Treat Options Oncol 2002;3:327–333.
Busam KJ, Iversen K, Coplan KA, et al. Immunoreactivity for A103, an antibody to melan-A (Mart-1), in adrenocortical and other steroid tumors. Am J Surg Pathol 1998;22:57–63.
Cordera F, Grant C, van Heerden J, et al. Androgen-secreting adrenal tumors. Surgery 2003;134:874–880.
Ganguly A. Primary aldosteronism. N Engl J Med 1998;339:1828–1834.
Heinz-Peer G, Honigschnabl S, Schneider B, et al. Characterization of adrenal masses using MR imaging with histopathologic correlation. AJR Am J Roentgenol 1999;173:15–22.

Kawashima A, Sandler CM, Fishman EK, et al. Spectrum of CT findings in nonmalignant disease of the adrenal gland. Radiographics 1998;18: 393–412.

McCluggage WG, Burton J, Maxwell P, Sloan JM. Immunohistochemical staining of normal, hyperplastic, and neoplastic adrenal cortex with a monoclonal antibody against alpha inhibin. J Clin Pathol 1998;51: 114–116.

Newhouse JH, Heffess CS, Wagner BJ, et al. Large degenerated adrenal adenomas: radiologic-pathologic correlation. Radiology 1999;210: 385–391.

NIH state-of-the-science statement on management of the clinically inapparent adrenal mass ('incidentaloma'). NIH Consens State Sci Statements. 2002 Feb 4–6;19:1–25.

Nishikawa T, Saito J, Omura M. Mini review: surgical indications for adrenal incidentaloma. Biomed Pharmacother 2002;56(Suppl 1):145s–148s.

Sasano H, Young WF Jr, Chrousos GP, Koch CA, Giordano TJ, Kawashima A. Adrenal cortical adenoma. In: DeLellis RA, Lloyd RV, Heitz PU, Eng C, eds. Pathology and Genetics of Tumours of Endocrine Organs. Kleihues P, Sobin LH, series eds. World Health Organization Classification of Tumours. Lyon, France: IARC Press, 2004:143–146.

Veglio F, Morello F, Rabbia F, et al. Recent advances in diagnosis and treatment of primary aldosteronism. Minerva Med. 2003;94:259–265.

Xiao XR, Ye LY, Shi LX, et al. Diagnosis and treatment of adrenal tumours: a review of 35 years' experience. Br J Urol. 1998;82:199–205.

Zhang PJ, Genega EM, Tomaszewski JE, et al. The role of calretinin, inhibin, melan-A, BCL-2, and C-kit in differentiating adrenal cortical and medullary tumors: an immunohistochemical study. Mod Pathol 2003;16: 591–597.

Pheochromocytoma

Bravo EL, Tagle R. Pheochromocytoma: state-of-the-art and future prospects. Endocr Rev 2003;24:539–553.

Bryant J, Farmer J, Kessler LJ, et al. Pheochromocytoma: the expanding genetic differential diagnosis. J Natl Cancer Inst 2003;95:1196–1204.

Ilias I, Pacak K. Current approaches and recommended algorithm for the diagnostic localization of pheochromocytoma. Clin Endocrinol Metab 2004;89:479–491.

Kaltsas GA, Papadogias D, Grossman AB. The clinical presentation (symptoms and signs) of sporadic and familial chromaffin cell tumours (phaeochromocytomas and paragangliomas). Front Horm Res 2004; 31:61–75.

McNicol AM, Young WF Jr, Kawashima A, Kominoth P, Tischler AS. Benign phaeochromocytoma. In: DeLellis RA, Lloyd RV, Heitz PU, Eng C, eds. Pathology and Genetics of Tumours of Endocrine Organs. Kleihues P, Sobin LH, series eds. World Health Organization Classification of Tumours. Lyon, France: IARC Press, 2004:151–155.

Manger WM, Eisenhofer G. Pheochromocytoma: diagnosis and management update. Curr Hypertens Rep 2004;6:477–484.

Neumann HP, Bausch B, McWhinney SR, et al. Germ-line mutations in nonsyndromic pheochromocytoma. N Engl J Med 2002;346:1459–1466.

Pacak K, Eisenhofer G, Ilias I. Diagnostic imaging of pheochromocytoma. Front Horm Res 2004;31:107–120.

Pederson LC, Lee JE. Pheochromocytoma. Curr Treat Options Oncol 2003; 4:329–337.

Ganglioneuroma

de Chadarevian JP, MaePascasio J, Halligan GE, et al. Malignant peripheral nerve sheath tumor arising from an adrenal ganglioneuroma in a 6-year-old boy. Pediatr Dev Pathol 2004;7:277–284.

Geoerger B, Hero B, Harms D, et al. Metabolic activity and clinical features of primary ganglioneuromas. Cancer 2001;91:1905–1913.

Lonergan GJ, Schwab CM, Suarez ES, Carlson CL. Neuroblastoma, ganglioneuroblastoma, and ganglioneuroma: radiologic-pathologic correlation. Radiographics 2002;22:911–934.

Shekitka KM, Sobin LH. Ganglioneuromas of the gastrointestinal tract. Relation to Von Recklinghausen disease and other multiple tumor syndromes. Am J Surg Pathol 1994;18:250–257.

Shimada H, Ambros IM, Dehner LP, et al. Terminology and morphologic criteria of neuroblastic tumors: recommendations by the International Neuroblastoma Pathology Committee. Cancer 1999;86:349–363.

Shimada H, Ambros IM, Dehner LP, et al. The International Neuroblastoma Pathology Classification (the Shimada system). Cancer 1999;86: 364–372.

Zhang Y, Nishimura H, Kato S, et al. MRI of ganglioneuroma: histologic correlation study. J Comput Assist Tomogr 2001;25:617–623.

Myelolipoma

Kenney PJ, Wagner BJ, Rao P, Heffess CS. Myelolipoma: CT and pathologic features. Radiology 1998;208:87–95.

Krebs TL, Wagner BJ. MR imaging of the adrenal gland: radiologic-pathologic correlation. Radiographics 1998;18:1425–1440.

Lack EE. Myelolipoma. In: Rosai J and Sobin LH, eds. Tumors of the adrenal gland and extra-adrenal paraganglia. Fascicle 19, third series. Washington DC: Armed Forces Institute of Pathology, 1997;174–180.

Lloyd RV, Kawashima A, Tischler AS. Adrenal soft tissue and germ cell tumours. In: DeLellis RA, Lloyd RV, Heitz PU, Eng C, eds. Pathology and Genetics of Tumours of Endocrine Organs. Kleihues P, Sobin LH, series eds. World Health Organization Classification of Tumours. Lyon, France: IARC Press, 2004:169–171.

Isayes KM, Mukundan G, Narra VR et al. Adrenal masses: MR imaging features with pathologic correlation. Radiographics 2004;24(Suppl 1): S73–86.

Settakorn J, Sirivanichai C, Rangdaeng S, Chaiwun B. Fine-needle aspiration cytology of adrenal myelolipoma: case report and review of the literature. Diagn Cytopathol 1999;21:409–412.

Composite Tumor

Franquemont DW, Mills SE, Lack EE. Immunohistochemical detection of neuroblastomatous foci in composite adrenal pheochromocytoma-neuroblastoma. Am J Clin Pathol 1994;102:163–170.

Lam KY, Lo CY. Composite Pheochromocytoma-Ganglioneuroma of the Adrenal Gland: An Uncommon Entity with Distinctive Clinicopathologic Features. Endocr Pathol 1999;10:343–352.

Satake H, Inoue K, Kamada M, et al. Malignant composite pheochromocytoma of the adrenal gland in a patient with von Recklinghausen's disease. J Urol 2001;165:1199–1200.

Tischler AS. Divergent differentiation in neuroendocrine tumors of the adrenal gland. Semin Diagn Pathol 2000;17:120–126.

Tischler AS, Kimura N, Lloyd RV, Komminoth P. Composite phaeochromocytoma or paraganglioma. In: DeLellis RA, Lloyd RV, Heitz PU, Eng C, eds. Pathology and Genetics of Tumours of Endocrine Organs. Kleihues P, Sobin LH, series eds. World Health Organization Classification of Tumours. Lyon, France: IARC Press, 2004:156–158.

Wieneke JA, Thompson LDR, Heffess CS. Corticomedullary mixed tumor of the adrenal gland. Ann Diagn Pathol 2001;5:304–305.

Adenomatoid Tumor

Cheng L, Ulbright TM. Adenomatoid tumour. In: DeLellis RA, Lloyd RV, Heitz PU, Eng C, eds. Pathology and Genetics of Tumours of Endocrine Organs. Kleihues P, Sobin LH, series eds. World Health Organization Classification of Tumours. Lyon, France: IARC Press, 2004:167.

Chung-Park M, Yang JT, McHenry CR, Khiyami A. Adenomatoid tumor of the adrenal gland with micronodular adrenal cortical hyperplasia. Hum Pathol. 2003;34:818–821.

Isotalo PA, Keeney GL, Sebo TJ, et al. Adenomatoid tumor of the adrenal gland: a clinicopathologic study of five cases and review of the literature. Am J Surg Pathol 2003;27:969–977.

9 Malignant Neoplasms of the Adrenal Gland

Ronald R de Krijger • *Paul Komminoth*

ADRENAL CORTICAL CARCINOMA

CLINICAL FEATURES

Adrenocortical carcinomas (ACC) account for about 0.2% of all cancers and about 3% of endocrine neo-

---

ADRENAL CORTICAL CARCINOMA
DISEASE FACT SHEET

Definition
▸ Malignant neoplasm arising from adrenal cortical cells

Incidence and Location
▸ About 0.2 % of all cancers
▸ 3 % of endocrine neoplasms
▸ About 1/1 000 000 population

Morbidity and Mortality
▸ Hormone production may cause significant morbidity
▸ Overall, about 70 % 5-year survival

Gender, Race and Age Distribution
▸ Equal gender distribution (although girls slightly more than boys in pediatric patients)
▸ Bimodal age peak: first and seventh decades

Clinical Features
▸ Symptoms related to hormone excess (glucocorticoid > androgen > mineralocorticoids >> estrogen)
▸ Abdominal mass
▸ Flank pain
▸ Incidental discovery is not uncommon

Radiographic Findings
▸ Large supra-renal masses with inhomogeneous enhancement
▸ Calcifications may be seen in 30 % of tumors
▸ High signal intensity on T2 weighted MR images
▸ PET scan may be useful

Prognosis and Therapy
▸ Age and stage dependent
▸ 5-year survival about 70 %
▸ Stage I/II have better prognosis than III/IV
▸ Radical surgery with complete resection of the tumor (including metastases and local recurrence)
▸ Chemotherapy has a limited role due to high drug resistance

---

plasms. The incidence of ACC is about 1 per 1 000 000 without a gender predilection. ACC occur in all age groups with its main incidence peak around 70 years of age and a second smaller peak in the first decade of life. Childhood ACC occur predominantly in females and almost always cause clinical signs and symptoms of endocrine abnormality (virilization or a mixed endocrine syndrome). If bilateral tumors are present, metastases from the opposite adrenal must be considered, a finding in about 10% of cases. Patients present with symptoms related to hormone overproduction by the tumor (glucocorticoids and/or androgen secretion; less frequently mineralocorticoids and rarely estrogen), an abdominal mass, flank pain (due to invasion of adjacent organs, tumor rupture or necrosis) or especially in the case of non-functioning tumors, may become symptomatic due to distant metastases to the lungs, liver, retroperitoneal lymph nodes or bone. An increasing number of tumors are discovered incidentally during radiographic studies for other reasons.

RADIOLOGIC FEATURES

On CT scan ACC present as suprarenal masses with inhomogeneous enhancement due to hemorrhage and necrosis and additional calcifications may be found in up to 30% of tumors. On MRI ACC usually appear heterogeneous on T1 weighted images and have a higher signal intensity than fat on T2 weighted images (Figure 9-1). Iodo-cholesterol scintigraphy and PET-scanning using (11)C-metomidate and (18)F-FDG may be useful to identify adrenocortical tumors and to localize distant metastases.

PATHOLOGIC FEATURES

GROSS FINDINGS

The left adrenal appears to be slightly more frequently affected than the right gland and bilateral ACC are extremely rare. ACC are usually bulky, large tumors with a weight >100 g in adults, although tumors as small as 12 g have metastasized. The average size is 12 cm with a range of 3–40 cm. Size and weight alone cannot be used to predict behavior of adrenal cortical neoplasms.

ADRENAL CORTICAL CARCINOMA
PATHOLOGIC FEATURES

Gross Findings

▶ Left slightly more common than right
▶ Usually large, bulky tumors
▶ Usually >100 g and mean diameter is 12 cm
▶ Lobulated, red-brown to yellow-orange (depending on lipid content)
▶ Cut surface is fleshy with a rubbery to firm consistency
▶ Hemorrhage, necrosis, fibrosis, calcification or cystic change may be noted
▶ Invasion into adjacent structures can be seen

Microscopic Findings

▶ Invasive growth (cortex, capsule, vessels, fat)
▶ Fibrous connective tissue bands
▶ Comedo- or confluent necrosis
▶ Cellular tumors with multiple patterns: trabecular, alveolar, solid, pseudoglandular and fascicular growth
▶ Increased nuclear to cytoplasmic ratio with uniform to profoundly pleomorphic, multinucleated neoplastic cells
▶ Cytoplasm is vacuolated or eosinophilic
▶ Mitotic activity is variable, but usually increased
▶ Atypical mitoses are seen

Immunohistochemical Results

▶ Positive for vimentin, inhibin, melan A, calretinin, SF-1 and D11
▶ Focal, weak reactions with cytokeratins, neurofilament, S-100 protein and IGF-II
▶ Negative with chromogranin, CEA, CD10, CD15, HMFG-2, HepPar-1, AFP

Fine Needle Aspiration

▶ Difficult to separate from benign adrenal cortical lesions
▶ Profound nuclear pleomorphism, nuclear chromatin irregularities, prominent nucleoli and mitotic figures may help

Pathologic Differential Diagnosis

▶ Adrenocortical adenoma, hepatocellular carcinoma, renal cell carcinoma, pheochromocytoma, and metastatic carcinomas

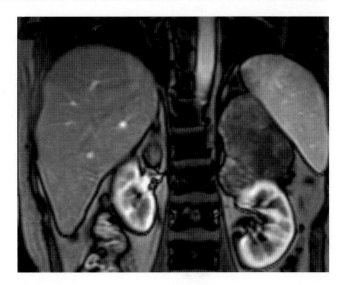

FIGURE 9-1

A MRI shows a heterogeneous mass displacing the left kidney, and focally invading into the kidney's superior pole.

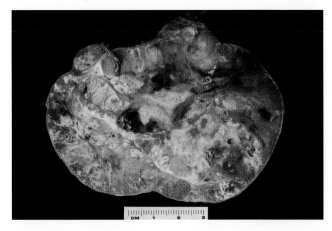

FIGURE 9-2

A variegated cut surface of a large adrenal cortical carcinoma. Lipid-rich cells give the yellow appearance, while necrosis gives areas of brown-red appearance.

ACC may appear encapsulated, are frequently lobular in appearance and red-brown to yellow-orange depending on lipid content (Figure 9-2). The cut surface is fleshy with a rubbery to firm consistency, frequently exhibiting hemorrhage, necrosis, cystic change, fibrosis or calcification, especially in larger tumors. Invasion into adjacent structures and large blood vessels can be seen (Figure 9-3). However, malignancy is not always macroscopically obvious.

MICROSCOPIC FINDINGS

Microscopically, ACC usually exhibit invasive growth, with capsular penetration and/or vascular invasion (Figures 9-4 to 9-6), while invasion into the adrenal cortex is more difficult to interpret. The tumors usually have a fibrous connective tissue capsule, often forming bands of fibrosis which separate the tumor into nodules (Figures 9-7 and 9-8). Comedo- or confluent necrosis is not identified in benign tumors (Figure 9-9). ACC are cellular tumors, composed of cells with an increased nuclear to cytoplasmic ratio (Figure 9-10), arranged in a variety of different growth patterns, frequently admixed in the same tumor. A trabecular growth with broad cords of cells is frequently seen (Figure 9-11), while alveolar, solid, pseudoglandular, and fascicular patterns can also be identified (Figure 9-12).

The cytoplasm of tumor cells may be vacuolated or eosinophilic dependent on their lipid content (Figure 9-13). The size and shape of nuclei may vary considerably with small and uniform nuclei to profoundly pleomorphic, multinucleated and giant nuclei with coarse

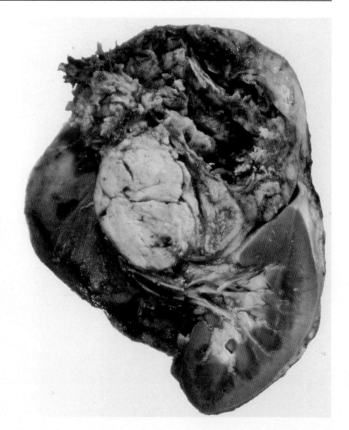

FIGURE 9-3

This adrenal cortical carcinoma has gross invasion of the surrounding organs with necrosis and cystic change.

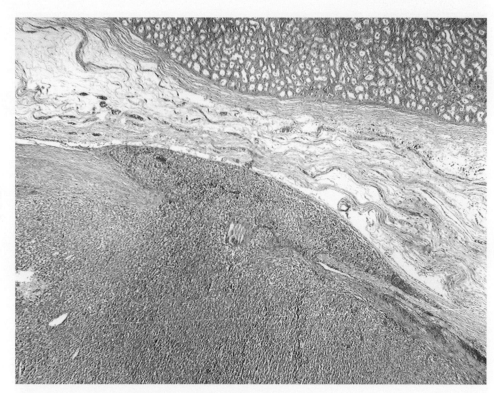

FIGURE 9-4

Extension of the tumor beyond the adrenal gland capsule and into the surrounding fat. Uninvolved kidney is present in the upper field.

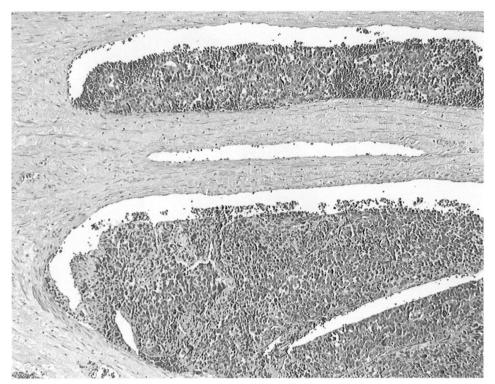

FIGURE 9-5
Large vessel invasion by the neoplastic cells identified beyond the
capsule of the adrenal gland.

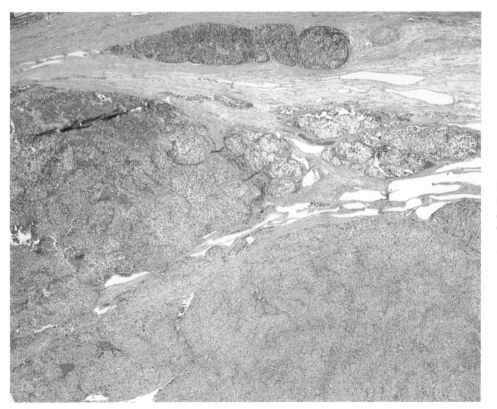

FIGURE 9-6
Nodular growth with invasion of the
capsule is seen in this adrenal cortical carcinoma.

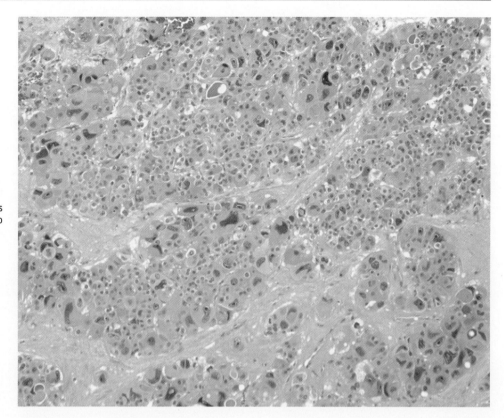

FIGURE 9-7

Fibrous bands separate this highly pleomorphic neoplasm into nodules.

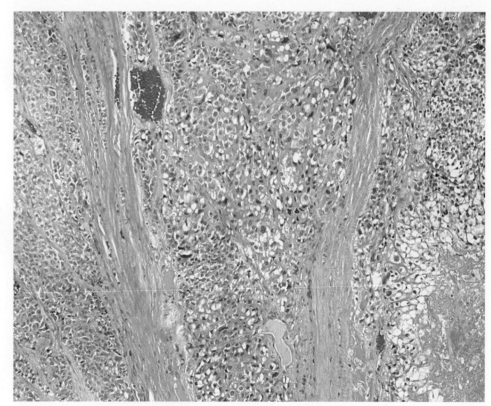

FIGURE 9-8

Heavy fibrous connective tissue bands are noted in this adrenal cortical carcinoma which is associated with necrosis (lower right corner).

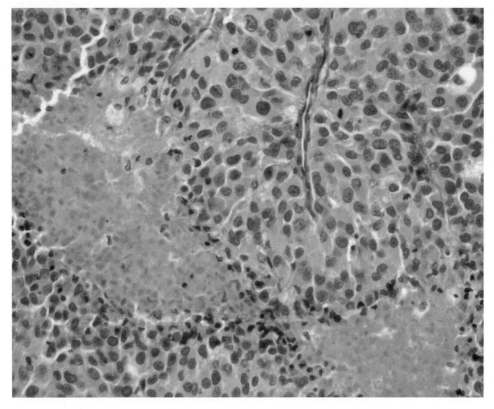

FIGURE 9-9

Confluent and comedo-necrosis in an adrenocortical carcinoma. Two mitotic figures are present.

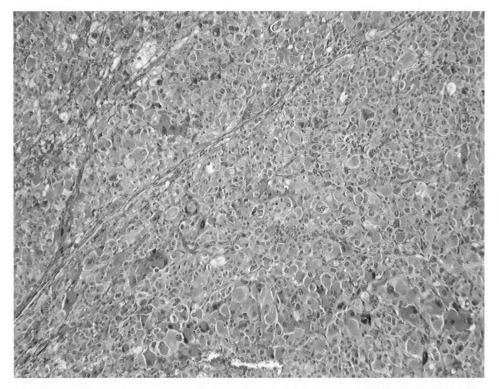

FIGURE 9-10

Highly cellular tumor with a vaguely trabecular pattern. Nuclear pleomorphism is noted even at this low power.

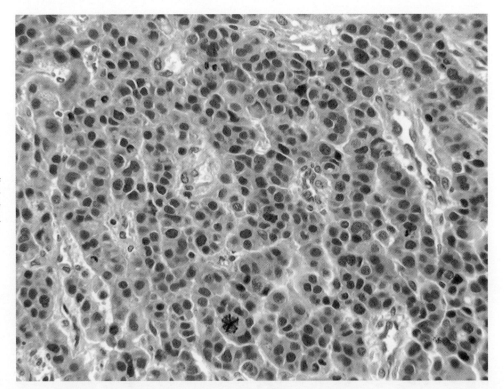

FIGURE 9-11

A trabecular to ribbon pattern of growth is quite characteristic for ACC. The cells have a high nuclear to cytoplasmic ratio and an atypical mitotic figure is present.

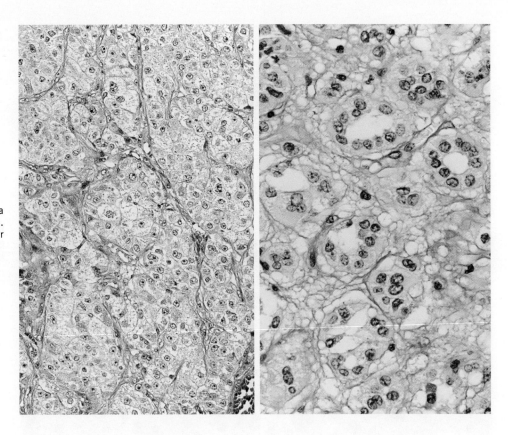

FIGURE 9-12

Right: Lipid rich tumor cells in a mixed alveolar-trabecular growth. Left: A focal pseudoglandular architecture.

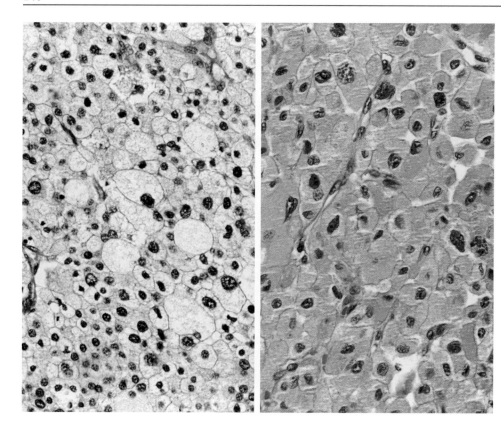

FIGURE 9-13
Left: Lipid rich cells in an ACC.
Right: Compact, eosinophilic cytoplasm in a different ACC.

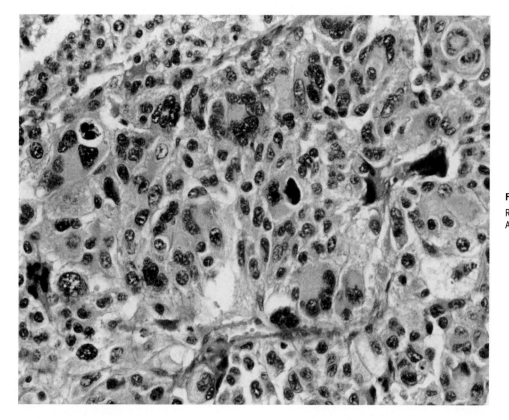

FIGURE 9-14
Remarkably pleomorphic cells in ACC.

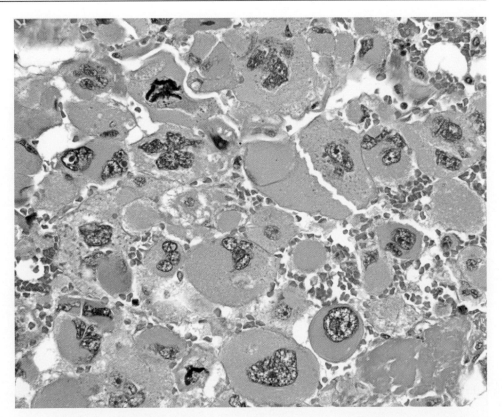

FIGURE 9-15

Compact eosinophilic cytoplasm surrounding profoundly pleomorphic nuclei. Atypical mitotic figures are noted.

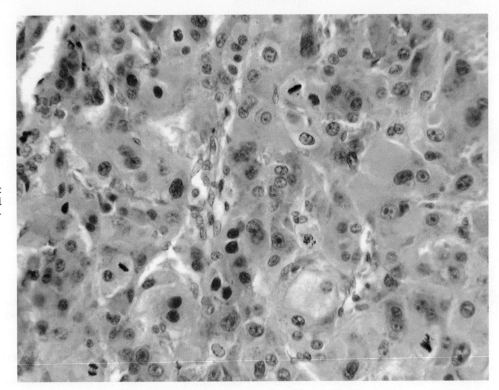

FIGURE 9-16

A remarkable number of mitotic figures are present in this adrenal cortical carcinoma, including atypical forms.

chromatin and prominent nucleoli (Figures 9-14 and 9-15). Eosinophilic globular inclusions and intranuclear cytopseudo inclusions may occasionally be seen. Rarely ACC are composed nearly exclusively of oncocytic cells. Mitotic activity in ACC is usually prominent when compared with adenomas and may include atypical forms (Figure 9-16), although the number of mitotic figures varies widely both within and between tumors. The most widely used scoring systems to diagnose ACC in adults are summarized in Table 9-1.

TABLE 9-1

Criteria for the Diagnosis of Adrenocortical Carcinomas

Feature	Qualifier	Hough	Van Slooten	Weiss	Aubert
Nuclear pleomorphism	High grade	0.39	2.1	1	
Nuclear hyperchromasia	Moderate/marked		2.6		
Abnormal nucleoli			4.1		
Mitotic activity	>5/50 HPF			1[1]	2[1]
	>10/100 HPF	0.60			
	>2/10 HPF		9.0		
Atypical mitotic figures	Present			1	1
Clear cells	<25 %			1[2]	2[2]
Architecture	Diffuse growth/sheets	0.92	1.6	1	
Necrosis	Present	0.69[3]		1[4]	1
Broad fibrous bands	Present	1.00			
Regressive changes	Extensive		5.7		
Venous invasion	Present			1[5]	
Sinusoidal invasion	Present	0.92[6]		1[7]	
Capsular invasion	Present	0.37	3.3[8]	1	1
Tumor mass	≥100 g	0.60			
Urinary 17-ketosteroids	≥10 mg/g creatinine/24 h	0.50			
Response to 50 μg ACTH	2× increase of 17-hydroxysteroids	0.42			
Endocrine syndrome	Cushing syndrome with virilism, virilism alone or no syndrome	0.42			
Weight loss	>10 pounds/3 months	2.00			
SUMMARY SCORE	Benign	0.17[9]	<8	1–2	1–2
	Indeterminate	1.00[10]			
	Malignant potential	2.91[11]	≥8	≥3	≥3

[1]Counting in areas with highest mitotic rate, 40× objective; [2]eosinophilic or compact tumor cell cytoplasm >75 % of tumor cells; [3]necrotic foci >2 HPF in diameter; [4]confluent necrosis; [5]smooth muscle in wall; [6]vascular invasion (sinusoidal or venous); [7]no smooth muscle in wall; [8]vascular and/or capsular invasion; [9]mean value = 0.17 ± 0.26; [10]mean value = 1.00 ± 0.58; [11]mean value = 2.91 ± 0.9. Hough et al. Am J Clin Pathol 1979;72:390–399; van Slooten et al. Cancer 1985;55:766–773; Weiss LM. Am J Surg Pathol 1984;8:163–169 and Weiss et al. 1989;13:202–206; Aubert et al. Am J Surg Pathol 2002;26:1612–1619.

ANCILLARY STUDIES

ULTRASTRUCTURAL FEATURES

Ultrastructural features vary widely among different neoplasms and within a tumor. Lipid-rich cells show intracytoplasmic lipid droplets while compact, eosinophilic cells show prominent smooth endoplasmic reticulum and abundant mitochondria. The majority of mitochondria are small and oval to round but may also be elongated and larger in size. Approximately 20 % of ACC may contain glycogen deposits (which may, when abundant, give rise to the erroneous diagnosis of renal cell carcinoma). About one-third of ACC lack convincing features of steroid cell differentiation, even rarely containing sparse dense-core granules.

IMMUNOHISTOCHEMICAL RESULTS

ACC are positive for vimentin, inhibin (Figure 9-17), melan A, (but not HMB45), and calretinin. Rarely, focal and weak reactions with cytokeratins, neurofilament or S-100 protein may be seen. Chromogranin, CEA, CD10, CD15, HepPar-1 and alpha-fetoprotein (AFP) are negative. p53 and MIB-1 (Ki-67) index (Figure 9-17) may help to discriminate malignant from benign adrenocortical neoplasms.

FINE NEEDLE ASPIRATION

Cytology usually fails to accurately separate benign from malignant adrenocortical lesions unless there is profound nuclear pleomorphism, nuclear chromatin irregularities and prominent nucleoli in cells arranged in vaguely acinar configurations (Figure 9-18). However, FNA may be helpful in diagnosing metastatic versus primary tumors, although renal cell carcinoma and hepatocellular carcinoma may be indistinguishable.

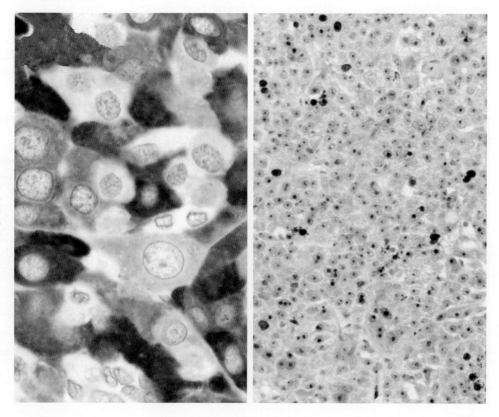

FIGURE 9-17

Left: ACC may react with inhibin, although the staining is often variable. Right: A high mitotic index in an adrenocortical carcinoma is highlighted with a MIB1 (Ki-67) immunoreaction.

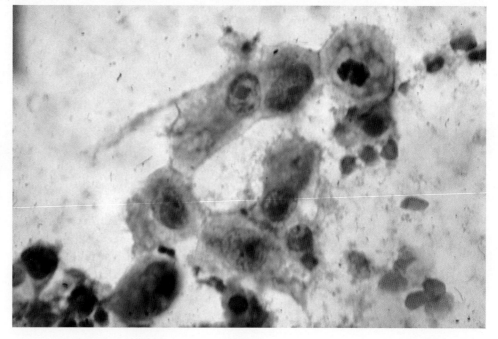

FIGURE 9-18

An atypical epithelial population with vague acinar patterns suggests an adrenal cortical carcinoma on this FNA, although it is not absolutely diagnostic (alcohol fixed, Papanicolau).

DIFFERENTIAL DIAGNOSIS

The major differential diagnostic considerations are between adrenal cortical adenoma and metastatic neoplasms. It may be very difficult to distinguish benign from malignant adrenocortical tumors especially when they are small and lack obvious signs of malignancy (Figure 9-19). Tumors in pediatric patients are particularly confounding, as they frequently exhibit a benign clinical course even when clearly adverse histological features are present. The most reliable predictive features for malignancy in pediatric tumors are: large tumor size (>11 cm) and weight (>400 g); older age at diagnosis (average 10 years); high mitotic count (average 31/50 HPF); vena cava invasion, and extensive tumor necrosis. Adequate sampling is mandatory in order to identify features that may be present only focally. The combined use of several scoring systems (Table 9.1) increases ones chances of yielding a definitive diagnosis. Core needle biopsies present a particular difficulty in separating hepatocellular carcinoma (HCC), renal cell carcinoma, metastatic carcinomas to the adrenal and pheochromocytoma from ACC. An extended, but pertinent immunohistochemistry panel (Table 9-2), will often resolve the differential.

TABLE 9-2
Differential Diagnosis of Adrenocortical Carcinoma: Immunohistochemistry

Tumor Type	CK	VIM	NF	S	EMA	CEA	CG	SYN	AFP	HEP	MA	CAL	INH
Cortical carcinoma	+/−	+	−/+	−/+	−	−	−	−/+	−	−	+	+	+
Pheochromocytoma	−	+/−	+	+	−	−	+	+	−	−	−	−	−
Renal cell carcinoma	+	+	−	−/+	+	−	−	−	−	−	−	−/+	−/+
Hepatocellular carcinoma	+	+/−	−	−/+	+/−	+	−	−	+	+	−	−	−/+
Metastatic adenocarcinoma	+	+/−	−	−/+	+	+	−	−	−	−	−	−/+	−
Liposarcoma	−	+	−	+	−	−	−	−	−	−	−/+	−	−

CK, cytokeratin; VIM, Vimentin; NF, neurofilament; S, S-100 protein; EMA, epithelial membrane antigen; CEA, carcinoembryonic antigen; CG, chromogranin A; SYN, synaptophysin; AFP, alpha-feto-protein; HEP, HepPar-1; MA, melan A; CAL, calretinin; INH, inhibin.

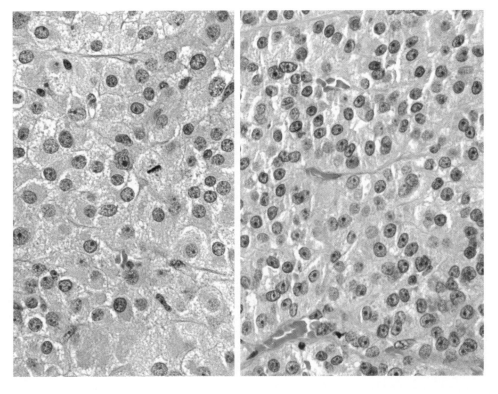

FIGURE 9-19

This tumor has increased mitotic figures and focal trabecular growth, but no other morphologic features of adrenal cortical carcinoma. This tumor would best be placed in the 'atypical adrenal cortical neoplasm' category.

PROGNOSIS AND THERAPY

Age and stage at diagnosis are the most important prognostic factors of ACC. Due to the detection of smaller lesions by advanced imaging techniques the 5-year survival is about 70%. Patients with stage I and II tumors have a better prognosis than stage III or IV patients, usually as a result of complete surgical resection. Radical surgery is the most effective treatment, including adjacent organs, solitary metastases and locoregional recurrence as clinically indicated. ACC are usually resistant to chemotherapy, possibly as a result of a high rate of multidrug-resistance gene *MDR-1* expression in ACC. If chemotherapy is used, the best results are achieved by the combination of etoposide, doxorubicin, and cisplatin associated with mitotane, achieving a response rate of 54%.

MALIGNANT PHEOCHROMOCYTOMA

CLINICAL FEATURES

Malignant pheochromocytomas (MPCC) are currently defined by the presence of metastases in locations where chromaffin tissue normally does not occur. This broad definition does not account for the potentially lethal behavior of tumors showing extensive local infiltration into adjacent organs or major blood vessels. About 10–15% of all pheochromocytomas are malignant by this definition. There is a nearly equal gender distribution for MPCC. The frequency of syndrome associated MPCC is usually lower than sporadic cases.

The clinical signs and symptoms of MPCC essentially do not differ from their benign counterparts and include catecholamine excess related symptoms (see Pheochromocytoma in Chapter 8, p. 210). These include sustained or intermittent hypertension associated with paroxysmal symptoms, headache, sweating, palpitation, tachycardia, and anxiety. Rarely, a mass effect attributable to the tumor may be present. Laboratory investigations will reveal remarkably elevated levels of serum and/or urine catecholamines, norepinephrine, epinephrine, metanephrine, dopamine, vanillylmandelic acid (VMA), or other catecholamine metabolites.

RADIOLOGIC FEATURES

MPCC are usually evaluated by CT, MRI and ^{131}I-metaiodobenzyl-guanidine (MIBG) scintigraphy. There are no radiologic features that can reliably distinguish benign from malignant, unless gross local invasion in neighboring organs is present (Figure 9-20) or if distant metastases are observed. MIBG may help identify a primary and metastases, but separation of multifocal disease versus metastasis is not always achieved.

MALIGNANT PHEOCHROMOCYTOMA DISEASE FACT SHEET

Definition
▸ A malignant tumor of chromaffin cells of the adrenal medulla

Incidence and Location
▸ Rare neoplasm, although about 10–15% of pheochromocytomas are malignant

Morbidity and Mortality
▸ Excess catecholamine secretion, with potential for strokes or myocardial infarction

Gender, Race and Age Distribution
▸ Nearly equal gender distribution
▸ All ages, although familial cases are usually younger

Clinical Features
▸ Sustained, labile, paroxysmal, episodic hypertension
▸ Headaches, diaphoresis, palpitations, tachycardia, anxiety
▸ Possible tumor mass
▸ Remarkably elevated levels of serum/urine catecholamines, norepinephrine, epinephrine, metanephrine, dopamine, vanillylmandelic acid

Radiographic Features
▸ Separation of benign and MPCC by invasion into the surrounding organs
▸ MIBG may identify multifocal or metastatic disease

Prognosis and Therapy
▸ 5-year survival 45–55%
▸ Long term follow-up advocated
▸ Surgery may cure, with ^{131}I-MIBG therapy, multidrug chemotherapy employed
▸ Newer treatments show promise

PATHOLOGIC FEATURES

GROSS FINDINGS

In general, malignant MPCC tend to be larger than their benign counterparts, although this criterion cannot be used in the individual case, as there is considerable overlap. Malignant MPCC may show local invasive growth into other organs, such as the liver, spleen, or kidney (Figure 9-21). The tumors also tend to be more nodular, lobulated or bosselated with a variegated cut surface.

MICROSCOPIC FINDINGS

Many studies have addressed the issue of the distinction between benign and malignant MPCC on histological criteria. In general, no single feature can be used to separate the two groups. However, an aggregation of histologic features has been identified in MPCC more

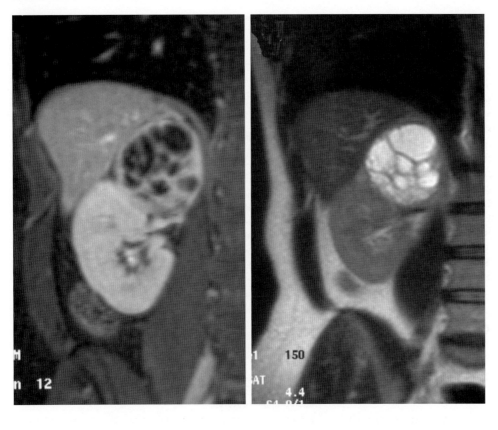

FIGURE 9-20

Right: A gadolinium MR image demonstrates a multilocular adrenal gland mass which invades into the kidney. Left: A T2 weighted MR images shows a bright signal intensity, suggesting the 'light-bulb' sign of a pheochromocytoma.

frequently than in benign pheochromocytoma. These criteria include:

- Capsular invasion (Figure 9-22);
- Vascular invasion (Figure 9-23);
- Extension into the periadrenal adipose tissue (Figure 9-24);
- Expanded, large, and confluent nests (Figures 9-25 and 9-26);
- Diffuse growth;
- Necrosis (Figure 9-27);
- Increased cellularity;
- Tumor cell spindling (Figure 9-28);
- Profound cellular and nuclear pleomorphism (Figure 9-29);
- Cellular monotony (usually with smaller cells having high nuclear to cytoplasmic ratio; Figure 9-30);
- Nuclear hyperchromasia;
- Macronucleoli;
- Increased mitotic figures (Figure 9-31);
- Any atypical mitotic figures (Figure 9-32); or
- Absence of hyaline globules.

A 'large nest' is defined as at least three times the size of the 'zellballen' in a normal paraganglion. For mitotic frequency, cut-offs of >3 per 10 or 20 HPFs have been used in different studies. Necrosis can be within the center of large nests, confluent, and/or diffuse. Needless to say, even using this cornucopia of criteria does not result in concordant results. More recently, a new

---

MALIGNANT PHEOCHROMOCYTOMA PATHOLOGIC FEATURES

Gross Findings

▶ Usually larger than benign tumors
▶ Locally invasive into adjacent organs
▶ More nodular, lobulated or bosselated

Microscopic Findings

▶ Invasive growth (capsular, vascular or periadrenal fat)
▶ Expanded, large, confluent nests and/or diffuse growth
▶ Necrosis
▶ Increased cellularity and cellular monotony
▶ Tumor spindling
▶ Profound pleomorphism, nuclear hyperchromasia, macronucleoli
▶ Increased mitotic figures and atypical forms
▶ Metastatic foci are histologically identical

Immunohistochemical Results

▶ Pheochromocytes stain with synaptophysin and chromogranin
▶ Reduced or absent S-100 protein positive sustentacular cells

Pathologic Differential Diagnosis

▶ Benign pheochromocytoma; adrenal cortical carcinoma

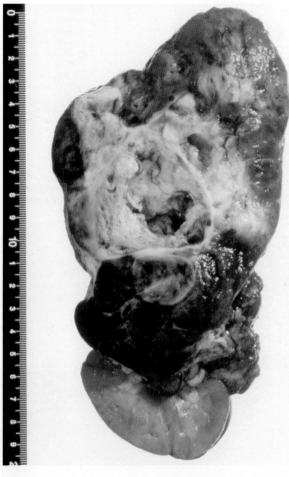

FIGURE 9-21

A MPCC with extensive local ingrowth into neighboring organs, including kidney (lower part) and liver (upper part).

scoring system called 'pheochromocytoma of the adrenal gland scaled score (PASS)' has been proposed (Table 9-3). A total score of ≥4 suggests malignant biologic behavior. The applicability and utility of this scoring system, however, has not yet been confirmed in the literature, nor is it universally accepted.

The histology of metastatic pheochromocytoma is similar to that of primary tumors (Figures 9-33 and 9-34).

ANCILLARY STUDIES

ULTRASTRUCTURAL FEATURES

Secretory granules (one type containing epinephrine and another with norepinephrine) will be identified in the neoplastic pheochromocytes, but there is no correlation between the ultrastructural findings and the biologic behavior.

IMMUNOHISTOCHEMICAL RESULTS

Chromogranin and synaptophysin will be present in the pheochromocytes of benign, malignant, and metastatic pheochromocytomas (Figure 9-34). While not absolutely diagnostic for MPCC, diminished or absent S-100 protein-reactive sustentacular cells correlates with large nests or diffuse growth (Figure 9-35), features related to malignancy. The lack of sustentacular component can be accentuated with a reticulin stain if S-100 protein is unavailable (Figure 9-36). MIB-1 labeling is valuable in identifying increased and/or atypical mitotic figures (see Figures 9-31 and 9-32), but an increased index is only 50% sensitive in detecting MPCC.

FIGURE 9-22

Capsular invasion through the adrenal gland capsule and into the adipose connective tissue suggests malignant pheochromocytoma.

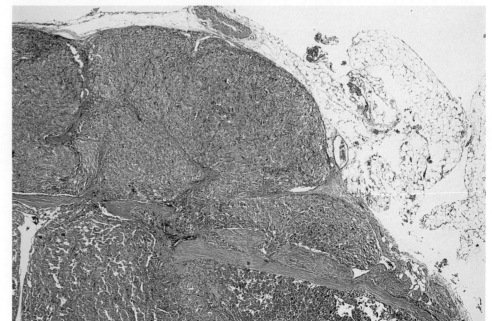

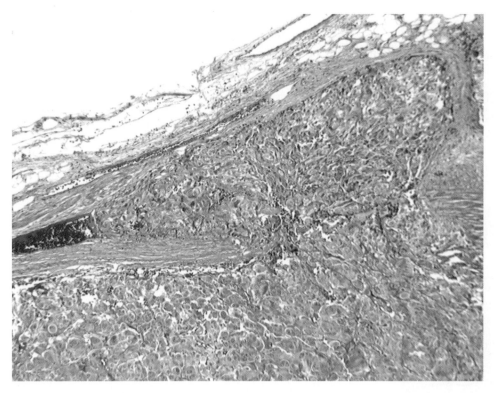

FIGURE 9-23
Vascular invasion, especially if extensive or involving large vessels suggests malignant pheochromo-cytoma.

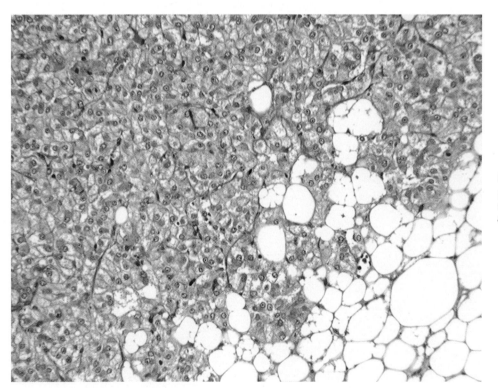

FIGURE 9-24
Extension of malignant pheochro-mocytes into the surrounding adrenal adipose connective tissue.

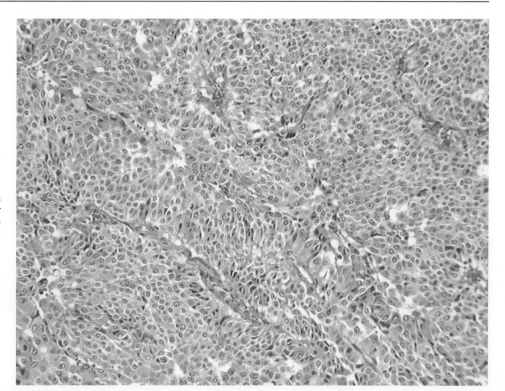

FIGURE 9-25

While nests are present, there is more of a diffuse and trabecular pattern with larger nests at the periphery of this malignant pheochromocytoma.

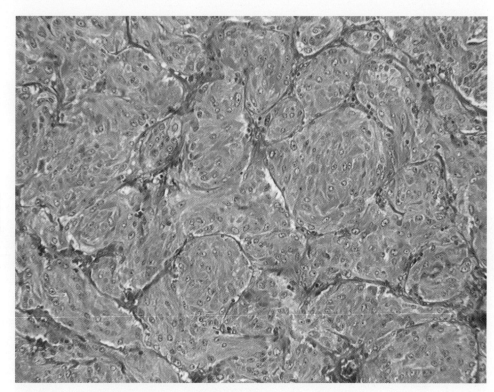

FIGURE 9-26

Nests are present, but they are larger than nests usually seen in benign pheochromocytoma. Large nests alone are not diagnostic of malignancy.

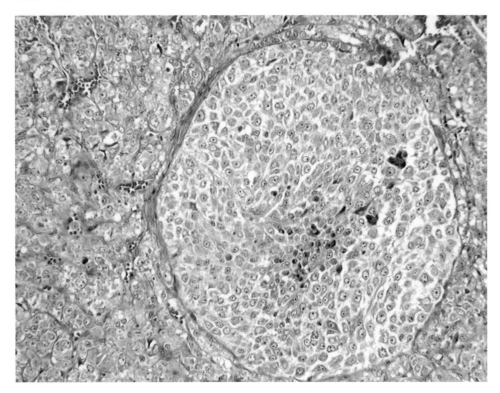

FIGURE 9-27
A large nest with central comedo-type necrosis in a malignant pheochromocytoma.

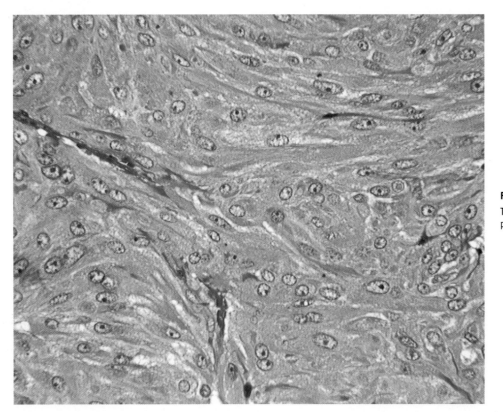

FIGURE 9-28
Tumor cell spindling in a malignant pheochromocytoma.

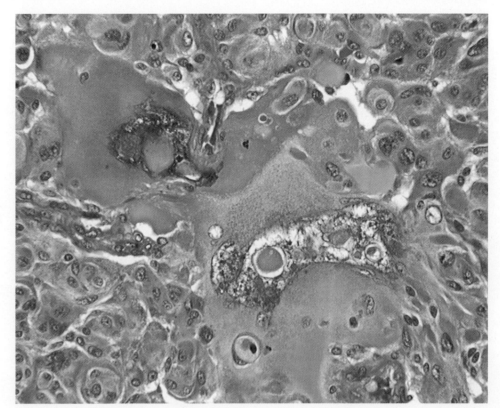

FIGURE 9-29

Profound pleomorphism with intranuclear cytoplasmic inclusions in a malignant pheochromocytoma.

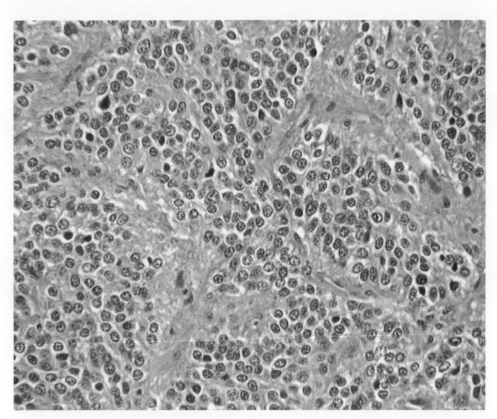

FIGURE 9-30

These small cells are arranged in large nests. The cells are monotonous, displaying a high nuclear to cytoplasmic ratio.

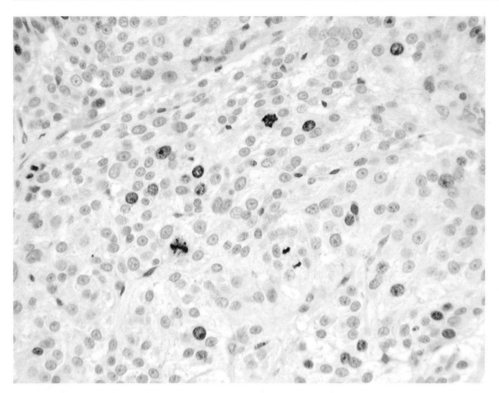

FIGURE 9-31
This Ki-67 immunohistochemistry stain highlights an increased number of mitotic figures in this malignant pheochromocytoma.

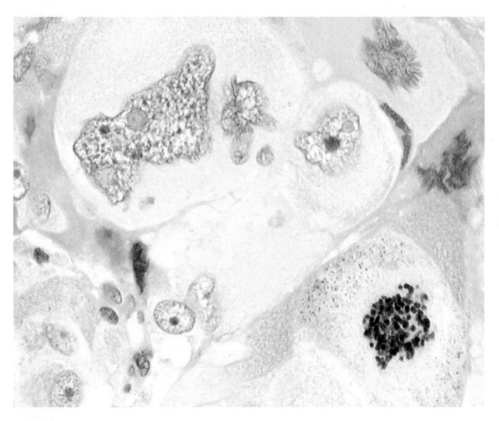

FIGURE 9-32
This atypical mitotic figure is highlighted by a Ki67 immunohistochemistry. Profound nuclear pleomorphism is also noted.

TABLE 9-3

Pheochromocytoma of the Adrenal Gland Scoring Scale (PASS)

Feature	Score if Present (Number of Points Assigned)
Large nests or diffuse growth (>10 % of tumor volume)	2
Central (middle of large nests) or confluent tumor necrosis (not degenerative change)	2
High cellularity	2
Cellular monotony	2
Tumor cell spindling (even if focal)	2
Mitotic figures >3/10 HPF	2
Atypical mitotic figure(s)	2
Extension into adipose tissue	2
Vascular invasion	1
Capsular invasion	1
Profound nuclear pleomorphism	1
Nuclear hyperchromasia	1
Total	20
≤3 Benign biologic behavior	
≥4 Malignant biologic behavior	

From: Thompson LDR. Pheochromocytoma of the adrenal gland scaled score (PASS) to separate benign from malignant neoplasms. Am J Surg Pathol 2002;26:551–566.

FINE NEEDLE ASPIRATION

Fine needle aspiration is usually contraindicated as the procedure may provoke hypertensive crisis. The smears do not separate benign from malignant pheochromocytomas.

OTHER ANCILLARY STUDIES

Ploidy studies do not correlate directly with behavior. Comparative genomic hybridization (CGH) studies suggest that the 6q, 11, and 17p regions may be implicated in tumor progression (Figure 9-37), but conflicting results force one to wait for better ancillary studies to resolve this issue.

DIFFERENTIAL DIAGNOSIS

The distinction between benign and MPCC is presently based on the detection of metastases or local, widely invasive disease, although histologic criteria may be useful as an adjunct to prospectively predict the behavior. Occasionally, MPCC may resemble an adrenal cortical carcinoma, but a small panel of immunohistochemical markers (inhibin, melan-A, chromogranin-A, S-100 protein) will usually resolve this issue.

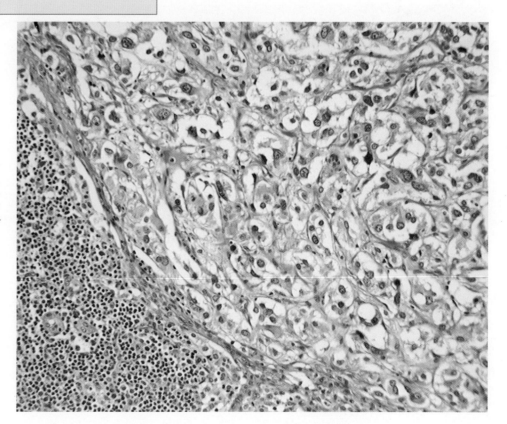

FIGURE 9-33

A focus of metastatic pheochromocytoma within a lymph node.

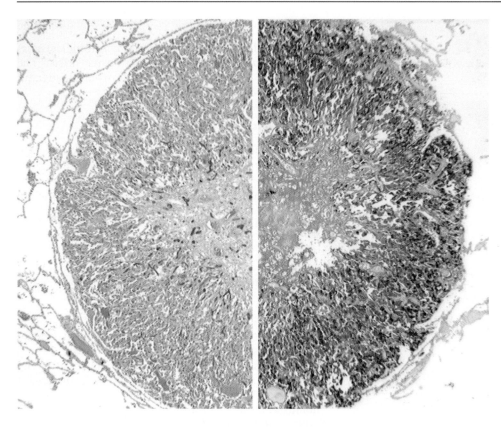

FIGURE 9-34
A focus of metastatic pheochromocytoma in the lung, highlighted
with a positive, strong immunoreaction with chromogranin
(right).

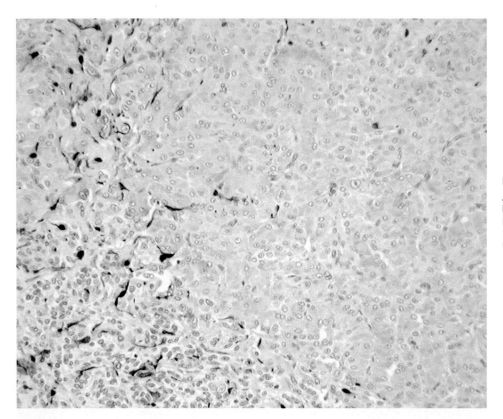

FIGURE 9-35
A transition from small nests to
large nests and diffuse growth is
highlighted with a decrease in S-
100 protein reaction in this malignant pheochromocytoma.

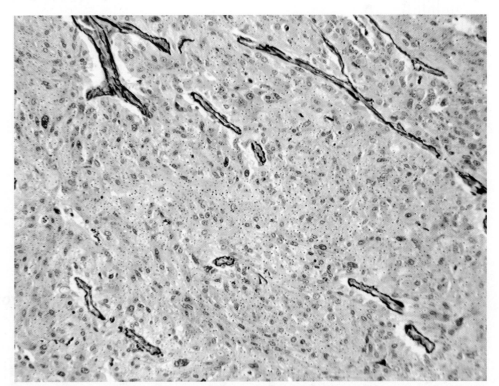

FIGURE 9-36
Large nests and a trabecular arrangement are accentuated by a reticulin stain in this malignant pheochromocytoma.

PROGNOSIS AND THERAPY

The prognosis of malignant MPCC is guarded, with 5-year survival figures between 45% and 55%, although there appears to be a subset of patients with superior survival. Irrespective of benign or malignant pheochromocytoma, long-term follow up is advocated for all patients. Surgery may cure patients, while ^{131}I-MIBG therapy may be employed in MIBG positive tumors and/or their metastases. Multidrug chemotherapy may be used in some patients, and radiation may be palliative. Embolization, radiofrequency ablation, cryotherapy, and percutaneous microwave coagulation are all promising therapies.

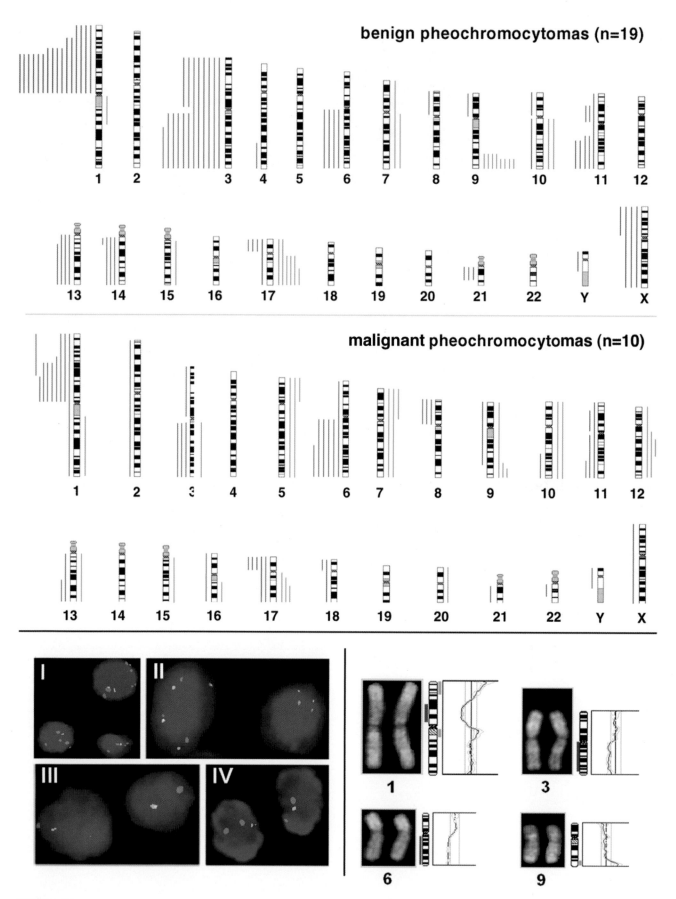

FIGURE 9-37

(A) Results of a comparison of 19 benign and 10 malignant PCC by comparative genomic hybridization (CGH), showing differential loss of 6q, 11, and 17p. (B) Fluorescent in situ hybridization (FISH) interface touch preparations confirming loss of 1p22–31 (I) but not of 1p36 (II), loss of the entire chromosome 3 (III) and loss of 6q (IV), as established before by CGH. (C) Details of CGH digital images of chromosomes 1, 3, 6, and 9, illustrating loss of 1p, 3q, 6q and gain of 9q. (With permission from Dannenberg H, et al. Am J Pathol 2000;157:353–359.)

NEUROBLASTOMA

CLINICAL FEATURES

Neuroblastomas are childhood tumors arising from cells in the sympathetic nervous system that originate from the neural crest. There is a spectrum from ganglioneuromas (GN) to ganglioneuroblastoma (GNB) to neuroblastomas (NB). NB constitute the most common extracranial solid childhood tumor, with an incidence of 1 per 7000 live births, constituting about 6% of all childhood malignancies; in fact, in the neonatal and infant period it may be the most common tumor.

NB are usually located in the adrenal medulla or in the paraspinal sympathetic ganglia of the abdomen and thorax. It is not uncommon to have an abdominal mass as the initial presentation. Additional symptoms include fever or pain, signs of spinal cord compression, the triad of iridal heterochromia, anisocoria and Horner's syndrome in up to 25% of patients with thoracic NB, or paraneoplastic syndromes, such as opsoclonus-myoclonus (ataxic eye movements and/or cerebellar ataxia), which occurs in 2% of patients.

Biochemistry is an important aid in the diagnosis of neuroblastoma, through the detection of urinary excretion of vanillylmandelic acid (VMA) and homovanillic acid (HVA).

A peculiar, unresolved aspect of neuroblastoma is their ability to mature or spontaneously regress. This feature is especially manifested in neonates and infants, and also in stage IV-S patients (see below). Through maturation NB develop into GN, which are benign neoplasms composed of mature ganglion cells and stroma. A few authors consider all GN to have developed from NB.

RADIOLOGIC FEATURES

Radiographic studies are important for the detection and precise identification of the site of neuroblastic tumors. Plain radiographs, echography, or CT scanning are all utilized in evaluation of a mass (Figure 9-38). Location with the adrenal gland or in areas of sympathetic ganglia, in addition to frequent calcifications may give a clue to establishing the diagnosis. Metaiodobenzylguanidine (MIBG) scanning, by selective take up of this radioactive compound in the tumor cells, serves both in the diagnosis and therapy of NB (Figure 9-39).

PATHOLOGIC FEATURES

GROSS FINDINGS

NB and GNB measure up to more than 10 cm in diameter. Many patients receive neoadjuvant chemo-

---

**NEUROBLASTOMA
DISEASE FACT SHEET**

Definition
▸ Tumor from neural-crest derived neuroblastic cells

Incidence and Location
▸ 1 in 7000 live births
▸ About 6% of all childhood malignancies
▸ Most common congenital neoplasm
▸ Adrenal gland > paraspinal ganglia in abdomen and thorax (mediastinum)

Morbidity and Mortality
▸ Morbidity due to compression of organs or structures by primary tumor or due to chemotherapy treatment

Gender, Race and Age Distribution
▸ Equal gender distribution
▸ Usually young children, with 25% presenting <1 year

Clinical Features
▸ Abdominal mass
▸ Fever, pain, spinal cord compression, paraneoplastic syndromes
▸ Overproduction of VMA and HVA detectable in urine
▸ May spontaneously mature or regress

Prognosis and Therapy
▸ Prognosis is risk group and age dependent (complex tables)
▸ Cure rate >90% for low-risk patients; 70–90% cure rate for intermediate-risk patients; 10–40% for high-risk patients
▸ Treatment is highly standardized, including surgery, chemotherapy, and radiotherapy; along with stem cell transplantation in high risk group

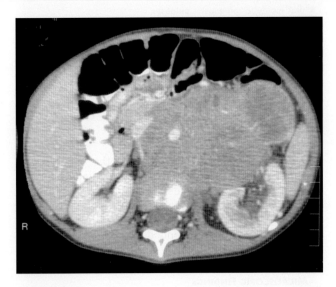

FIGURE 9-38

CT scan of massive abdominal neuroblastoma with typical encasement of aorta and caval vein.

NEUROBLASTOMA
PATHOLOGIC FEATURES

Gross Findings

▸ Firm gray to white tumor up to 10 cm
▸ Post-chemotherapy changes, include hemorrhage, cystic change, calcification
▸ Nodular appearance requires additional sampling

Microscopic Findings

▸ Sub-grouping of tumors according to Shimada classification, based on presence of stroma and ganglion cells
  – *Undifferentiated*: small blue round cell neoplasm
  – *Poorly differentiated*: scant neuropil and <5 % ganglion cells
  – *Differentiating*: 5–50 % ganglion cells with abundant neuropil
  – *Ganglioneuroblastoma*: >50 % ganglion-like cells, but still with primitive cells present
    ▹ Intermixed and nodular subgroups also identified
▸ MKI index used for prognostication

Ultrastructural Features

▸ Axonal processes, small secretory granules and synaptic-like vesicles

Immunohistochemical Results

▸ Positive with NSE, synaptophysin, CD56, chromogranin-A, tyrosine hydroxylase, PGP9.5, NB84
▸ Negative with actin, desmin, CD99, CD45RB, vimentin

Fine Needle Aspiration

▸ Cellular smears
▸ Small cells with high nuclear to cytoplasmic ratio, hyperchromatic nuclei and coarse chromatin
▸ Background fibrillar matrix material
▸ Small clusters, rosettes or single cells
▸ Ganglion-cells may be present

Ancillary Studies

▸ Amplification of *MYCN* oncogene (FISH technique)
▸ Loss of heterozygosity of 1p
▸ Gain of 17q
▸ DNA ploidy for prognostic purposes

Pathologic Differential Diagnosis

▸ Dependent on type of neuroblastoma; includes 'small blue round cell neoplasms', rhabdomyosarcoma, lymphoma, Ewing/PNET, Wilms tumor, osteosarcoma, malignant peripheral nerve sheath tumor, desmoplastic small blue round cell tumor

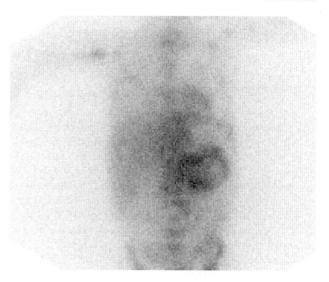

FIGURE 9-39

^{123}I-MIBG scan of neuroblastoma shows abnormal uptake in skeletal bones and in the left sided abdominal mass. Normal uptake in heart, liver and bladder.

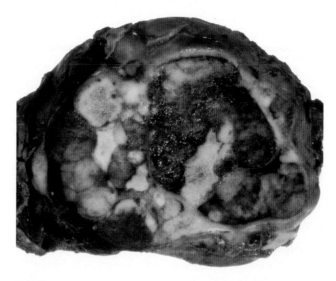

FIGURE 9-40

Gross picture of neuroblastoma, showing hemorrhagic and cystic change.

therapy, which significantly alters the macroscopic appearance of the tumor. Tumors are usually firm and light gray to tan brown, depending on the amount of hemorrhage, with areas of calcification and cystic change (Figure 9-40). If a nodular appearance is seen, additional sampling is recommended to diagnose the nodular variant of GNB.

MICROSCOPIC FINDINGS

Microscopically, it is important to separate NB and GNB into their subtypes as they have important biologic, therapeutic, and prognostic implications. NB and GNB present a range of growth patterns. In principle, the international neuroblastoma pathology classification recommends classification of NB only on pre-chemotherapy specimens. At the *undifferentiated* end of the spectrum is the small blue round cell tumor, which cannot be identified as a neuroblastoma by conventional light microscopy, but instead needs ancillary techniques (see below) to be confirmed as a neuroblastoma (Figure 9-41). These tumors are composed of small to medium-sized cells with very little cytoplasm and do not contain identifiable background neuropil (thin neuritic processes; Figure 9-42). The *poorly differentiated* NB is usually recognized by the presence of varying amounts of neuropil (Figure 9-43). Less than 5 % of tumor cells

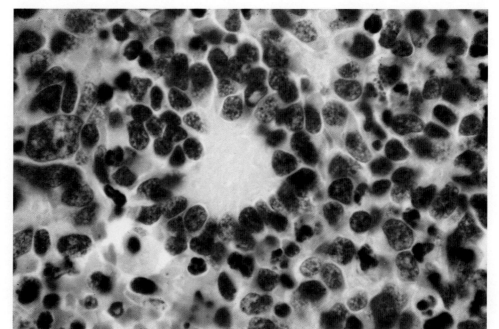

FIGURE 9-41

This 'small blue round cell neoplasm' shows a rosette pattern identified in an undifferentiated NB.

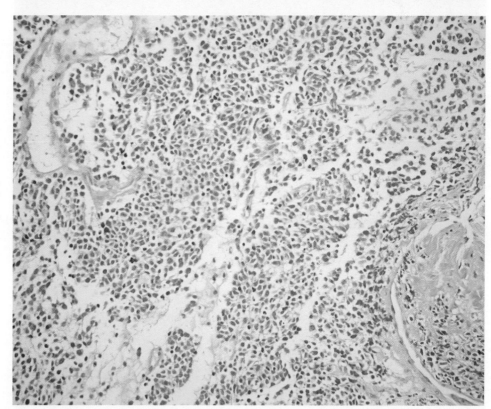

FIGURE 9-42

A 'small blue round cell tumor', showing no histological clues to the diagnosis; because of positive immunostaining for synaptophysin and CD56 and negative staining for other markers, this tumor was classified as an undifferentiated neuroblastoma, in accordance with the clinical findings.

show differentiation towards ganglion cells, which separates this category from the *differentiating subtype* of NB, which have more than 5% but less than 50% of such cells (Figure 9-44). This subgroup has abundant neuropil. The differentiating cells in the latter two groups usually have substantial cytoplasm (in contrast to the neuroblasts in the undifferentiated subtype), and eccentric large nuclei.

In GNB, there is a mixture of primitive, small neuroblastic cells and large ganglion or ganglion-like cells, the latter constituting more than 50% of the tumor volume

(Figure 9-45). The *intermixed subgroup* has gradual transitions between the various components of the lesion, whereas in the *nodular subgroup* (as the name implies) there are abrupt transitions from well-differentiated areas with ganglion cells to nodules of primitive neuroblasts (hemorrhagic appearance on gross inspection).

A scoring of the mitosis-karyorrhexis index (MKI; number of mitotic and/or karyorrhectic nuclei per 5000 cells) is also used for prognostication, with an index above 200 (>4%) imparting a poor prognosis.

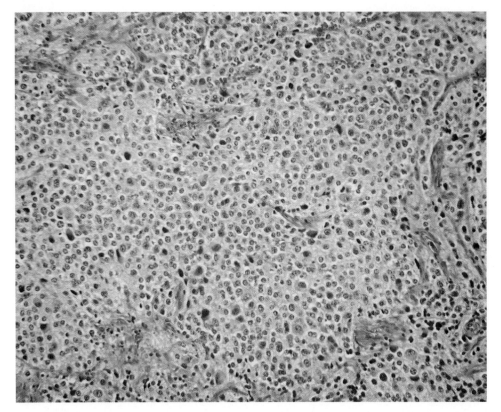

FIGURE 9-43

Poorly differentiated neuroblastoma, showing signs of differentiation of some cells in the direction of ganglion cells (<5 %), and the presence of stroma.

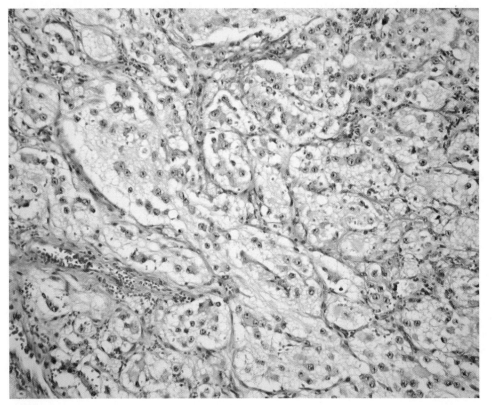

FIGURE 9-44

Differentiating neuroblastoma, with clear-cut differentiation in the direction of ganglion cells, comprising <50% of the tumor volume, and extensive stroma.

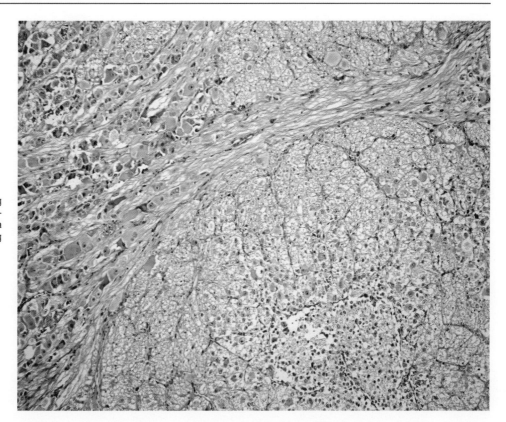

FIGURE 9-45
Ganglioneuroblastoma, consisting almost entirely of well differentiated ganglion cells and stroma (>50 %), but with a few remaining foci of neuroblasts.

ANCILLARY STUDIES

ULTRASTRUCTURAL FEATURES

Distinctive ultrastructural features of NB include axonal processes, small secretory granules and synaptic-like vesicles. The most relevant subgroup of neuroblastoma in which electron microscopy might play a role is that of undifferentiated neuroblastoma. However, other ancillary studies have largely supplanted the role of electron microscopy.

IMMUNOHISTOCHEMICAL RESULTS

The main purpose of immunohistochemistry for NB is generally in the undifferentiated or poorly differentiated category, where other 'small blue round cell neoplasms' come into play. NB show immunoreactivity with neuron-specific enolase, chromogranin-A, synaptophysin, CD56 (Figure 9-46), tyrosine hydroxylase, protein gene product 9.5, and NB84. NB84, while positive in nearly 100 % of cases, may also be reactive in Ewing sarcoma (20–65 %) and desmoplastic small blue round cell tumor (30–50 %). NB usually do not react with actin, desmin, CD45RB, vimentin, or CD99.

FINE NEEDLE ASPIRATION

Smears are usually cellular, composed of cells with a very high nuclear to cytoplasmic ratio, small, round, hyperchromatic nuclei with coarsely clumped, dense chromatin, and a background of fibrillar matrix material. Cells may be arranged in small clusters, rosettes, or singly (Figure 9-47). Occasionally, ganglion-type cells may be appreciated. Additional studies can be performed on the aspirated material which will help with the differential diagnosis.

MOLECULAR STUDIES

Molecular analysis provides a key role in therapy and prognosis. Specifically, amplification of the *MYCN* oncogene is investigated by fluorescence in situ hybridization. When normal, i.e. not amplified, this adds to a favorable prognosis, whereas amplification (>10 copies) is unfavorable (Figure 9-48). Other molecular analyses that are required for NB are loss of heterozygosity of 1p or a gain of 17q, both of which are unfavorable. DNA ploidy may also be used, with hyperdiploid tumors having a favorable prognosis. Molecular studies require fresh tumor tissue, which should be procured with minimal delay.

DIFFERENTIAL DIAGNOSIS

The differential diagnosis of neuroblastic tumors is dependent on the tumor subgroup. Undifferentiated NB raises the broadest differential with the 'small blue round cell neoplasms' category, which includes rhabdomyosarcomas (RMS), lymphomas, Ewing/primitive neuroectodermal tumor (PNET), osteosarcomas, Wilms tumors, and desmoplastic small blue round cell tumors. Clinical, biochemical, and immunohistochemistry used

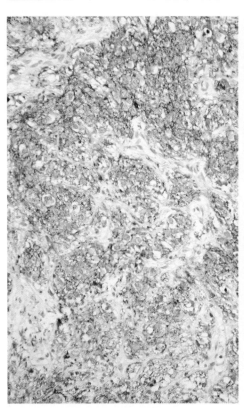
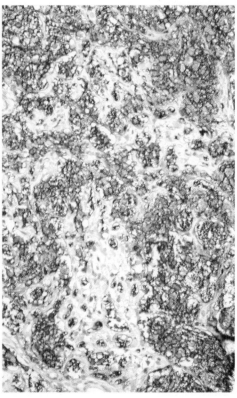

FIGURE 9-46

A poorly differentiated neuroblastoma showing strong uniform cytoplasmic immunoreactivity for synaptophysin (left) and CD56 (right).

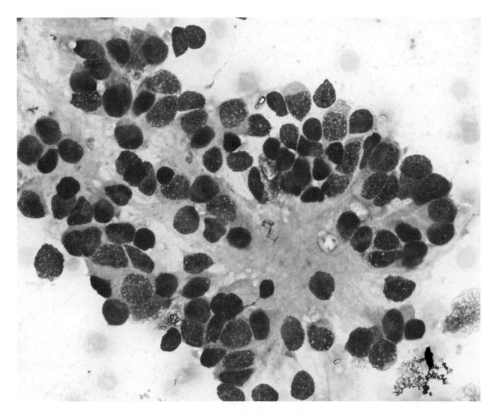

FIGURE 9-47

A loose aggregate of small cells with a high nuclear to cytoplasmic ratio, arranged in a pseudorosette with dendritic, fibrillar matrix between the cells. Nuclear hyperchromasia is noted in this neuroblastoma, poorly differentiated type.

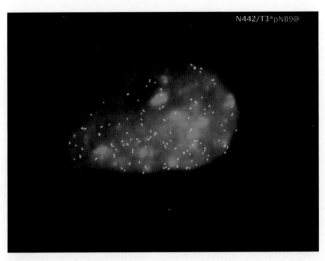

FIGURE 9-48
Fluorescent *in situ* hybridization (FISH), showing amplification of the *MYCN* gene.

TABLE 9-4

Prognostic Criteria in Neuroblastoma Staging Criteria for Neuroblastoma

Prognostic Factor	Favorable	Unfavorable
Stage	1, 2, 4S	3, 4
Age	<1 year	>1 year
Ferritin, LDH	Low	High
NSE	Low	High
Histology	Favorable	Unfavorable
MYCN oncogene	Normal copy	Amplified (>10 copies)
DNA index	Hyperdiploid	Diploid
Chromosome 1p	Normal	Deletion

TABLE 9-5

Staging System for Neuroblastomas, Proposed by the International Staging System Working Party

Stage	Features
Stage 1	Localized tumor, completely excised, with or without microscopic residual disease and negative lymph nodes
Stage 2A	Localized tumor, incompletely excised; negative lymph nodes
Stage 2B	Same as stage 2A, with positive ipsilateral nodes; negative contralateral lymph nodes
Stage 3	Unresectable tumor, crossing midline with or without lymph node involvement; midline tumor with bilateral lymph node involvement
Stage 4	Dissemination to distant lymph nodes, bone, bone marrow, liver, skin or other
Stage 4S	Localized primary tumor, dissemination limited to skin, liver and/or bone marrow, <1 year of age

in conjunction will help with this distinction. Occasionally, specific chromosomal translocations in alveolar RMS and Ewing/PNET may make a definitive separation. Poorly differentiated and differentiating NB or GNB are usually straight forward, requiring only confirmatory immunohistochemistry.

PROGNOSIS AND THERAPY

Prognosis in NB is based on several factors, which are listed in Table 9-4. Risk groups are well established based on stage, age, *MYCN* status, histology, and DNA index. Staging criteria are listed in Table 9-5. Prognosis depends on many factors, histology representing only one. However, the pathologist plays a key role by dividing tumor material for molecular studies, creating imprints, fixing for ultrastructure and/or freezing material for a tissue bank.

Unfavorable prognosis subsets include: undifferentiated NB and GNB nodular type for any patient age; poorly differentiated NB > 1.5 years; differentiating NB > 5 years; and high MKI. A low MKI is favorable with age < 5 years, and intermediate MKI is favorable with <1.5 year old patients.

Treatment is based on tumor classification, with surgery alone for low risk group patients. Intermediate-risk group patients receive pre-operative chemotherapy followed by surgery. Depending on the specific grading and staging, chemotherapeutic regimens may differ and additional radiotherapy may be applied. Standard treatment for high-risk group patients is pre-operative chemotherapy, followed by surgery, if possible. Subsequently, myeloablative chemotherapy with stem cell rescue (i.e., bone marrow and/or peripheral blood stem cell transplantation) and the tumor site is irradiated. Finally, retinoic acid is given for 6 months. Many regimens are used, but are beyond the scope of this chapter. While cure rates are >90% for low-risk patients and 70–90% for intermediate-risk patients, they are considerably lower for high-risk group patients, who experience a 50% relapse due to drug resistance and 10–40% long-term survival.

UNCOMMON PRIMARY MALIGNANT NEOPLASMS

PRIMARY MALIGNANT MELANOMA

True primary adrenal malignant melanomas are extremely rare, with adrenal metastases from occult or skin primaries much more frequent. A primary mela-

UNCOMMON PRIMARY MALIGNANT NEOPLASMS

Malignant Melanoma

▸ True primary malignant melanoma is rare requiring that only one adrenal gland be affected, no extra-adrenal primary, and no removal of a pigmented skin, mucous membrane or eye lesion
▸ Metastases are more common
▸ Tumors are brown to black if melanin producing
▸ Protean histologic manifestations as their cutaneous counterparts
▸ S-100 protein, HMB45, melan-A and tyrosinase positive
▸ Differential diagnosis includes other pigmented adrenal gland primaries
▸ Usually fatal in <2 years

Angiosarcoma

▸ Rare vascular neoplasm affecting elderly patients who present with abdominal mass or flank pain
▸ Arsenicals and radiotherapy are possible etiologic factors
▸ Macroscopic tumors are reddish and ill-demarcated
▸ Epithelioid appearance to richly anastomosing vascular channels
▸ Endothelial cells are pleomorphic and epithelioid with neolumen formation and mitotic figures
▸ FVIIIR-Ag, CD34, CD31, keratin, EMA positive
▸ Must exclude metastatic neoplasms, organizing thrombus/hemorrhage
▸ Surgery and chemotherapy may palliate otherwise lethal outcome

Leiomyosarcoma

▸ Arising from the central vein, patients present with a large, unilateral adrenal gland mass, which may invade the IVC
▸ Atypical spindle cells with hyperchromatic nuclei seen scrolling off central vein and invading between adrenal gland parenchyma
▸ Necrosis, increased mitotic figures and hemorrhage
▸ Desmin and actin are positive
▸ Metastatic neoplasms must be excluded
▸ Radical surgery and adjuvant multimodality therapy may alter otherwise guarded patient prognosis

noma is defined as only one adrenal gland involved, exclusion of an extra-adrenal primary (clinically or at autopsy) and, no history of removal of a pigmented lesion of the skin, mucous membranes or eye. MRI may show high signal intensity on T1 weighted images and low signal intensity on T2 weighted images possibly reflecting melanin production. The tumors are brown to black, although they may not be pigmented. The histologic findings mimic their cutaneous counterparts (Figure 9-49). A variety of histologic patterns are seen, with prominent nucleoli and intranuclear cytoplasmic inclusions a helpful hint to the diagnosis (Figure 9-50). Melanosomes or premelanosomes may be seen by electron microscopy. The tumor cells exhibit immunoreactivity for S-100 protein, HMB45, melan-A, and tyrosinase. The differential diagnosis includes metastatic melanoma, melanotic pheochromocytoma, GN or GNB, pigmented (black) adrenocortical adenomas and adrenal hematoma with hemosiderin-laden macrophages. Primary malignant melanomas are highly malignant and usually lethal within 2 years.

ANGIOSARCOMA

Primary adrenal angiosarcoma is extremely rare. It usually affects elderly patients who present with an abdominal mass, flank pain or is detected incidentally. Direct exposure to arsenicals (vineyard cultivators) and abdominal radiotherapy have been reported as possible causative factors. CT generally shows a heterogeneous mass with frequent necrosis, contrast-enhancement, and occasional calcifications. Grossly, tumors are reddish and ill demarcated. Histologically, the tumors frequently exhibit a predominantly epithelioid differentiation (Figure 9-51). The neoplasms are invasive and mostly arranged in solid sheets, nests and anastomosing cords (Figure 9-52). Endothelial cells line dilated, anastomosing vascular spaces, display pleomorphism, intracytoplasmic neolumen formation, and mitotic figures (Figure 9-53). Ultrastructural findings include the identification of rod-shaped microtubulated bodies and intracytoplasmic lumen formation. The neoplastic cells are immunoreactivity for Factor VIII-RAg, CD34, CD31, Ulex europaeus agglutinin-1 lectin (UEA-1), and epithelial markers, including cytokeratin (Figure 9-53), epithelial membrane antigen, and B72.3. The differential diagnosis includes metastatic angiosarcoma (about 20% of angiosarcomas metastasize to the adrenal), organizing thrombus/hemorrhage within an adrenal adenoma, intravascular papillary endothelial hyperplasia, and occasionally other neoplasms. Surgical resection with chemotherapy may alter the aggressive clinical course which ends in a usually fatal outcome.

LEIOMYOSARCOMA

Leiomyosarcoma is thought to arise from the large central vessels of the adrenal gland. These tumors are rare, unilateral, and large (>10 cm). Patients usually present with signs and symptoms of a large retroperitoneal mass, with tumor extension into the inferior vena cava as a direct extension from the adrenal vasculature. Histologically, atypical neoplastic cells are noted scrolling off the central vein's wall and infiltrating into the surrounding parenchyma (Figure 9-54). The neoplastic cells are spindled with tapered nuclei and small vacuoles (Figure 9-55). There is associated necrosis, increased mitotic activity and frequent hemorrhage. The cells are desmin and actin positive (Figure 9-56). The differential diagnosis includes metastatic neoplasms. Radical surgery with adjuvant multimodality therapy may alter an otherwise guarded patient outcome.

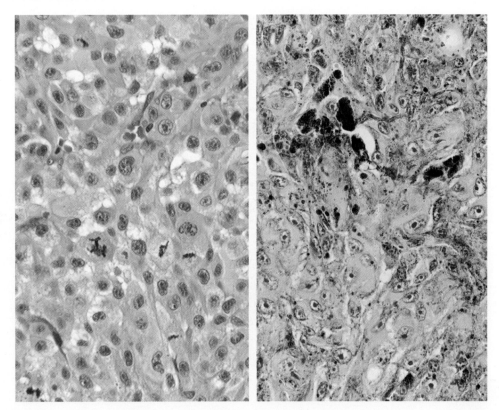

FIGURE 9-49

Left: A primary adrenal gland melanoma demonstrates an epithelioid pattern with numerous atypical mitotic figures. Right: Heavy melanin pigment is present in this adrenal gland melanoma.

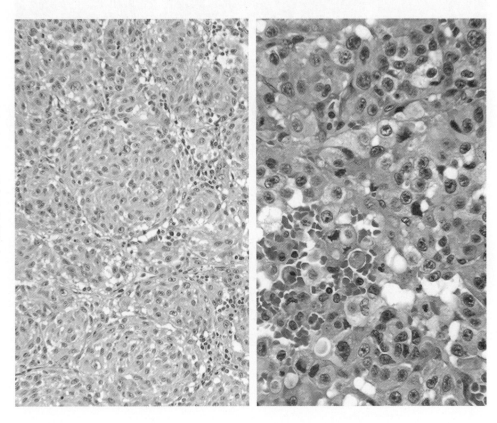

FIGURE 9-50

Left: A whorled or meningothelial pattern was seen in this primary adrenal gland melanoma. Right: An epithelioid pattern with eccentric nuclei and prominent nucleoli is noted in this primary adrenal gland melanoma. Erythrocytes extravasation is also present.

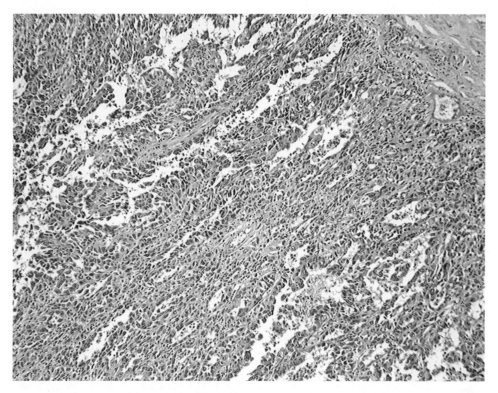

FIGURE 9-51

This primary angiosarcoma has multiple spaces lined by epithelioid cells. Note areas of degeneration.

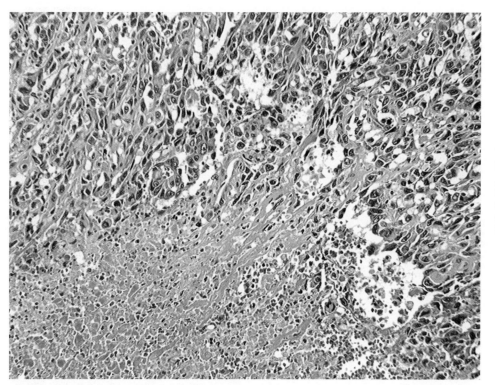

FIGURE 9-52

Areas of necrosis are associated with an arborizing vascular pattern to this primary angiosarcoma of the adrenal gland. Erythrocytes are noted.

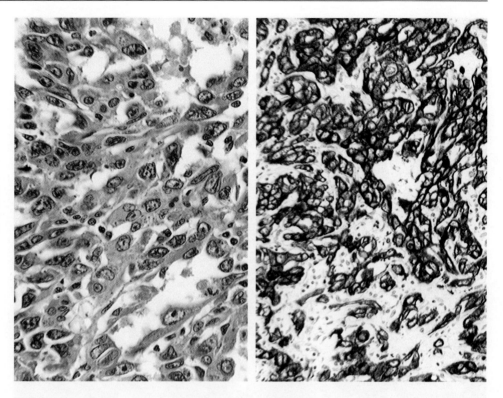

FIGURE 9-53

Left: An anastomosing and arborizing vascular pattern is noted, lined by atypical endothelial cells with a hobnail and epithelioid appearance. Right: The neoplastic cells are strongly keratin immunoreactive.

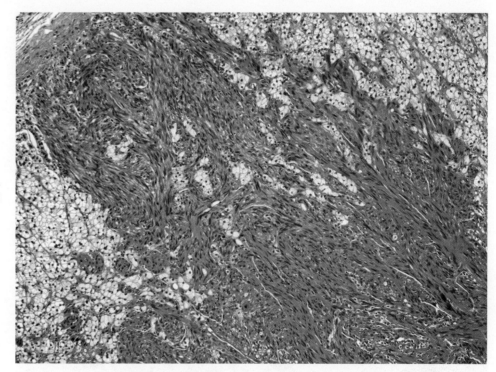

FIGURE 9-54

A primary adrenal gland leiomyosarcoma invades into the surrounding adrenal cortical tissue.

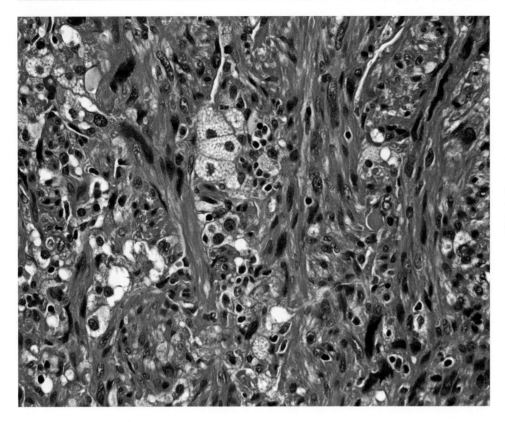

FIGURE 9-55
The atypical spindle cells of a primary leiomyosarcoma invade between adrenal cortical cells.

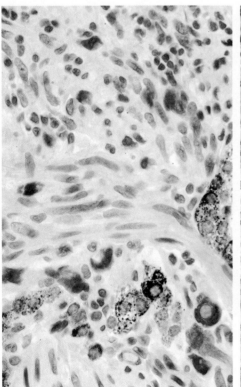
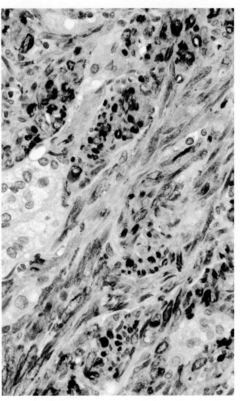

FIGURE 9-56
Right: The benign adrenal gland is melan A immunoreactive while the leiomyosarcoma is negative. Left: The leiomyosarcoma cells are strongly and diffusely desmin immunoreactive while the adrenal cortical cells are negative.

METASTATIC TUMORS

CLINICAL FEATURES

Adrenal glands are frequently involved by metastases and constitute the fourth most common site of metastases after lung, liver and bone. This is probably due to the rich blood supply of the organ. Up to one-third of cancer patients have adrenal metastases; 40–50% are bilateral; >90% are carcinomas and about half of these are adenocarcinomas. The most common primary tumor sites are lung and breast (together up to 80%) followed by gastrointestinal tract (stomach, pancreas, colon, liver), kidney, skin (melanoma) and ovary. Rarely, metastases may also occur to primary tumors of the adrenals (pheochromocytomas and adrenocortical adenomas). Secondary involvement of the adrenals by malignant lymphomas may be seen in up to 25% of patients with disseminated disease. Patients with adrenal metastases are usually older and rarely do they present with symptoms referable to the adrenal gland. More than 90% of the adrenal parenchyma must be destroyed by the neoplasm before functional adrenal insufficiency (Addison's disease) is noted.

**METASTATIC TUMORS
DISEASE FACT SHEET**

Definition
▶ Adrenal mass caused by metastatic tumor

Incidence and Location
▶ Adrenal gland is the fourth most common site of metastatic disease
▶ Up to one-third of cancer patients have adrenal metastases
▶ 40–50% have bilateral disease
▶ >90% are carcinomas (about 50% of these are adenocarcinoma)
▶ Secondary involvement by lymphomas (25% of patients)

Morbidity and Mortality
▶ Depends on extent of adrenal gland replacement and underlying primary tumor type

Gender, Race and Age Distribution
▶ Equal gender distribution
▶ Usually elderly patients

Clinical Features
▶ Rarely present with adrenal gland symptoms
▶ If >90% of parenchyma destroyed; functional adrenal insufficiency (Addison's disease) may occur

Prognosis and Therapy
▶ Prognosis depends on extent of systemic disease, with long term survival rare
▶ Median survival with symptomatic adrenal metastases, 3 mo
▶ Surgery is of limited value

RADIOLOGIC FEATURES

On CT scans involved adrenals usually exhibit soft tissue density and may appear like an adrenocortical lesion. On MRI adrenals with metastases show a heterogeneous signal intensity on T2 weighted images but in case of hemorrhage or necrosis high signals on both T1 and T2 weighted images may be seen.

PATHOLOGIC FEATURES

GROSS FINDINGS

Adrenal metastases may appear as single or multiple firm gray-white masses that replace part or all of the affected gland (Figure 9-57). Large metastases usually exhibit foci of hemorrhage and necrosis and may therefore grossly imitate primary adrenocortical carcinoma. However, metastases usually lack the yellow color of adrenocortical primaries.

MICROSCOPIC FINDINGS

The microscopic appearance of the metastases varies according to the nature of the primary tumor. However, difficulty may be encountered with metastases of undifferentiated tumors. Furthermore, some metastases, such as large cell carcinoma (lung; Figure 9-58), renal cell carcinoma (Figures 9-59 and 9-60) or hepatocellular carcinoma (Figure 9-61) histologically may mimic an adrenocortical primary.

**METASTATIC TUMORS
PATHOLOGIC FEATURES**

Gross Findings
▶ Single or multiple usually gray-white and firm masses
▶ When large, necrosis and/or hemorrhage may be seen

Microscopic Findings
▶ Identical to primary tumor
▶ Large cell carcinoma, renal cell carcinoma and hepatocellular carcinoma are frequently mimics of adrenal primaries

Immunohistochemical Results
▶ Discriminating markers depend on the type of primary tumor

Fine Needle Aspiration
▶ May be valuable in identifying 'non-adrenal' primary lesions, although full separation may require clinical, radiographic, and immunohistochemical studies

Pathologic Differential Diagnosis
▶ Adrenal (cortical) primaries

ANCILLARY STUDIES

IMMUNOHISTOCHEMICAL RESULTS

Immunohistochemistry is helpful to define the origin of metastases of an unknown primary and to distinguish metastases from an adrenal primary. Discriminating markers depend on the suspected primary tumor and are not different from those used for tumors of the primary sites. Metastases of carcinomas are usually clearly positive for cytokeratin while primary adrenocortical tumors are usually negative or only focally positive for these markers and in addition are immunoreactive for inhibin, melan A, calretinin and vimentin.

FINE NEEDLE ASPIRATION

Cytological and immunocytochemical features of metastatic tumors are similar to those of the primary, although occasionally difficulties may be encountered in separating metastatic from primary adrenal tumors. Clinical and radiographic correlation is necessary.

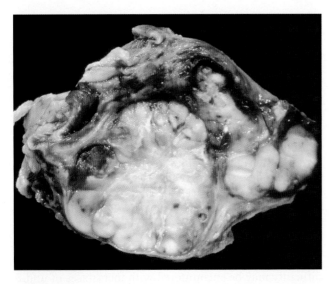

FIGURE 9-57
Adrenocortical metastasis of a primary large cell lung carcinoma.

DIFFERENTIAL DIAGNOSIS

The main differential diagnosis is separating metastases and primary adrenal tumors. Clinical information, radiographic findings, histology, and special studies will aid with this distinction in most cases.

PROGNOSIS AND THERAPY

The prognosis of adrenal metastases is mainly dependent on the extent of systemic disease. The overall

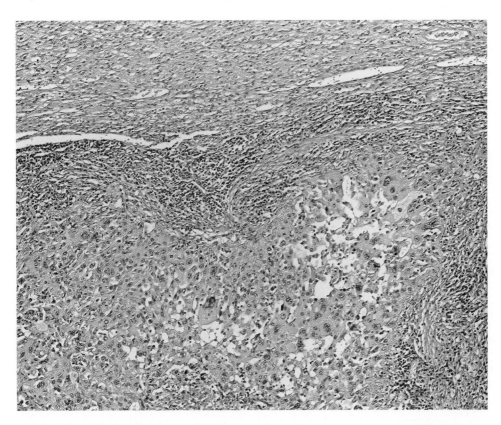

FIGURE 9-58

A metastasis from a large cell lung carcinoma mimic an adrenal cortical neoplasm, although the presence of a lymphoid infiltrate is not common in adrenal gland primaries.

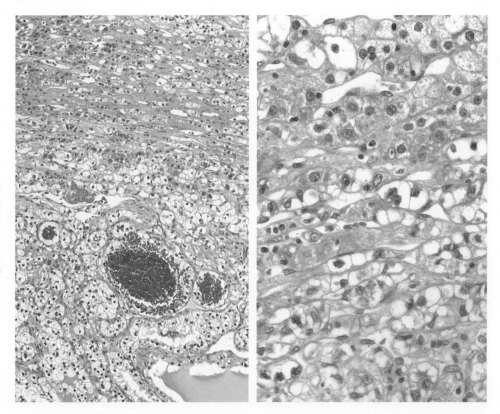

FIGURE 9-59

Left: A metastatic renal cell carcinoma imitating a primary adrenocortical tumor, although the clear cell nature and pseudoglandular vascular arrangement is characteristic for a renal cell carcinoma. Right: High-power shows microvacuolated adrenal cortical cells (upper) while the prominent cellular borders and cleared cytoplasm of the metastatic renal cell carcinoma are seen in the lower half.

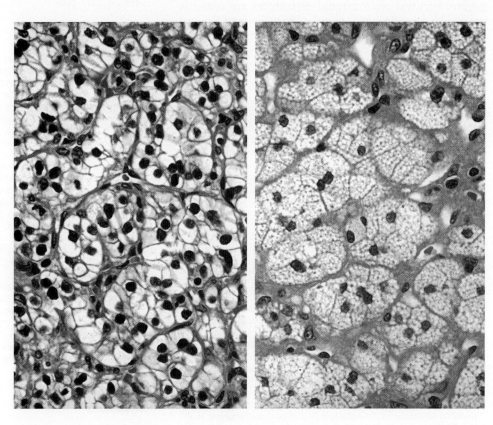

FIGURE 9-60

Left: An alveolar or nests pattern of cells with prominent and accentuated intercellular borders with clear cytoplasm surrounding small dark nuclei are seen in this renal cell carcinoma. Right: In contrast to the renal cell carcinoma, the cytoplasm of adrenal cortical tissue is microvescicular with nuclei that are not as hyperchromatic.

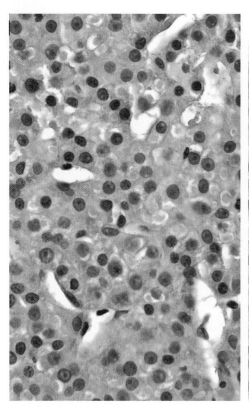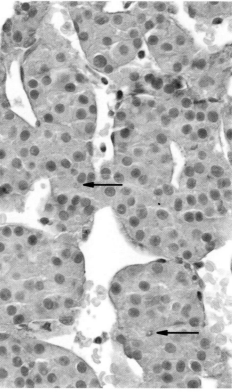

FIGURE 9-61

Left: The trabecular and cord-like growth of this metastatic hepato-cellular carcinoma mimics a primary adrenal cortical lesion. However, there are small canals. Right: The canalicular pattern of a hepatocel-lular carcinoma is highlighted by immunoreactivity with polyclonal CEA (arrows).

prognosis is determined by the primary type, but in general survival once adrenal metastases are noted is limited to a median of 3 months. Surgery is of limited value.

SUGGESTED READING

Adrenal Cortical Carcinoma

Boscaro M, Fallo F, Barzon L, et al. Adrenocortical carcinoma: epidemiology and natural history. Minerva Endocrinol 1995;20:89–94.

Cagle PT, Hough AJ, Pysher TJ, et al. Comparison of adrenal cortical tumors in children and adults. Cancer 1986;57:2235–2237.

Hough AJ, Hollifield JW, Page DL, Hartmann WH. Prognostic factors in adrenal cortical tumors. A mathematical analysis of clinical and mor-phologic data. Am J Clin Pathol 1979;72:390–399.

Narasimhan KL, Samujh R, Bhansali A, et al. Adrenocortical tumors in childhood. Pediatr Surg Int 2003;19:432–435.

Stojadinovic A, Brennan MF, Hoos A, et al. Adrenocortical adenoma and carcinoma: histopathological and molecular comparative analysis. Mod Pathol 2003;16:742–751.

van Slooten H, Schaberg A, Smeenk D, Moolenaar AJ. Morphologic char-acteristics of benign and malignant adrenocortical tumors. Cancer 1985;55:766–773.

Weiss LM, Bertagna X, Chrousos GP, et al. Adrenal cortical carcinoma. *In*: DeLellis RA, Lloyd RV, Heitz PU, Eng C, eds. Pathology and Genetics of Tumours of Endocrine Organs. Kleihues P, Sobin LH, series eds. World Health Organization Classification of Tumours. Lyon, France: IARC Press, 2004:139–142.

Weiss LM, Medeiros LJ, Vickery AL, Jr. Pathologic features of prognostic significance in adrenocortical carcinoma. Am J Surg Pathol 1989;13:202–206.

Wieneke JA, Thompson LDR, Heffess CS. Adrenal cortical neoplasms in the pediatric population: a clinicopathologic and immunophenotypic analy-sis of 83 patients. Am J Surg Pathol 2003;27:867–881.

Zhao J, Speel EJ, Muletta-Feurer S, Rutimann, et al. Analysis of genomic alterations in sporadic adrenocortical lesions. Gain of chromosome 17 is an early event in adrenocortical tumorigenesis. Am J Pathol 1999;155:1039–1045.

Malignant Pheochromocytoma

Boltze C, Mundschenk J, Unger N, et al. Expression profile of the telomeric complex discriminates between benign and malignant pheochromocy-toma. J Clin Endocrinol Metab 2003;88:4280–4286.

Dannenberg H, Speel EJ, Zhao J, Saremaslani P, et al. Losses of chromo-somes 1p and 3q are early genetic events in the development of sporadic pheochromocytomas. Am J Pathol 2000;157:353–359.

Eisenhofer G, Bornstein SR, Brouwers FM, et al. Malignant pheochromocy-toma: current status and initiatives for future progress. Endocr Relat Cancer 2004;11:423–436.

Gimenez-Roqueplo AP, Favier J, Rustin P, et al. Mutations in the SDHB gene are associated with extra-adrenal and/or malignant phaeochromo-cytomas. Cancer Res. 2003;63:5615–5621.

Ilias I, Pacak K. Anatomical and functional imaging of metastatic pheo-chromocytoma. Ann NY Acad Sci 2004;1018:495–504.

Lehnert H, Mundschenk J, Hahn K. Malignant pheochromocytoma. Front Horm Res 2004;31:155–162.

Ohta S, Lai EW, Pang AL, Brouwers FM, et al. Downregulation of metastasis suppressor genes in malignant pheochromocytoma. Int J Cancer 2005;114:139–143.

Thompson LDR, Young WF Jr., Kawashima A, et al. Malignant adrenal pha-eochromocytoma. *In*: DeLellis RA, Lloyd RV, Heitz PU, Eng C, eds. Pathology and Genetics of Tumours of Endocrine Organs. Kleihues P, Sobin LH, series eds. World Health Organization Classification of Tumours. Lyon, France: IARC Press, 2004:147–150.

Thompson LDR. Pheochromocytoma of the adrenal gland scaled score (PASS) to separate benign from malignant neoplasms. Am J Surg Pathol 2002;26:551–566.

Neuroblastoma

Laprie A, Michon J, Hartmann O, et al; Neuroblastoma Study Group of the French Society of Pediatric Oncology. High-dose chemotherapy followed by locoregional irradiation improves the outcome of patients with international neuroblastoma staging system stage II and III neuroblastoma with MYCN amplification. Cancer 2004;101:1081–1089.

Levitt GA, Platt KA, De Byrne R, et al. 4S neuroblastoma: the long-term outcome. Pediatr Blood Cancer 2004;43:120–125.

Miettinen M, Chatten J, Paetau A, Stevenson A. Monoclonal antibody NB84 in the differential diagnosis of neuroblastoma and other small blue round cell tumors. Am J Surg Pathol 1998;22:327–332.

Peuchmaur M, d'Amore ES, Joshi VV, et al. Revision of the International Neuroblastoma Pathology Classification: confirmation of favorable and unfavorable prognostic subsets in ganglioneuroblastoma, nodular. Cancer 2003;98:2274–2281.

Riley RD, Heney D, Jones DR, et al. A systematic review of molecular and biological tumor markers in neuroblastoma. Clin Cancer Res 2004;10:4–12.

Shimada H, Ambros IM, Dehner LP, et al. The international neuroblastoma pathology classification (the Shimada system). Cancer 1999;86:364–372.

Shimada H, Ambros IM, Dehner LP, et al. Terminology and morphologic criteria of neuroblastic tumors. Cancer 1999;86:349–363.

Simon T, Spitz R, Faldum A, et al. New definition of low-risk neuroblastoma using stage, age, and 1p and MYCN status. J Pediatr Hematol Oncol 2004;26:791–796.

Uncommon Primary Neoplasms

Amerigo J, Roig J, Pulido F, et al. Primary malignant melanoma of the adrenal gland. Surgery 2000;127:107–111.

Croitoru AG, Klausner AP, McWilliams G, Unger PD. Primary epithelioid angiosarcoma of the adrenal gland. Ann Diagn Pathol 2001;5:300–303.

Dao AH, Page DL, Reynolds VH, Adkins RB, Jr. Primary malignant melanoma of the adrenal gland. A report of two cases and review of the literature. Am Surg 1990;56:199–203.

Kareti LR, Katlein S, Siew S, Blauvelt A. Angiosarcoma of the adrenal gland. Arch Pathol Lab Med 1988;112:1163–1165.

Kato T, Kato T, Sakamoto S, et al. Primary adrenal leiomyosarcoma with inferior vena cava thrombosis. Int J Clin Oncol 2004;9:189–192.

Kruger S, Kujath P, Johannisson R, Feller AC. Primary epithelioid angiosarcoma of the adrenal gland case report and review of the literature. Tumori 2001;87:262–265.

Lack EE, Graham CW, Azumi N, et al. Primary leiomyosarcoma of adrenal gland. Case report with immunohistochemical and ultrastructural study. Am J Surg Pathol. 1991;15:899–905.

Livaditou A, Alexiou G, Floros D, et al. Epithelioid angiosarcoma of the adrenal gland associated with chronic arsenical intoxication? Pathol Res Pract 1991;187:284–289.

Lloyd RV, Kawashima A, Tischler AS. Adrenal soft tissue and germ cell tumours. In: DeLellis RA, Lloyd RV, Heitz PU, Eng C, eds. Pathology and Genetics of Tumours of Endocrine Organs. Kleihues P, Sobin LH, series eds. World Health Organization Classification of Tumours. Lyon, France: IARC Press, 2004:169–171.

Thamboo TP, Liew LC, Raju GC. Adrenal leiomyosarcoma: a case report and literature review. Pathology. 2003;35:47–49.

Wenig BM, Abbondanzo SL, Heffess CS. Epithelioid angiosarcoma of the adrenal glands. A clinicopathologic study of nine cases with a discussion of the implications of finding 'epithelial-specific' markers. Am J Surg Pathol 1994;18:62–73.

Zalatnai A, Szende B, Toth M, Racz K. Primary malignant melanoma of adrenal gland in a 41-yr-old woman. Endocr Pathol 2003;14:101–105.

Metastatic Tumors

Lack EE. Tumors of the adrenal gland and extra-adrenal paraganglia. 3rd ed. In: Rosai J, Sobin LH, series eds. Atlas of tumor pathology, Vol 19. Washington DC: AFIP, 1997.

Lam KY, Lo CY. Metastatic tumours of the adrenal glands: a 30-year experience in a teaching hospital. Clin Endocrinol 2002;56:95–101.

Lee JE, Evans DB, Hickey RC, Sherman et al. Unknown primary cancer presenting as an adrenal mass: frequency and implications for diagnostic evaluation of adrenal incidentalomas. Surgery 1998;124:1115–1122.

Lloyd RV, Kawashima A, Tischler AS. Secondary tumours. In: DeLellis RA, Lloyd RV, Heitz PU, Eng C, eds. Pathology and Genetics of Tumours of Endocrine Organs. Kleihues P, Sobin LH, series eds. World Health Organization Classification of Tumours. Lyon, France: IARC Press, 2004:172–173.

Lo CY, van Heerden JA, Soreide JA, et al. Adrenalectomy for metastatic disease to the adrenal glands. Br J Surg 1996;83:528–531.

10 Non-neoplastic Lesions of the Pituitary Gland

Lester DR Thompson • Clara S Heffess

INFLAMMATORY LESIONS

A number of different inflammatory lesions can affect the pituitary gland, although granulomatous and auto-immune are the most common. Sarcoid will be high-lighted, although infections (*Mycobacterium tuberculosis*, *Treponema pallidum*, and fungi) and giant cell idio-pathic granulomatous inflammation also occurs.

GRANULOMATOUS INFLAMMATION

CLINICAL FEATURES

Sarcoidosis is a granulomatous disease of unknown etiology with focal or generalized multiorgan involve-

ment. It is slightly more common in women than in men and generally affects younger patients (20 to 40 years). There is a high association with Black people. Less than 10% of sarcoidosis patients have central nervous system involvement, with the posterior pitu-itary affected more commonly than the anterior; diabe-tes insipidus results. The diagnosis is confirmed by a combination of clinical, radiographic and histologic results; skin anergy is typical, but non-diagnostic. The sellar may be enlarged, but this is a non-specific radio-graphic findings.

PATHOLOGIC FEATURES

MICROSCOPIC FINDINGS

Multiple non-caseating granulomas composed of epi-thelioid histiocytes are associated with a mixed inflam-matory cell infiltrate with occasional Langhans type giant cells (Figure 10-1). Rarely, intracytoplasmic aster-oid and/or Schaumann bodies may be present. All special stains for microorganisms are negative. Although histologic evidence is necessary for diagnosis, the find-ings are not specific for the disease and definite diagno-sis is only rendered based on clinical history, radiographs, blood tests, and lack of identification of an infectious agent; in this regard, a diagnosis of sarcoidosis is one of exclusion.

GRANULOMATOUS INFLAMMATION
DISEASE FACT SHEET

Definition
▸ Sarcoidosis is a granulomatous disease of unknown etiology with focal or generalized multiorgan involvement

Incidence and Location
▸ <10% of sarcoid patients
▸ Uncommon, but if involved, posterior pituitary involvement

Gender, Race and Age Distribution
▸ Females slightly more common than males
▸ Black people >>> White people (10–17:1)
▸ Young patients (20–40 years)

Clinical Features
▸ Usually referable to respiratory system
▸ If pituitary involvement, usually diabetes insipidus

Prognosis and Therapy
▸ Dependent upon systemic involvement
▸ 50% may have permanent organ dysfunction
▸ 10% have a waxing and waning clinical course
▸ Glucocorticoids generally used

GRANULOMATOUS INFLAMMATION
PATHOLOGIC FEATURES

Microscopic Findings
▸ Multiple, tight, non-caseating granulomas
▸ Epithelioid histiocytes
▸ Mixed inflammatory cells
▸ Langhans type giant cells

Pathologic Differential Diagnosis
▸ Infectious agents (mycobacterial, fungal), giant cell granuloma

---

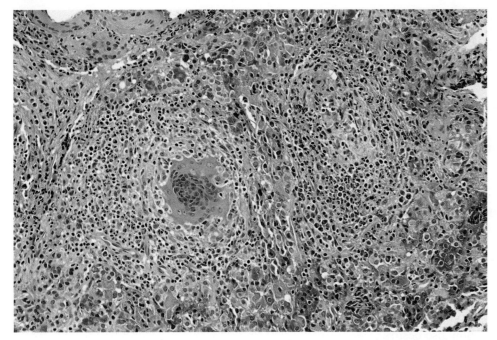

FIGURE 10-1
Langhans type giant cells are associated with a mixed inflammatory infiltrate in this example of a granulomatous hypophysitis.

DIFFERENTIAL DIAGNOSIS

The differential diagnosis for granulomatous inflammation includes infectious agents (mycobacteria, fungi, spirochetes) along with the non-specific giant cell granuloma.

PROGNOSIS AND THERAPY

The overall prognosis is good, although approximately 50% of patients may have permanent organ dysfunction. A prolonged remitting and relapsing course may be seen in about 10% of patients. The treatment of choice is glucocorticoids, although dependent upon systemic manifestations.

AUTOIMMUNE (LYMPHOCYTIC) INFLAMMATION

This is a rare, destructive, inflammatory infiltration of the pituitary resulting in pituitary insufficiency, and most often occurring in late pregnancy or the postpartum period. An autoimmune etiology is favored, especially in light of antipituitary antibodies.

CLINICAL FEATURES

The disorder affects predominantly young females during late pregnancy or puerperium, with symptoms

---

AUTOIMMUNE (LYMPHOCYTIC) INFLAMMATION DISEASE FACT SHEET

Definition
▶ A destructive, inflammatory infiltrate resulting in pituitary insufficiency most often associated with pregnancy/post-partum

Incidence and Location
▶ Rare

Gender, Race and Age Distribution
▶ Female >>> Male
▶ Usually young

Clinical Features
▶ Headache, visual disturbances
▶ Amenorrhea, galactorrhea
▶ Variable degrees of hypopituitarism or hyperprolactinemia
▶ Antipituitary antibodies
▶ Men have decreased libido, impotence, and low testosterone levels

Prognosis and Therapy
▶ Pituitary may regain size and function
▶ Surgery and hormone replacement

---

including headache and visual disturbances, amenorrhea, galactorrhea, and varying degrees of hypopituitarism. Laboratory investigation demonstrates marked reduction in hormone function of one or more pituitary hormones. Serologic antipituitary antibodies may be seen in up to 20% of patients. Other endocrine organs may be affected by inflammation concurrently (Hashimoto's thyroiditis, adrenalitis). Men are rarely affected, and present with headaches, impotence and diminished libido with decreased serum testosterone levels.

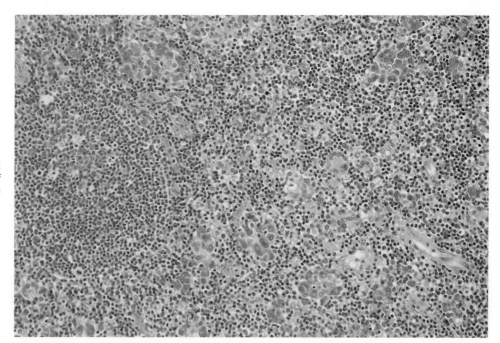

FIGURE 10-2

The pituitary parenchyma is effaced by an extensive cellular infiltrate of plasma cells and lymphocytes. Note the follicle formation on the left.

RADIOLOGIC FEATURES

CT scan and MRI show pituitary enlargement and demonstrate a contrast-enhanced intrasellar mass with suprasellar extension, simulating the appearance of a macroadenoma.

AUTOIMMUNE (LYMPHOCYTIC) INFLAMMATION PATHOLOGIC FEATURES

Gross Findings

▸ Enlarged, yellow, firm gland

Microscopic Findings

▸ Lymphocytes and plasma cells effacing pituitary
▸ Lymphoid follicles with germinal centers
▸ Fibrosis to a variable degree
▸ Epithelioid histiocytes but not granulomas

Pathologic Differential Diagnosis

▸ Pituitary adenoma, granulomatous inflammation, non-specific lymphocytic infiltrate

PATHOLOGIC FEATURES

The gland is enlarged, yellow and firm. The normal architecture is effaced by an extensive cellular infiltrate composed of lymphocytes and plasma cells (Figure 10-2). Lymphoid follicles with germinal centers may be evident. Fibrosis is present to a variable degree, although complete replacement by fibrosis can be identified (Figure 10-3). Well-formed granulomas are not present although epithelioid histiocytes may be seen.

DIFFERENTIAL DIAGNOSIS

The differential diagnosis includes a pituitary adenoma, granulomatous inflammation and non-specific lymphocytic infiltrate. Clinical and histologic correlation is required to render a definitive diagnosis.

PROGNOSIS AND THERAPY

The pituitary gland may regain normal size and endocrine function after surgical decompression and hormone replacement. If the diagnosis is suspected, a steroid trial may be therapeutic.

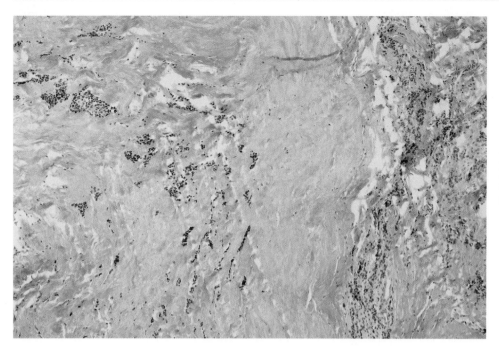

FIGURE 10-3
Late in the disease process of autoimmune hypophysitis, extensive fibrosis remains.

CIRCULATORY

A variety of circulatory disturbances may affect the pituitary gland, including infarction of a neoplasm (apoplexy), infarction (no tumor present) and necrosis.

CIRCULATORY
DISEASE FACT SHEET

Definition
▶ Hemorrhage followed by infarction and complete destruction of the pituitary gland or adenoma

Incidence and Location
▶ Rare

Morbidity and Mortality
▶ A neurologic emergency requiring immediate intervention

Clinical Features
▶ Sudden severe headache, nausea, vomiting, consciousness alterations and visual disturbances

Prognosis and Therapy
▶ Good, but a neurologic emergency requiring immediate surgery

INFARCTION (APOPLEXY)

CLINICAL FEATURES

Pituitary apoplexy is a major hemorrhagic event that results when there is rapid enlargement with hemorrhage, often accompanied with infarction, and complete destruction of a pituitary neoplasm (adenoma). Symptoms include sudden severe headache, nausea, vomiting, consciousness alterations, visual disturbances and ophthalmoplegia. Etiologic factors that may precipitate hemorrhage include head trauma, anticoagulation, thrombosis, bromocriptine and radiation therapy. Generally, large, non-functioning adenomas are affected, with approximately 10 percent of adenomas clinically presenting with apoplexy. Curiously, endocrinopathy may ameliorate or improve after hemorrhagic infarction.

PATHOLOGIC FEATURES

The specimen consists of necrotic tumor or blood, with the necrotic tissue often obscuring the underlying neoplasm (Figure 10-4). The underlying tumor can be accentuated with a reticulum stain, while immunohistochemical studies can 'prove' the underlying neoplasm.

DIFFERENTIAL DIAGNOSIS

Separation from infarction by histology alone is difficult, unless the underlying tumor is present. Infarction

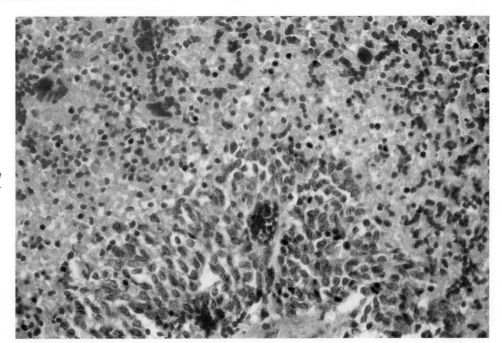

FIGURE 10-4
A pituitary adenoma is partially infarcted in this example of pituitary apoplexy.

CIRCULATORY PATHOLOGIC FEATURES

Gross Findings
▸ Blood clot and necrotic tumor

Microscopic Findings
▸ Pituitary adenoma is obscured by blood and necrosis
▸ Reticulum stain accentuates tumor growth pattern

Immunohistochemical Results
▸ Immunohistochemical studies prove adenoma type

Differential Diagnosis
▸ Infarction (no tumor present), Sheehan's syndrome (postpartum uterine hemorrhage Leading to vascular collapse which results in anterior pituitary ischemia and necrosis – pan hypopituitarism)

of the pituitary gland occurs with diabetes mellitus, sickle cell disease, increased intracranial pressure of any etiology, cerebrovascular accidents, and transection of the pituitary stalk. The inadequate perfusion of the pituitary gland leads to ischemia with subsequent necrosis. Hypopituitarism develops only after massive destruction of the anterior pituitary gland.

PROGNOSIS AND THERAPY

This is considered a neurologic emergency and requires immediate surgical intervention, as sudden death can occur without appropriate therapy.

NECROSIS (SHEEHAN'S SYNDROME)

Pituitary infarction associated with postpartum uterine hemorrhage resulting in permanent hypopituitarism is referred to as Sheehan's syndrome. It has been postulated that vasospasm in response to vascular collapse (shock) leads to pituitary ischemia and thrombosis. The posterior lobe is usually spared, since it is not dependent on the portal system for its blood supply. With time there is replacement of the necrotic tissue by fibrosis and atrophy of the anterior pituitary gland (Figure 10-5). resulting in marked pituitary insufficiency. Replacement hormone therapy is requisite.

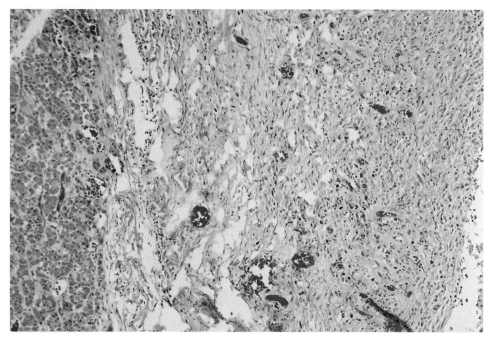

FIGURE 10-5
Scarring is nearly all that remains in this Sheehan's syndrome pituitary gland.

CYSTS

DERMOID

Slow growing cystic lesions in the sellar region (supra or intrasellar) resulting from inclusion of epithelial elements during closure of the neural tube.

CLINICAL FEATURES

This uncommon cyst usually occurs in childhood equally in boys and girls. Patients may be asymptomatic or present with headache and visual disturbances. Typically it arises in the midline in the posterior cranial fossa with a relationship to the fontanelle or the fourth ventricle.

RADIOLOGIC FEATURES

Computed tomography scan shows a low density mass, while MRI shows a heterogeneous signal intensity due to the presence of sebaceous material and hair in association with the cyst, along with a high signal intensity on T1 weighted imaging as a result of the increased lipid content (Figure 10-6).

**DERMOID
DISEASE FACT SHEET**

Definition
▶ Slow growing cystic lesion in the sellar region resulting from inclusion of epithelial elements during closure of the neural tube

Incidence and Location
▶ Rare
▶ Supra- or intrasellar, usually midline

Morbidity and Mortality
▶ Chemical meningitis with cyst leakage
▶ Rarely death related to malignant transformation

Gender, Race and Age Distribution
▶ Equal gender distribution
▶ Usually childhood

Clinical Features
▶ Headaches and visual disturbances

Prognosis and Therapy
▶ Recurrence will result if incompletely excised, with increased risk of infection
▶ Leakage of cyst contents may cause chemical meningitis
▶ Rare transformation into squamous cell carcinoma
▶ Surgery

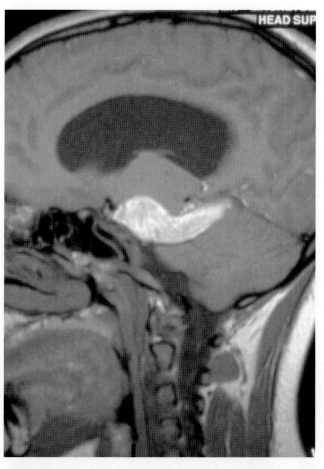

FIGURE 10-6
Mid-saggital MRI shows a mass with a high signal intensity on T1 weighted imaging as a result of the increased lipid content (Courtesy of Dr A Levy).

PATHOLOGIC FEATURES

GROSS FINDINGS

A thick walled, well delineated, encapsulated mass contains yellowish, greasy material, occasionally with hair and/or calcifications.

MICROSCOPIC FINDINGS

Desquamated epithelium and sebaceous secretions fill the cystic spaces which are lined by stratified squamous epithelium that may include cutaneous adnexal structures (sebaceous glands or hair follicles). A foreign body giant cell reaction (secondary to the cyst content) may be seen in and surrounding the thick fibrous connective tissue capsule. Mature bone is uncommon.

ANCILLARY STUDIES

While unnecessary for the diagnosis, epithelial markers (cytokeratin, epithelial membrane antigen) are present,

---

> **DERMOID**
> **PATHOLOGIC FEATURES**
>
> **Gross Findings**
> ▸ Encapsulated and well delineated mass
> ▸ Greasy cystic content, hair and/or calcifications
>
> **Microscopic Findings**
> ▸ Cystic spaces lined by stratified squamous epithelium
> ▸ Includes cutaneous adnexal structures
> ▸ Foreign body giant cell reaction and bone can be seen
>
> **Immunohistochemical Results**
> ▸ Positive epithelial markers
> ▸ CEA in adnexal structures
>
> **Pathologic Differential Diagnosis**
> ▸ Epidermoid cyst, craniopharyngioma

with adnexal structures reacting identically to their cutaneous counterparts.

DIFFERENTIAL DIAGNOSIS

The differential diagnosis includes epidermoid cysts and craniopharyngioma. Epidermoid cysts lack sebaceous differentiation, containing only keratinaceous debris. Craniopharyngioma has a stellate reticulum, basaloid cells, inflammatory debris and calcifications.

PROGNOSIS AND THERAPY

Incomplete resection results in recurrence, and with recurrence, there is an increased risk of infection. Occasionally, leakage of the cyst content may result in chemical meningitis. There are isolated reports of malignant transformation of the cystic epithelium into a squamous cell carcinoma. Surgical removal is the treatment of choice.

EPIDERMOID CYST

CLINICAL FEATURES

Also called a 'pearly tumor' and cholesteatoma, epidermoid cysts are more common than dermoid cysts. With a peak incidence in the fifth decade, there is an equal gender distribution. Patients may be asymptomatic or may present with headache and visual disturbances. The typical sites of occurrence are suprasellar and parasellar locations and is most frequent in the cerebellopontine angle. It is presumed to be of developmental origin although there are rare examples of iatrogenic 'implantation' of cutaneous epithelium secondary to lumbar puncture.

RADIOLOGIC FEATURES

Computed tomography scan shows a low density mass while MRI has a variable signal intensity dependent on the cyst content: high lipid content: bright (white) signal intensity on T1 weighted images; low lipid content: dark (black) signal intensity on T1 weighted images.

PATHOLOGIC FEATURES

GROSS FINDINGS

Most lesions are thin-walled, unilocular cysts with a smooth capsule, although a multilocular cystic mass is described. The contents are flaky, white ('pearly tumor'). They are often larger than dermoid cysts.

MICROSCOPIC FINDINGS

The capsule is usually thin, surrounding a cyst lined by a stratified squamous epithelium and filled with degenerating squames, cholesterol clefts and cellular debris (Figures 10-7 and 10-8). Skin adnexal structures are not present.

DIFFERENTIAL DIAGNOSIS

The differential diagnosis includes dermoid cysts and craniopharyngioma. Dermoid cysts have adnexal structures. Craniopharyngiomas have stellate reticulum, basaloid cells and calcification.

PROGNOSIS AND THERAPY

Incomplete resection results in recurrence, and with recurrence, there is an increased risk of infection. Occasionally, leakage of the cyst content may result in chemical meningitis. There are isolated reports of malignant transformation of the cystic epithelium into a squamous cell carcinoma. Surgical removal is the treatment of choice.

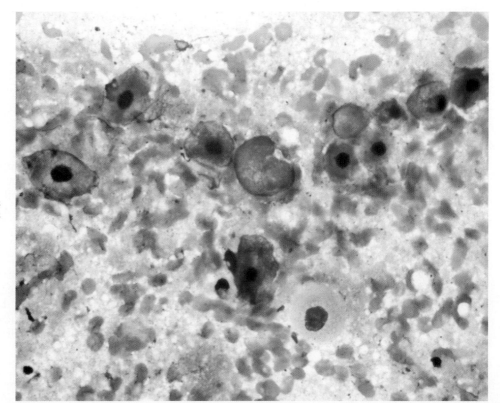

FIGURE 10-7

Smears show mature squamous cells in a backround of keratinaceous debris.

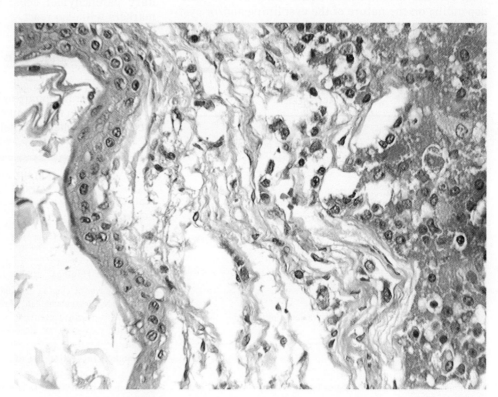

FIGURE 10-8

A squamous epithelial lined cyst is immediately adjacent to benign pituitary parenchyma in this epidermoid cyst. No adnexal structures were identified.

RATHKE'S POUCH CYST

Non-neoplastic intrasellar or suprasellar cystic mass derived from the remnants of Rathke's pouch lying between the developing anterior and intermediate lobes of the pituitary gland.

CLINICAL FEATURES

The clinically significant incidence is unknown, but up to 20% of patients will have a Rathke's pouch cyst at autopsy. There is no gender predilection with an occurrence over a wide age range although most common in adults. The symptoms vary according to size and location with most lesions being asymptomatic. If large enough, they impinge on the optic chiasm, resulting in disturbances of the visual fields or hypothalamic/pituitary function.

RADIOLOGIC FEATURES

All techniques demonstrate sellar enlargement and erosion; CT shows an intrasellar cystic mass with or without suprasellar extension that does not enhance with contrast media; MRI's signal intensity will vary depending on the nature of the cyst lining and/or cyst content: simple cyst with clear fluid has a signal inten-

sity of cerebrospinal fluid; high protein content in the fluid appear hyperintense (white) on nonenhanced T1 weighted imaging.

PATHOLOGIC FEATURES

GROSS FINDINGS

They are generally composed of a thin walled cystic structure with variable cyst content, usually <1 cm in diameter. An epithelial lining may be difficult to appreciate macroscopically and a few cases have mucin filling the cyst.

MICROSCOPIC FINDINGS

A single layer of ciliated cuboidal or columnar epithelium with mucus secretory cells is characteristic (Figure 10-9), but may be replaced by metaplastic squamous epithelium. Mucus is usually seen in the cyst. Pituitary parenchymal cells are variably present.

ANCILLARY STUDIES

The cyst lining is cytokeratin and EMA positive, with chromogranin/synaptophysin highlighting the pituitary parenchymal cells; pituitary peptide hormone markers will also react.

DIFFERENTIAL DIAGNOSIS

Suprasellar craniopharyngiomas, arachnoid cysts and mucoceles from the paranasal sinuses. Arachnoid cysts are lined by meningothelial cells which are S-100

RATHKE'S POUCH CYST
DISEASE FACT SHEET

Definition
▸ Cystic mass derived from remnants of Rathke's pouch between the anterior and intermediate lobes of the pituitary

Incidence and Location
▸ Up to 20% of patients (in autopsy series)

Gender, Race and Age Distribution
▸ Equal gender distribution
▸ Usually adults

Clinical Features
▸ Most are asymptomatic
▸ If large (>1 cm), visual field or hypothalamic/pituitary function alterations

Radiologic Findings
▸ Sellar enlargement and erosion
▸ Intrasellar cystic mass, with signal intensity varying based on cyst content (MRI)

Prognosis and Therapy
▸ Benign lesions usually cured with surgery

RATHKE'S POUCH CYST
PATHOLOGIC FEATURES

Gross Findings
▸ Thin walled cyst with a variable cyst content, usually <1 cm
▸ Thick mucus may fill the cyst

Microscopic Findings
▸ Single layer of ciliated cuboidal to columnar epithelium
▸ Squamous metaplasia can be seen
▸ Mucus is usually present
▸ Pituitary parenchymal cells are variably present

Immunohistochemical Results
▸ Cyst lining is keratin and EMA reactive
▸ Pituitary parenchymal cells will be chromogranin/synaptophysin and peptide hormone marker positive

Pathologic Differential Diagnosis
▸ Craniopharyngioma, arachnoid cysts, mucoceles

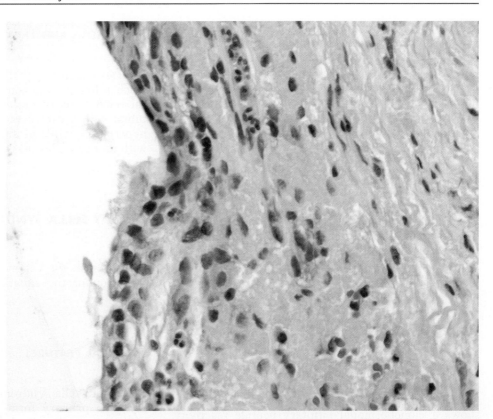

FIGURE 10-9
The left part of the field demonstrates a ciliated epithelium subtended by a few pituitary parenchymal cells, with fibrosis occupying the majority of the sample in this Rathke's pouch cyst.

protein positive. The separation of sinonasal tract mucocele from Rathke's pouch cyst requires radiographic identification of direct extension from the paranasal sinuses into the intracranial cavity: histology is identical.

PROGNOSIS AND THERAPY

These benign lesions are usually cured with surgery.

HYPERPLASIA

Nodular or diffuse, focal or multifocal abnormal increase in the number of parenchymal pituicytes; in general, only a single cell type predominates in pituitary hyperplasia.

CLINICAL FEATURES

This is a rare disorder without a gender predilection, occurring in a wide age range. It may be primary or may be secondary to ectopic hormone-related substances produced by extrapituitary neoplasms or by loss of the negative feedback to the pituitary gland in various chronic hypofunctioning endocrine conditions, such as:

HYPERPLASIA
DISEASE FACT SHEET

Definition
▶ Nodular/diffuse, focal or multifocal abnormal increase in the number of endocrine cells

Incidence and Location
▶ Rare

Gender, Race and Age Distribution
▶ Equal gender distribution
▶ Wide age range

Clinical Features
▶ Depends upon loss of negative feedback in chronic hypofunctioning endocrine conditions and which hormone is affected (ACTH, Prolactin, TSH, FSH, LH)
▶ Ectopic hormone production by an extrapituitary neoplasm

Prognosis and Therapy
▶ Medical management of the underlying endocrinopathy
▶ Resection of the extrapituitary hormone secreting tumor
▶ Pituitary surgery if primary

• Adenocorticotroph cell (ACTH) hyperplasia in untreated Addison's disease and in association with ectopic production of ACTH releasing substances by extrapituitary (neuroendocrine) tumors;
• Prolactin cell hyperplasia during pregnancy and lactation, estrogen therapy, or in the pituitary immediately adjacent to a prolactin cell adenoma;

- Thyrotroph cell hyperplasia (TSH) in patients with long-standing hypothyroidism.

Interestingly, in postmenopausal women, the pituitary tends to be small without gonadotroph hyperplasia despite the decreased production of follicle stimulating hormone (FSH) or luteinizing hormone (LH) and increased secretion of FSH and LH by the pituitary gonadotrophic cells.

PATHOLOGIC FEATURES

A definitive diagnosis is impossible on a small biopsy, as the process may be a focal or multifocal, nodular or diffuse hyperplastic proliferation of pituitary cells. Special studies are necessary to aid in diagnosis.

ANCILLARY STUDIES

In the nodular form, a reticulin stain shows acinar expansion while still retaining the acinar configuration of the gland, while immunohistochemistry usually shows a monohormonal pituitary peptide reactivity. Rarely, there is plurihormonal pituitary peptide reactivity.

In the diffuse form, while very difficult to separate from a pituitary adenoma, there is a retention of the delicate reticulin fibers throughout the cellular proliferation (similar to normal pituitary). In tumors, there is a disruption or loss of the reticulin pattern.

DIFFERENTIAL DIAGNOSIS

The separation from a microadenoma versus adenoma can be difficult. However, reticulin and immunohistochemical studies can help.

HYPERPLASIA
PATHOLOGIC FEATURES

Microscopic Findings
- Focal or multifocal
- Nodular or diffuse proliferation
- Special studies needed to confirm

Ancillary Studies
- Nodular: reticulin shows acinar expansion but architectural retention and usually a monohormonal peptide reactivity
- Diffuse: reticulin shows delicate reticulin fibers throughout the proliferation and usually a monohormonal peptide reactivity

Pathologic Differential Diagnosis
- Microadenoma, adenoma

PROGNOSIS AND THERAPY

Medical treatment of the underlying endocrinopathy (such as hypothyroidism or Addison's disease) or surgical removal of an extrapituitary hormone producing tumor will treat cases causing secondary pituitary hyperplasia, while pituitary surgery is used for those with an intrasellar mass lesion.

EMPTY SELLA SYNDROME

Reduction in the volume of sellar content due to the extension of the subarachnoid space into the sella turcica.

CLINICAL FEATURES

The empty sella syndrome can be primary or secondary. The primary form is due to an incomplete or incompetent sellar diaphragm, with downward herniation of the arachnoid membrane (intrasellar arachnoidocele) resulting in pituitary compression. While nearly 50% of adults have a diaphragmatic defect by autopsy studies, primary empty sella syndrome is uncommon. Women are disproportionately affected.

EMPTY SELLA SYNDROME
DISEASE FACT SHEET

Definition
- Reduction in volume of sellar content

Incidence and Location
- While a diaphragmatic defect is present in nearly 50% of adults, primary empty sellar is uncommon

Gender, Race and Age Distribution
- Both forms affect women more commonly than men
- Usually middle aged

Clinical Features
- Primary or secondary forms are separated
- Incidental radiographic finding
- Headache of long-standing duration
- Visual field defects and impaired pituitary function
- CSF rhinorrhea into sphenoid sinus

Prognosis and Therapy
- Good, with most cases requiring no treatment
- If there is a CSF leak, surgery may be necessary

The secondary form results from surgery, irradiation and hemorrhage/infarction (see circulatory section) and usually occurs in middle age, hypertensive, obese women.

Frequently an incidental radiographic finding, patients often complain of headache of long-standing duration. Visual field defects or impaired pituitary function may also be present, although not usually a clinical endocrine-related syndrome. While infrequent, rhinorrhea of the cerebrospinal fluid into the sphenoid sinuses through an eroded sella floor due to increased intracranial pressure is noteworthy.

RADIOLOGIC FEATURES

Computed tomography shows an intrasellar low density area consistent with empty sella syndrome.

PATHOLOGIC FEATURES

The arachnoid membrane may be the only tissue identified, although an adenoma may be present in secondary cases.

EMPTY SELLA SYNDROME
PATHOLOGIC FEATURES

Microscopic Findings
▸ Arachnoid membrane in primary cases
▸ Adenoma may be seen in secondary cases

Pathologic Differential Diagnosis
▸ Pituitary tumor

DIFFERENTIAL DIAGNOSIS

A pituitary tumor may be present, especially in secondary form.

PROGNOSIS AND THERAPY

Uncomplicated empty sella syndrome requires no treatment, although spontaneous leak of CSF is usually an indication for surgical management.

SUGGESTED READING

Inflammatory Lesions

Asa SL. Tumor-like lesions of the sella turcica. Tumors of the Pituitary Gland. Atlas of Tumor Pathology, Third Series, Fascicle 22. Washington, DC: Armed Forces Institute of Pathology, 1998:191–210.

Beressi N, Beressi J-P, Cohen R, Modigliani E. Lymphocytic hypophysitis. A review of 145 cases. Ann Med Interne 1999;150:327–341.

Lloyd RV, Douglas BR, Young WF Jr. Pituitary gland. Endocrine Diseases. Atlas of Nontumor Pathology, First Series, Fascicle 1. Washington, DC: Armed Forces Institute of Pathology, 2002:1–44.

Missler U, Mack M, Nowack G, et al. Pituitary sarcoidosis. Klin Wochenschr 1990;68:342–345.

Pestell RG, Best JD, Alford FP. Lymphocytic hypophysitis. The clinical spectrum of the disorder and evidence for an autoimmune pathogenesis. Clin Endocrinol 1990;33:457–466.

Tashiro T, Sano T, Xu B, Wakatsuki S, et al. Spectrum of different types of hypophysitis: a clinicopathologic study of hypophysitis in 31 cases. Endocr Pathol 2002;13:183–195.

Tindall GT, Barrow L. Pituitary deficiency states. In: Tindall GT, Barrow L, eds. Disorders of the pituitary. St. Louis: The C. V. Mosby Co., 1986;455–456.

Circulatory

Asa SL. Tumor-like lesions of the sella turcica. Tumors of the Pituitary Gland. Atlas of Tumor Pathology, Third Series, Fascicle 22. Washington, DC: Armed Forces Institute of Pathology, 1998:191–210.

Berthelot JL, Rey A. [Pituitary apoplexy.] Presse Med 1995;24:501–503.

Goswami R, Kochupillai N, Crock PA, et al. Pituitary autoimmunity in patients with Sheehan's syndrome. J Clin Endocrinol Metab 2002;87: 4137–4141.

Lloyd RV. Non-neoplastic lesions, including hyperplasia. In: Surgical pathology of the pituitary gland. Vol. 27, In: Major problems in pathology. Philadelphia: W. B. Saunders Co., 1993;26–28.

Lloyd RV, Douglas BR, Young WF Jr. Pituitary gland. Endocrine Diseases. Atlas of Nontumor Pathology, First Series, Fascicle 1. Washington, DC: Armed Forces Institute of Pathology, 2002:1–44.

Prager D, Braunstein GD. Pituitary disorders during pregnancy. Endocrinol Metab Clin North Am 1995;24:1–14.

Cysts

Asa SL. Tumor-like lesions of the sella turcica. Tumors of the Pituitary Gland. Atlas of Tumor Pathology, Third Series, Fascicle 22. Washington, DC: Armed Forces Institute of Pathology, 1998:191–210.

Hirano A, Hirano M. Benign cysts in the central nervous system: neuropathological observations of the cyst walls. Neuropathology 2004;24: 1–7.

Ikeda H, Yoshimoto T. Clinicopathological study of Rathke's cleft cysts. Clin Neuropathol 2002;21:82–91.

Kasperbauer JL, Orvidas LJ, Atkinson JL, Abboud CF. Rathke cleft cyst: diagnostic and therapeutic considerations. Laryngoscope 2002;112: 1836–1839.

Lloyd RV, Douglas BR, Young WF Jr. Pituitary gland. Endocrine Diseases. Atlas of Nontumor Pathology, First Series, Fascicle 1. Washington, DC: Armed Forces Institute of Pathology, 2002:1–44.

Lunardi P, Missori P, Gagliardi FM, Firtuna A. Dermoid cysts of the posterior cranial fossa in children. Report of nine cases and review of the literature. Surg Neurol 1990;34:39–42.

Teramoto A, Hirakawa K, Sanno N, Osamura Y. Incidental pituitary lesions in 1,000 unselected autopsy specimens. Radiology 1994;193:161–164.

Hyperplasia

Asa SL. Tumor-like lesions of the sella turcica. Tumors of the Pituitary Gland. Atlas of Tumor Pathology, Third Series, Fascicle 22. Washington, DC: Armed Forces Institute of Pathology, 1998:191–210.

Jay V, Kovacs K, Horvath E, et al. Idiopathic prolactin cell hyperplasia of the pituitary mimicking prolactin cell adenoma: a morphological study including immunocytochemistry, electron microscopy, and in situ hybridization. Acta Neuropathol 1991;82:147–151.

Kovacs K, Horvath E. Hyperplasia. In: Tumors of the pituitary gland. Atlas of tumor pathology. Fascicle 21, second series. Armed Forces Institute of Pathology. Washington, 1986:210–216.

Lloyd RV. Non-neoplastic pituitary lesions, including hyperplasia. In: Surgical pathology of the pituitary gland. Major problems in pathology, Vol. 27. Philadelphia: W. B. Saunders Co., 1993;28.

Lloyd RV, Douglas BR, Young WF Jr. Pituitary gland. Endocrine Diseases. Atlas of Nontumor Pathology, First Series, Fascicle 1. Washington, DC: Armed Forces Institute of Pathology, 2002:1–44.

Moran A, Asa SL, Kovacs K, et al. Gigantism due to pituitary mammosomatotroph hyperplasia. N Engl J Med 1990;323:322–327.

Scheithauer BW, Sano T, Kovacs K, et al. The pituitary gland in pregnancy: a clinicopathologic and immunohistochemical study of 69 cases. Mayo Clin Proc 1990;65:461–474.

Empty Sellar Syndrome

Asa SL. Tumor-like lesions of the sella turcica. Tumors of the Pituitary Gland. Atlas of Tumor Pathology, Third Series, Fascicle 22. Washington, DC: Armed Forces Institute of Pathology, 1998:191–210.

Bakiri F, Bendib SE, Maoui R, et al. The sella turcica in Sheehan's syndrome: computerized tomographic study in 54 patients. J Endocrinol Invest 1991;14:193–196.

Bergeron C, Kovacs K, Bilbao JM. Primary 'empty sella.' A histologic and immunologic study. Arch Intern Med 1979;139:248–249.

Bergland RM, Ray BS, Torack RM. Anatomical variations in the pituitary gland and adjacent structures in 225 human autopsy cases. J Neurosurg 1968;28:93–99.

Gharib H, Frey HM, Laws ER Jr, et al. Co-existent primary empty sella syndrome and hyperprolactinemia: report of 11 cases. Arch Intern Med 1983;143:1383–1386.

Lloyd RV, Douglas BR, Young WF Jr. Pituitary gland. Endocrine Diseases. Atlas of Nontumor Pathology, First Series, Fascicle 1. Washington, DC: Armed Forces Institute of Pathology, 2002:1–44.

Benign Neoplasms of the Pituitary Gland

Lester DR Thompson • Clara S Heffess

GENERAL CONSIDERATIONS

Pituitary tumors represent about 15% of all intracranial tumors. They are divided into benign and malignant, primary and secondary, epithelial and non-epithelial. The vast majority arise from hormone-producing cells. The adenomas are classified by size (< or >1 cm), function (hormone producing or not), immunophenotype (various hormone markers), cell type (chromophobe, basophilic, acidophilic), quantity of hormone (mono- or plurihormonal), secretory granule content (sparsely or densely granulated), and biologic behavior (benign, invasive, malignant). Most pituitary adenomas were subclinical and null cell type. With more sophisticated radiographic imaging and more sensitive laboratory studies (radioimmunoassay) smaller and smaller tumors are being detected.

The clinical manifestations are exceedingly important, with symptoms and laboratory studies suggesting the diagnosis in most cases. Therefore, since this book is not a clinical endocrinology text, only key clinical and laboratory features will be highlighted in each tumor type. Adenomas in general are more common in women than men, but is partly cell type dependent (growth hormone-secreting tumors are more common in males). Patients are affected in the third to sixth decades, although growth hormone-secreting tumors are more common in children than adults. Tumors in children seem to be more aggressive than those of adults. Endocrinopathy manifestations are dependent upon the cell type(s), but increasing tumor size results in headaches and visual field disturbances due to compression of the optic chiasm. Only about 3% of pituitary adenomas are associated with a multiple endocrine neoplasia (MEN) syndrome.

Computed tomography (CT) scans (coronal specifically) and magnetic resonance imaging (MRI) is used to define the exact location and extent of the tumor, with MRI resulting in better images (bone artifacts in CT obscure the lesion). Contrast enhanced CT or MRI scans show hypodense/hypointense microadenomas, while macroadenomas have uniform enhancement, with T1 weighted imaging producing an isointense, strong enhancement (Figure 11-1). Pituitary adenomas have been classified according to their radiologic findings into grades I–IV lesions, based on size and presence of bone erosion.

The immunohistochemical features identified in all pituitary adenomas include reactivity with cytokeratin and various neuroendocrine markers (chromogranin [Figure 11-2], synaptophysin and neuron specific enolase). This immunoreactivity is not specific but confirms a diagnosis in conjunction with the clinical, radiographic and other pathologic (light microscopy) findings. Whereas the ultrastructural features of pituitary adenomas vary according to cell type, nearly all have intracytoplasmic electron dense neurosecretory granules that vary in size from 100 to >1000 nm in diameter.

Treatment options include surgery (trans-sphenoidal approach), pharmacotherapy and radiation. Most patients have an excellent prognosis. The most common malignant pituitary tumor is a metastasis to the gland.

PROLACTIN CELL ADENOMA

A benign, well-differentiated neoplasm composed of lactotroph cells.

CLINICAL FEATURES

Prolactinomas are the most common pituitary adenoma, accounting for about 25% of all adenomas. The vast majority are microadenomas (<1 cm; Figures 11-3 and 11-4). Women are affected more commonly than men, with a peak incidence between 20–30 years. Women tend to have microadenomas (<1 cm) and hyperprolactinemia which results in amenorrhea, galactorrhea and infertility. About 30% of women with amenorrhea and galactorrhea have a prolactin secreting tumor. Men tend to have macroadenomas (>1 cm) and present with gonadal dysfunction, decreased libido and impotence; gynecomastia is rare. The macroadenomas tend to be more aggressive or invasive, which result in mass symptoms (headache, visual field disturbances), while also yielding a higher prolactin level (serum prolactin levels appear to parallel tumor size). Whereas there are many causes for increased prolactin levels (pregnancy, nursing, hypothyroidism, drugs [antidepressants, antihypertensives, estrogen], stress, sarcoid, metastatic tumors, other pituitary tumors), a serum prolactin

PROLACTIN CELL ADENOMA
DISEASE FACT SHEET

Definition

▶ Benign neoplasm composed of lactotroph cells

Incidence and Location

▶ About 25% of all pituitary adenomas
▶ Lateral or posterior anterior pituitary gland

Morbidity and Mortality

▶ Hormone excess
▶ No mortality identified

Gender, Race and Age Distribution

▶ Female > Male
▶ Peak between 20–30 years

Clinical Features

▶ Women: amenorrhea, galactorrhea and infertility
▶ Men: gonadal dysfunction, decreased libido and impotence
▶ Serum prolactin level >250 ng/mL
▶ Thyrotropin releasing hormone (TRH) stimulation: decreased prolactin response

Prognosis and Therapy

▶ Good, although recurrences develop more frequently in large tumors, patients with exceptionally high serum prolactin levels, and men
▶ Surgery and pharmacotherapy (Bromocriptine)
▶ Radiation for recurrent or persistent disease

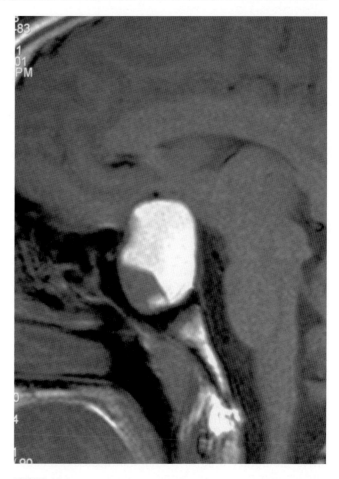

FIGURE 11-1

T1 weighted MR image produces an isointense, strong enhancement within this pituitary adenoma (courtesy of Dr A Levy).

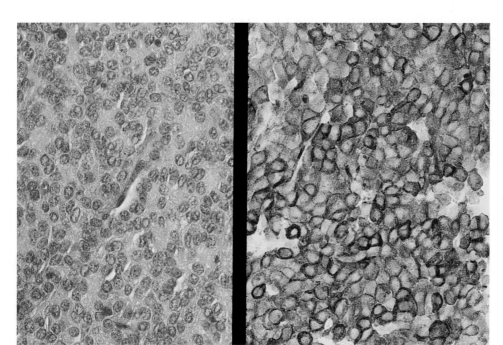

FIGURE 11-2

The growth of pituitary adenomas can be quite variable (solid, left), but the neuroendocrine nature of the neoplasm is confirmed with a neuroendocrine marker (chromogranin, right).

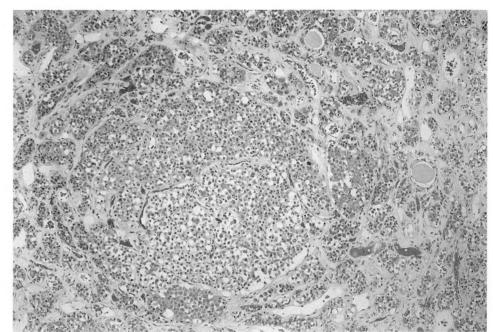

FIGURE 11-3

A microadenoma is a well formed nodule of neoplastic cells in the pituitary parenchyma.

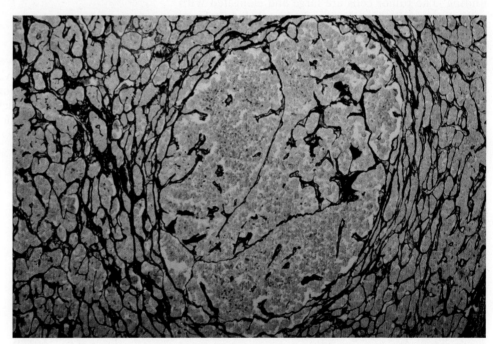

FIGURE 11-4

A microadenoma displays disruption of the reticulin fibers (reticulin stain).

level of over 250 ng/mL is diagnostic of pituitary adenoma (although several separate samples should be tested to be certain). Separation from hypothalamic disease can be attempted with the thyrotropin releasing hormone (TRH) stimulation, followed by measuring the prolactin response (diminished response in adenoma patients). However, the findings are inconsistent in some cases.

RADIOLOGIC FEATURES

The size of a tumor and the degree of extension can be determined, along with contrast enhancement and gland homogeneity. Gadolinium coronal T1 MR images show a dynamic relationship, with microadenomas initially (first minute) showing less contrast enhancement than the surrounding pituitary. However, radiology evaluation is not always helpful.

PATHOLOGIC FEATURES

Most tumors involved the lateral or posterior parts of the anterior pituitary gland. Diffuse, papillary and fibrotic patterns are seen, the latter usually an autopsy finding. The tumor cells are large and elongated with irregular nuclei, prominent nucleoli and slightly basophilic cytoplasm. Cell membranes are indistinct (Figure 11-5). Calcifications are common, including psammoma bodies (about 20%). Amyloid is less frequent (up to 10%). Cyst formation is present in the fibrotic type. Tumors are separated into the most common 'sparsely granulated' (chromophobe) adenoma, and the much less common 'densely granulated' (acidophil) adenoma.

PROLACTIN CELL ADENOMA PATHOLOGIC FEATURES

Gross Findings
- Microadenomas (<1 cm) in females
- Macroadenomas (>1 cm) in males

Microscopic Findings
- Diffuse, papillary or fibrotic patterns of growth
- Large cells with slightly basophilic cytoplasm and prominent nucleoli
- Calcification (including psammoma bodies) is common
- Sparsely granulated (chromophobic) adenoma is much more common than densely granulated (acidophil) adenoma
- About 50% are invasive at the time of surgery

Ultrastructural Features
- Numerous electron dense 200 to 300 nm granules
- Prominent rough endoplasmic reticulum forming concentric whorls (Neberkerns)
- Misplaced granule exocytosis

Immunohistochemical Results
- Prolactin positive, accentuated in the Golgi region
- Chromogranin B reactive (absent chromogranin A)

Pathologic Differential Diagnosis
- Other pituitary adenomas, sphenoid or nasopharyngeal neoplasms

---

The latter has irregular ovoid nuclei in polyhedral cells which are separated by a vascular stroma. Nearly 50% of prolactinomas have bone erosion and suprasellar growth at presentation, including elevation of the sellar diaphragm, rostral extension into the sphenoid sinus or

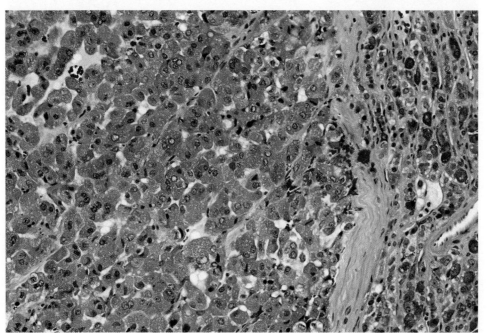

FIGURE 11-5

Prolactin adenomas have large cells with slightly basophilic cytoplasm and indistinct cell membranes. Separation from the surrounding parenchyma is noted.

lateral extension into the cavernous sinus. Treatment effects after dopamine agonists include decreased cell size, increased nuclear to cytoplasmic ratio and perivascular and interstitial fibrosis.

ANCILLARY STUDIES

ULTRASTRUCTURAL FEATURES

Large, lactotroph cells with round to oval cytoplasmic electron dense granules averaging 200–300 nm in diameter (slightly smaller than normal lactotrophs of 350 nm), prominent rough endoplastic reticulum forming concentric whorls (Neberkerns; Figure 11-6), large Golgi apparatus, and misplaced, lateral cell wall granule exocytosis (Figure 11-7) are helpful in confirming the diagnosis.

IMMUNOHISTOCHEMICAL RESULTS

In addition to the epithelial markers, there is strong and diffuse immunoreactivity with prolactin, specifically accentuated in the Golgi region in the sparsely granulated adenomas (Figure 11-8). This tumor type *does not* react with chromogranin A, but reacts with chromogranin B and synaptophysin.

DIFFERENTIAL DIAGNOSIS

Other pituitary adenomas and tumors of the sphenoid, pharynx and nasopharynx can sometimes cause confusion. However, histology and special studies will separate these lesions.

PROGNOSIS AND THERAPY

The goal of the treatment is the suppression of excessive hormone production with decrease of prolactin levels, decrease of the size of any demonstrable tumor, restoration of normal function and prevention of recurrence or progression of the disease. Surgery is the mainstay of therapy, although usually only successful in microadenomas and patients with serum prolactin levels <250 ng/mL. Bromocriptine (an inhibitor of prolactin secretion) decreases serum prolactin levels and gives symptomatic relief, but symptoms reappear with discontinuance of use. Radiation is usually employed for recurrent or persistent disease, which develops in up to 20% of patients, more often men.

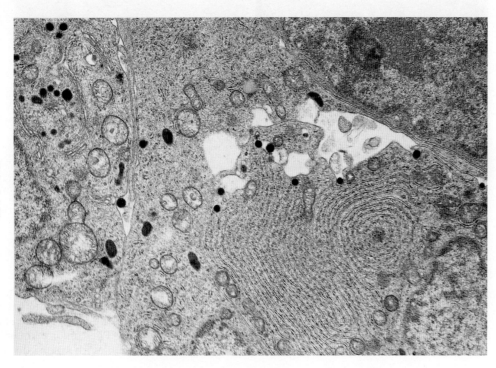

FIGURE 11-6
This prolactin cell adenoma has extensively developed, highly organized RER forming concentric whorls. Exocytoses are also seen (magnification 8100×) (courtesy of Dr E Horvath).

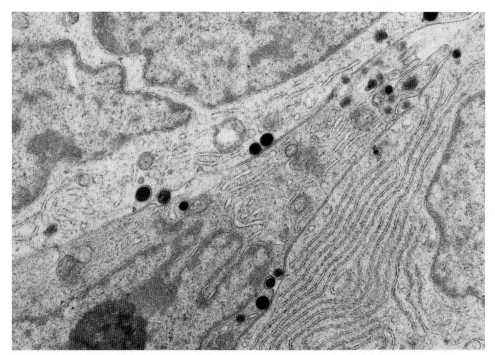

FIGURE 11-7
A prolactin cell adenoma with 'misplaced' exocytosis. Identified along the lateral cell membranes, this is the ultrastructural marker of prolactin differentiation. Two extruded granules are well defined while others are already fading (magnification 10 400×) (courtesy of Dr E Horvath).

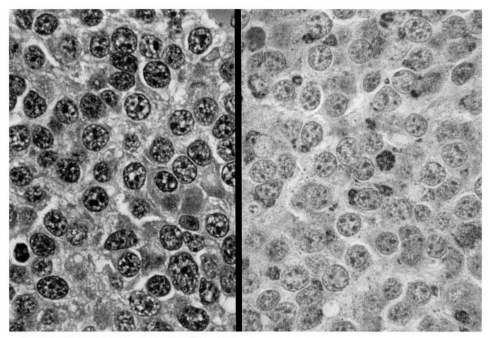

FIGURE 11-8
Monotonous neoplastic cells of a prolactin producing adenoma (left) demonstrate strong, perinuclear 'Golgi region' prolactin immunoreactivity (right).

GROWTH HORMONE-PRODUCING ADENOMA

A benign neoplasm composed of somatotrophs causing either acromegaly or gigantism depending upon whether the epiphyseal plate is closed.

CLINICAL FEATURES

Growth hormone (GH) producing adenomas are the second most common type of pituitary adenoma accounting for approximately 25% of all pituitary adenomas. The tumor primarily affects middle age women and men, with an insidious onset and slow progression.

GROWTH HORMONE-PRODUCING ADENOMA DISEASE FACT SHEET

Definition
▸ Benign neoplasm composed of somatotrophs causing acromegaly or gigantism

Incidence and Location
▸ Second most common adenoma
▸ About 25% of pituitary adenomas

Morbidity and Mortality
▸ Post-operative complications (rhinorrhea, visual loss, infection)

Gender, Race and Age Distribution
▸ Equal gender distribution
▸ Middle age

Clinical Features
▸ Slowly progressive
▸ Bone enlargement with increased hand, foot and hat size
▸ Paresthesias of the hands, muscle weakness, joint pain
▸ Hypertension, sleep apnea and voice changes
▸ Depression in women and change in libido in men
▸ Elevated GH levels, non-suppressed by oral glucose

Prognosis and Therapy
▸ Good, although cardiovascular disease is most common cause of death
▸ Surgery is potentially curative, although radiation and pharmacotherapy is employed with variable results

GROWTH HORMONE-PRODUCING ADENOMA PATHOLOGIC FEATURES

Microscopic Findings
▸ Depends upon which type is identified by immunohistochemistry and ultrastructural features
▸ *Sparsely granulated*: irregular, pleomorphic nuclei with a pale, spherical intracytoplasmic inclusion body
▸ *Acidophil stem cell*: often invasive, contains diagnostic large cytoplasmic vacuoles

Ultrastructural Features
▸ *Densely granulated GH cell adenoma*: Cytoplasm contains numerous round or fusiform granules 300–400 nm in diameter
▸ *Sparsely granulated GH cell adenoma*: 200 nm secretory granules, parallel RER arrays, and 'fibrous body'
▸ *Mixed GH cell and prolactin cell adenoma*: Lactotroph and somatotroph cells
▸ *Mammosomatotroph cell adenoma*: Small (400 nm) and large (2000 nm), pleomorphic granules; electron dense intercellular material (extruded secretory granules)
▸ *Acidophil stem cell adenoma*: Giant, abnormal mitochondria and sparse secretory granules <200 nm

Immunohistochemical Results
▸ GH immunoreactive in all
▸ Sparsely granulated has peri-fibrous body reactivity
▸ Plurihormonal tumors have two co-existing cell populations or a single cell population producing two hormones (mammosomatotroph and acidophil stem cell types)

Pathologic Differential Diagnosis
▸ Clinically between Beckwith-Wiedemann syndrome, cerebral gigantism, Paget's disease and prognathism (all have normal GH levels)

However, mammosomatotroph adenomas occur in younger patients who present with gigantism.

Clinical manifestations are based on excess hormone (with somatomedin effect), mass effect or adenohypophyseal hypofunction. GH is controlled by a complex feedback inhibition hypothalamic regulation, working through somatomedins or insulin-like growth factors to achieve its effect. Symptoms include increased hand, foot and hat size (acromegaly), prognathism, paresthesias of the hands, muscle weakness, joint pain, sleep apnea (tongue and uvula enlargement), hypertension and cardiovascular disease (left ventricular hypertrophy), menstrual alterations (amenorrhea), depression, change in libido or impotence, and diabetes mellitus. Elevation of serum or plasma levels of GH that do not suppress with the administration of oral glucose is most helpful.

RADIOLOGIC FEATURES

Skull radiographs showing thickening of the skull, increased bone density and sinus enlargement (frontal bossing) show the *effects* of GH rather than the small pituitary adenoma demonstrated by CT or MR.

PATHOLOGIC FEATURES

Five different types of adenomas are recognized in association with acromegaly with the various adenomas differing in cellular and morphological composition, hormonal production and biologic behavior. Monohormonal variants are more common than bi-hormonal variants, although three of the GH producing tumor types are plurihormonal. While immunohistochemistry confirms the presence of GH, ultrastructural studies are necessary to determine the morphologic type. Space limitations preclude an exhaustive discussion, but key differences are highlighted:

• *Densely granulated GH cell adenoma*: Also called an acidophilic adenoma it is a vascular tumor with diffuse, trabecular or sinusoid patterns. The cells are medium sized, polyhedral with round nuclei and granular acidophilic cytoplasm.

• *Sparsely granulated GH cell adenoma*: This chromophobic cell adenoma has variably sized cells with irregular, pleomorphic, eccentric, single or multiple nuclei. There is a pale, spherical intracytoplasmic

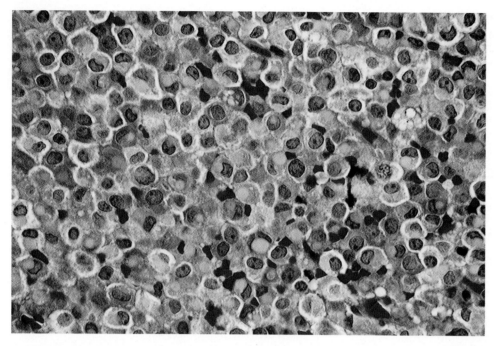

FIGURE 11-9

A sparsely granulated GH cell adenoma demonstrates a fibrous body or intracytoplasmic spherical inclusion in many of the tumor cells (pale staining body).

inclusion (fibrous body), diagnostic for this tumor type (Figure 11-9).

- *Mixed GH cell and prolactin cell adenoma*: Two distinct cell populations.
- *Mammosomatotroph cell adenoma*: Derived from mammosomatotroph cells, there is a diffuse growth of a single cell type which produce both hormones along with extracellular growth hormone deposits.
- *Acidophil stem cell adenoma*: Also called an 'invasive adenoma', it is a stem cell derived, predominantly prolactin-producing with only limited GH reaction neoplasm arranged in a diffuse pattern. Large cytoplasmic vacuoles may reach the size of the nucleus and are diagnostic. It is important to recognize as it tends to be more aggressive, invading local structures and reaching a larger size.

ANCILLARY STUDIES

ULTRASTRUCTURAL FEATURES

- *Densely granulated GH cell adenoma:* cytoplasm contains numerous round or fusiform granules (crystallization of secretory material) ranging from 350–500 nm in diameter, prominent Golgi apparatus and well developed rough endoplasmic reticulum (RER) (Figure 11-10).
- *Sparsely granulated GH cell adenoma:* small, sparse secretory granules averaging 200 nm in diameter and parallel RER arrays (Figure 11-11).
- *Mixed GH cell and prolactin cell adenoma:* contain two populations comprised of lactotroph and somatotroph cells.
- *Mammosomatotroph cell adenoma:* variably sized cytoplasmic secretory granules: smaller, round granules up to 400 nm in diameter; larger, pleomorphic

granules up to 2000 nm in diameter. Electron dense intercellular material (extruded secretory granules) is diagnostic (Figure 11-12).
- *Acidophil stem cell adenoma:* giant, abnormal mitochondria visible by light microscopy as vacuoles are diagnostic (Figure 11-13); small, sparse secretory granules <200 nm, along with misplaced exocytosis and fibrous bodies.

IMMUNOHISTOCHEMICAL RESULTS

All of the GH cell adenomas have GH immunoreactivity. Specifically, the sparsely granulated type has accentuated reactivity in the Golgi region and around fibrous bodies (which are keratin reactive [Figure 11-14]). The plurihormonal tumors have two co-existing cell populations, with the staining density and pattern depending upon the proportion of each population. In the mammosomatotroph cell and acidophil stem cell types, both hormones are found in the same tumor cell (confirmed by electron-gold immunohistochemistry).

DIFFERENTIAL DIAGNOSIS

The differential diagnosis is a clinical one, with separation of cerebral gigantism, Beckwith-Wiedemann syndrome, Paget's disease, and simple prognathism from a pituitary adenoma by normal GH levels.

PROGNOSIS AND THERAPY

Densely granulated GH adenomas are slow growing tumors with a better prognosis than the sparsely

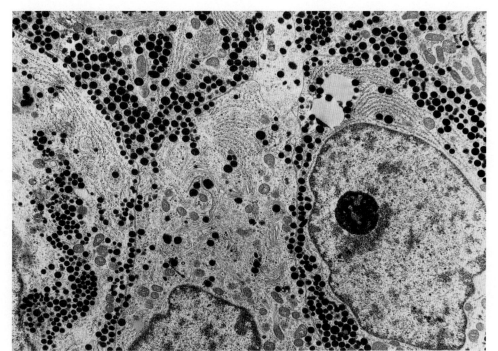

FIGURE 11-10

Densely granulated GH cell adenoma. The centrally placed nucleus, parallel arrays of often peripherally placed RER, prominent Golgi region and numerous large (chiefly 350–500 nm) secretory granules are typical for this neoplasm (magnification, 5300×). (Courtesy of Dr E Horvath.)

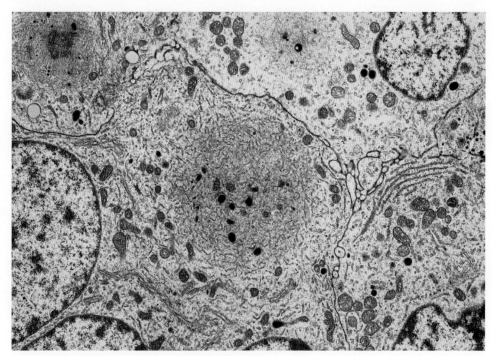

FIGURE 11-11

Sparsely granulated GH cell adenoma. The eccentric, often flattened or crescent nucleus, variably developed RER seen in small scattered profiles, a less than prominent Golgi apparatus displaced by the fibrous bodies, and the scant, small secretory granules are notable features (magnification, 6450×). (Courtesy of Dr E Horvath.)

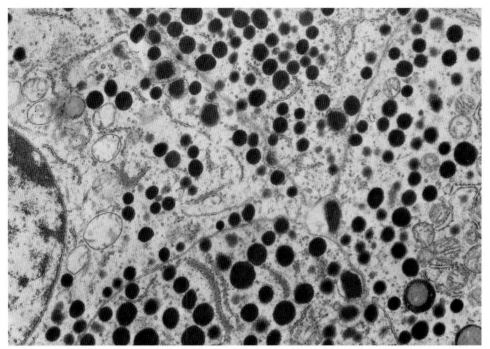

FIGURE 11-12

Mammosomatotroph cell adenoma. The EM findings are similar to densely granulated GH cell adenoma, although the secretory granules tend to be larger (they may measure up to 1200–1500 nm) and more irregular with variable texture and electron density. Exocytosis is an important marker, with the extruded secretory material remaining visible in the extracellular space longer than in prolactin cell adenomas (magnification 9680×). (Courtesy of Dr E Horvath.)

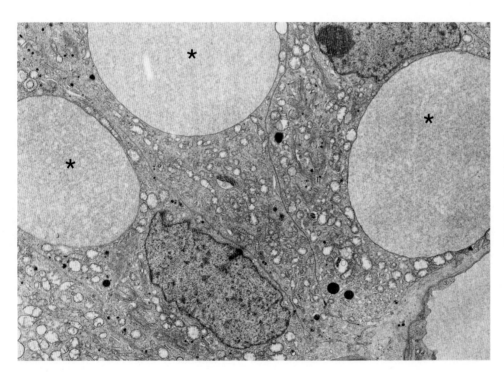

FIGURE 11-13

Acidophilic stem cell adenoma. The tumor is characterized by the formation of giant mitochondria (*). Bundles of electron dense tubular structures occur mainly in the small mitochondria (magnification 3840×). (Courtesy of Dr E Horvath.)

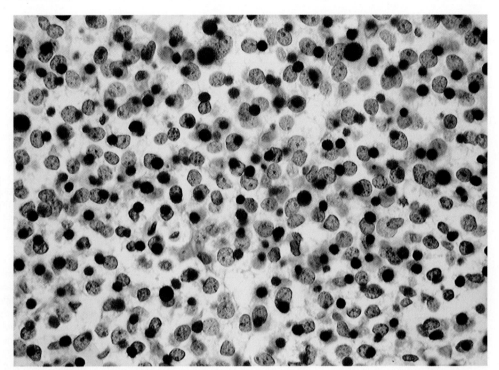

FIGURE 11-14
The fibrous bodies of the sparsely granulated GH cell adenoma have a characteristic globular keratin immunoreactivity.

granulated tumors that seem to be more aggressive. Surgery is potentially curative, although post-operative complications include CSF rhinorrhea, hemorrhage, visual loss and infection. Radiation is usually used in patients with 'incurable' tumors. Pharmacotherapy will yield symptomatic improvement, but requires high doses and is not curative; withdrawal results in elevated GH levels. If patients die from disease, it is usually from cardiovascular disease. It is also important to note that ectopic GH hormone can be produced by other non-pituitary neoplasms; and patients with acromegaly are susceptible to colon polyps and carcinoma.

CORTICOTROPHIC CELL-PRODUCING ADENOMA

A neoplastic proliferation of adrenocorticotropin secreting cells producing ACTH. Cushing disease is a pituitary ACTH dependent disease, while Cushing syndrome usually has a non-pituitary etiology.

CLINICAL FEATURES

About 15% of all pituitary tumors are corticotroph cell (ACTH) tumors. There is a marked female predominance with a wide age range at presentation (20–60 years). Most of these adenomas are functional, falling into three categories: ACTH adenoma with Cushing syndrome (67%); ACTH adenoma with Nelson syndrome (13%); and non-functional adenoma (20%). Over 80% of the adenomas are microadenomas (4–6 mm), requiring a vigilant MRI examination.

Hypercortisolism is caused by many things, including pituitary tumors, adrenal tumors, and ectopic neoplasms, among others. ACTH is cleaved from pro-opiomelanocortin in the anterior pituitary. ACTH concentration is diurnal, controlled by corticotropin-releasing factor (CRF), and ACTH controls the release of cortisol from the adrenal cortex. Because pituitary ACTH producing tumors still have some intact feedback inhibition pathways, the excess cortisol or 17-hydroxy-corticosteroids in the urine is associated with excess plasma ACTH (although usually <200 pg/ml). While dexamethasone stimulation tests can be performed, direct ACTH measurements seem to be superior. Cushing disease is produced by microadenomas in about 90% of patients, who complain of centripetal and nuchal obesity, facial plethora (moon facies), muscle weakness and atrophy, purple stria, hirsutism, hypertension, amenorrhea, osteoporosis, fatigue, psychiatric abnormalities and diabetes mellitus.

The rare clinically silent ACTH-producing tumors are endocrinologically inactive, perhaps due to an inability of the tumor to secrete ACTH, quantitative levels too low to produce symptoms, or it is an abnormal form of ACTH. The tumors tend to be large and more aggressive, with infarction common.

Nelson syndrome is characterized by hyperpigmentation of exposed skin areas due to a large ACTH producing adenoma following bilateral adrenalectomy for a pre-existing Cushing disease. These large adenomas tend to be invasive in up to 25% of patients. The hyperpigmentation is related to increased levels of ß melanocyte-stimulating hormone. By definition, there are elevated plasma ACTH levels.

CORTICOTROPHIC CELL-PRODUCING ADENOMA
DISEASE FACT SHEET

Definition
▸ Neoplastic proliferation of adrenocorticotropin secreting cells

Incidence and Location
▸ Approximately 15% of adenomas
▸ About 5 cases per million population per year

Morbidity and Mortality
▸ Cardiovascular disease from excess cortisol is most significant
▸ Approximately 20% of Nelson syndrome patients die of their tumor

Gender, Race and Age Distribution
▸ Female >>> Male (8 : 1)
▸ 20–60 years

Clinical Features
▸ ACTH production associated with Cushing syndrome or Nelson syndrome
▸ *Cushing syndrome*: centripetal and nuchal obesity, moon facies, muscle weakness, purple stria, hypertension, hirsutism, osteoporosis, fatigue, amenorrhea, psychiatric abnormalities, diabetes mellitus
▸ *Nelson syndrome*: hyperpigmentation in association with an ACTH producing tumor following bilateral adrenalectomy
▸ Elevated plasma ACTH levels

Prognosis and Therapy
▸ ACTH producing tumors can be cured by surgery in about 80% of patients, with follow-up radiation and/or pharmacotherapy
▸ Recurrences are frequent (20%)
▸ Nelson syndrome managed by surgery, radiation and pharmacotherapy, but poor control and uncommon long-term cures; 20% of patients die with disease

CORTICOTROPHIC CELL-PRODUCING ADENOMA
PATHOLOGIC FEATURES

Gross Findings
▸ Slight preference for the median portion of anterior pituitary

Microscopic Findings
▸ *Functioning corticotroph cell adenoma, densely granulated*: Follicle and sinusoidal growth of medium to large monotonous cells with strongly basophilic cytoplasm and prominent nucleoli. Non-tumorous corticotrophs show acidophilic hyaline-like, keratin positive material in the cytoplasm (Crooke's hyaline change), considered diagnostic
▸ *Functioning corticotroph cell adenoma, sparsely granulated*: Diffuse histology with a negative PAS reaction

Ultrastructural Features
▸ *Functioning corticotroph cell adenoma, densely granulated*: Densely granulated with pleomorphic secretory granules from 250–500 nm. Perinuclear bundles of 7 nm, intermediate filaments (keratin; Crooke's change) is diagnostic
▸ *Functioning corticotroph cell adenoma, sparsely granulated*: Only sparse, 200 nm secretory granules without keratin filaments
▸ *Silent corticotroph adenoma*: Three different types, with basophilic, chromophobic, and acidophilic

Immunohistochemical Results
▸ *Functioning corticotroph cell adenoma, densely granulated*: ACTH, α and β endorphins, α-melanocytic-stimulating hormone
▸ *Functioning corticotroph cell adenoma, sparsely granulated*: Faint ACTH reaction
▸ *Silent corticotroph adenoma*: Weak ACTH, α and β endorphin, GH, prolactin reaction

PATHOLOGIC FEATURES

GROSS FINDINGS

The adenoma is usually in the median portion of the anterior pituitary. It is usually readily distinguished from the surrounding parenchyma, but is not encapsulated.

MICROSCOPIC FINDINGS

Tumors are separated into functioning and non-functioning as well as by degree of granularity.
- *Functioning corticotroph cell adenoma, densely granulated:* Medium to large monotonous cells with strongly basophilic cytoplasm and prominent nucleoli. The cells are arranged in follicles and rosette-like structures, especially accentuated around capillaries (Figure 11-15). Non-tumorous corticotrophs show acidophilic hyaline-like, keratin positive material in the cytoplasm (Crooke's hyaline change), diagnostic of hypercorticism (Figure 11-16 and 11-17). There is

a strong PAS reaction around the cell membrane (Figure 11-17).
- *Functioning corticotroph cell adenoma, sparsely granulated:* Diffuse histology with a negative PAS reaction.
- *Silent corticotroph adenoma:* Morphology is similar to functional tumors.

ANCILLARY STUDIES

ULTRASTRUCTURAL FEATURES

- *Functioning corticotroph cell adenoma, densely granulated:* Densely granulated with pleomorphic secretory granules from 250–500 nm. Perinuclear bundles of 7 nm, intermediate filaments (keratin; Crooke's change) is diagnostic (Figure 11-18).
- *Functioning corticotroph cell adenoma, sparsely granulated:* Only sparse, 200 nm secretory granules without keratin filaments.
- *Silent corticotroph adenoma:* Three different types, with basophilic, chromophobic, and acidophilic

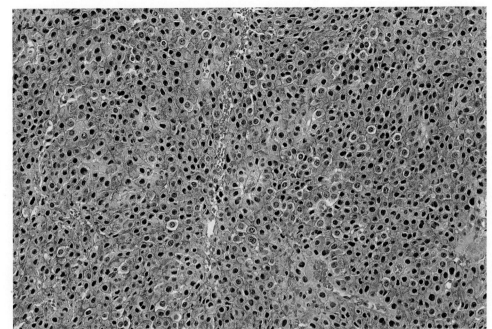

FIGURE 11-15

Basophilic, densely granulated monotonous cells with prominent perivascular cellular accentuation.

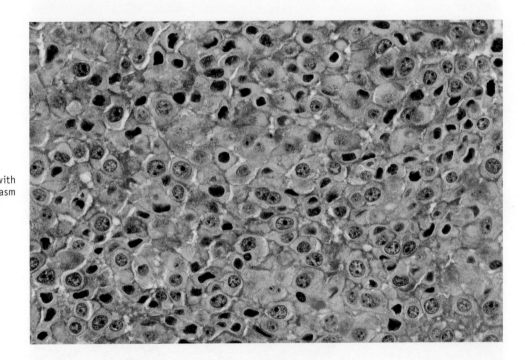

FIGURE 11-16

Non-tumorous corticotrophs with acidophilic hyaline-like cytoplasm (Crooke's hyaline change).

(latter has segmented Golgi and small peripherally located secretory granules).

IMMUNOHISTOCHEMICAL RESULTS

- *Functioning corticotroph cell adenoma, densely granulated:* ACTH positive, but also react with α and β endorphins and melanocytic-stimulating hormone.
- *Functioning corticotroph cell adenoma, sparsely granulated:* Only a faint ACTH reaction.

- *Silent corticotroph adenoma:* Weak reaction for ACTH, but α and β endorphin reactivity and GH and prolactin may be seen.

PROGNOSIS AND THERAPY

ACTH producing tumors which are functional can be cured in 75–90% of patients by surgery, with radiation employed for the remainder. Various drugs have

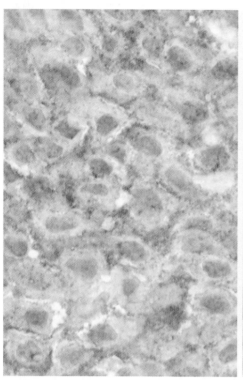
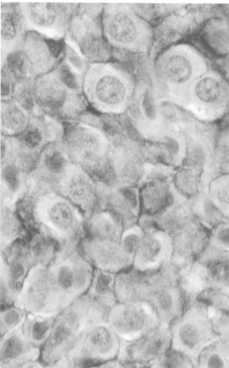

FIGURE 11-17
Left: Crooke's hyaline is accentuated with keratin immunohistochemistry. Right: A strong cytoplasmic PAS reaction is noted, accentuated along the cell membrane.

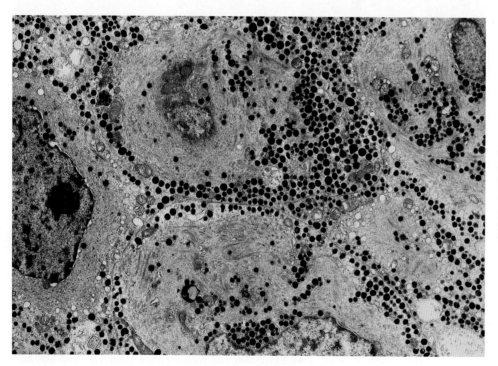

FIGURE 11-18
Corticotroph cell (Crooke's cell) adenoma. Cells display massive accumulation of cytokeratin filaments (Crooke's hyaline substance). The membranous organelles are largely obscured by the filamentous mass (magnification 5400×). (Courtesy of Dr E Horvath.)

been employed to treat Cushing disease and include Mitotane, Metyrapone, and dopamine agonists. Patients frequently develop recurrence, especially with macroadenomas (up to 20%). The silent corticotroph adenoma tends to be more aggressive, with a tendency to recur based on larger size. Patients with Nelson syn-

drome do not have a good response to therapy, with long-term cures uncommon. Surgery, irradiation, and Cyproheptadine (pharmacotherapy) may achieve symptomatic relief and control. However, approximately 20% of patients with Nelson syndrome die of their disease.

GLYCOPROTEIN HORMONE-PRODUCING ADENOMA

Tumors are separated into thyrotroph cell adenoma and gonadotroph cell adenoma.

GLYCOPROTEIN HORMONE-PRODUCING ADENOMA DISEASE FACT SHEET

Definition
▸ Thyrotroph and gonadotroph cell adenomas

Incidence and Location
▸ TSH secreting adenoma is rare
▸ FSH/LH adenomas account for about 10 % of all adenomas

Morbidity and Mortality
▸ Significant invasion (brain) with common recurrence

Gender, Race and Age Distribution
▸ Equal gender distribution
▸ Wide age distribution

Clinical Features
▸ *Thyrotroph*: Visual field defects due to frequent invasion; long standing hypo- or hyperthyroidism and goiter

Prognosis and Therapy
▸ *Thyrotroph*: Good with surgery, although recurrences develop, especially if there has been a long pre-operative history of hyperthyroidism
▸ *Gonadotroph*: Morbidity due to brain invasion; recurrence common

---

THYROTROPH CELL ADENOMA (TSH SECRETING ADENOMA)

Thyrotroph cell adenomas are extremely rare tumors representing the least common pituitary tumor type and account for 1% of all pituitary adenomas. They are usually large adenomas causing visual field defects and are frequently invasive. They are most commonly associated with long-standing hyperthyroidism (hypermetabolic state, tachycardia, tremor), hypothyroidism and goiter. Most tumors are chromophobic with solid growth (Figure 11-19), indistinct cell borders and a weak PAS reaction. They are thyroid stimulating hormone (TSH)

GLYCOPROTEIN HORMONE-PRODUCING ADENOMA PATHOLOGIC FEATURES

Microscopic Findings
▸ *Thyrotroph*: Most are chromophobic with indistinct cell borders; weak PAS reaction
▸ *Gonadotroph*: Large size with frequent hemorrhagic necrosis; perivascular pseudorosettes, small to medium polygonal or elongated cells, chromophobic

Ultrastructural Features
▸ *Thyrotroph*: Lysozymes and sparse electron dense secretory granules along the membrane
▸ *Gonadotroph*: Spherical 50–150 nm granules with vacuolar degeneration of the Golgi apparatus

Immunohistochemical Results
▸ *Thyrotroph*: TSH reactivity
▸ *Gonadotroph*: Patchy, uneven FSH > LH reactivity

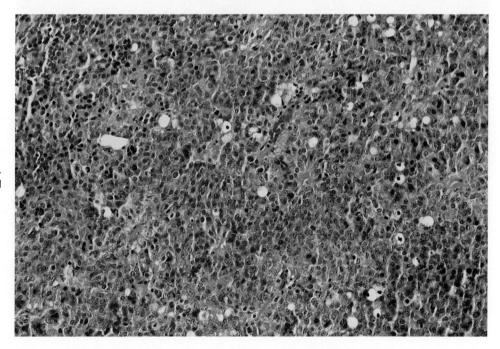

FIGURE 11-19

A thyrotroph cell adenoma is a chromophobic adenoma with a solid pattern.

reactive, and lysozymes and sparse electron dense secretory granules are accumulated along the cell membrane (Figure 11-20). Surgery for large size adenomas and thyroid hormone replacement treatment for hypothyroid patients. Follow-up is necessary, especially if there is a long preoperative history of either hyperthyroidism or hypothyroidism.

GONADOTROPH CELL ADENOMA (FSH AND LH HORMONE-PRODUCING ADENOMAS)

The true incidence is unknown, probably representing about 10% of all pituitary adenomas, although they are thought to represent the majority of clinically nonfunctional adenomas. About a quarter of these tumors are clinically non-functional, even though producing gonadotropins. Functional tumors are more common in men, with a wide age range. Most tumors are of large size (macroadenomas) with significant suprasellar or parasellar extension, causing visual disturbance and headaches. Women have amenorrhea and/or galactorrhea while men have decreased libido. Hemorrhagic necrosis is more common than in other adenoma types. Most of the tumors are arranged in perivascular pseudorosettes (Figure 11-21), comprised of small to medium, polygonal or elongated cells (Figure 11-22) which are mostly chromophobic with limited PAS positivity, although oncocytic variants are frequent (Figure 11-23). The cells are immunoreactive with FSH and/or LH, although patchy and uneven in distribution. FSH tends to be stronger and more widely distributed than LH. The cytoplasm by EM contains 50–150 nm spherical secretory granules, the majority of which are distributed along the cell membrane and within cell processes (Figure 11-24). A vacuolar degeneration of the Golgi apparatus is seen in tumors from female patients (Figure 11-25). Surgery is the treatment of choice, although morbidity due to invasion of critical brain structures is common. Recurrence is common.

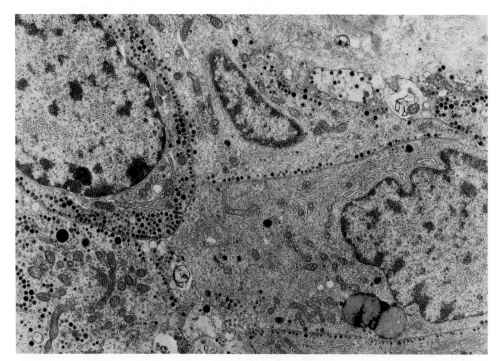

FIGURE 11-20

TSH cell adenoma. The sparse, small (here less than 200 nm) secretory granules often form a single layer under the plasmalemma (magnification 6600×). (Courtesy of Dr E Horvath).

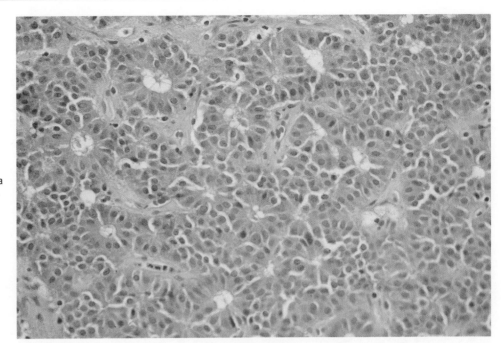

FIGURE 11-21
This gonadotroph adenoma has a remarkable pseudorosette pattern.

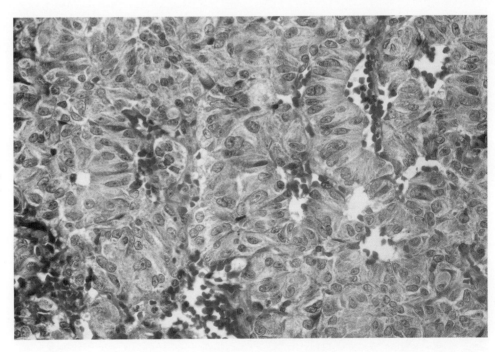

FIGURE 11-22
This gonadotroph adenoma is comprised of moderately pleomorphic, elongated tumor cells.

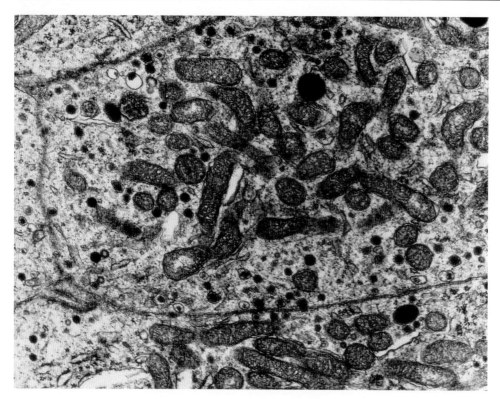

FIGURE 11-23
Irregular and enlarged mitochondria are the clue to this oncocytic gonadotroph cell adenoma.

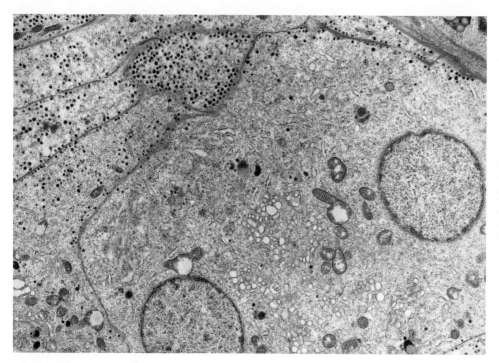

FIGURE 11-24
Gonadotroph cell adenoma. There is a polarity of the adenoma cells as well as an uneven distribution of secretory granules (scarcity within the nuclear pole, accumulation within the cell processes) (magnification 6000×). (Courtesy of Dr E Horvath.)

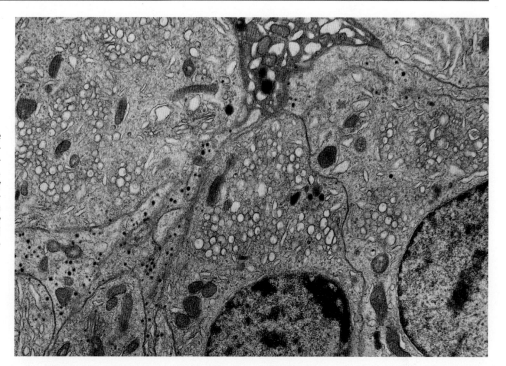

FIGURE 11-25
Gonadotroph cell adenoma, female type. The complete vacuolar transformation of the large Golgi apparatus is seen ('honeycomb Golgi'). The vacuoles are not optically empty, but are filled with a proteinaceous substance of low electron density. No immature secretory granules are apparent in the Golgi region (magnification 5900×) (courtesy of Dr E Horvath).

PLURIHORMONAL ADENOMA

A pituitary adenoma with multiple hormonal functions clinically and/or consisting of more than one hormone and/or cell type as detected by immunohistochemistry and electron microscopy, but not including the combinations of GH, PRL and TSH, or of FSH and LH.

**PLURIHORMONAL ADENOMA
DISEASE FACT SHEET**

Definition
▶ Pituitary neoplasm with multiple hormones identified clinically, immunohistochemically, or by ultrastructure

Incidence and Location
▶ Unknown incidence

Morbidity and Mortality
▶ Occasionally invasive with recurrences

Gender, Race and Age Distribution
▶ Equal gender distribution
▶ Women are usually younger than men (mean, 30 years)

Clinical Features
▶ Variable clinical presentation based on hormone production
▶ Visual disturbances

Prognosis and Therapy
▶ Good, similar to adenomas of other types
▶ Recurrences develop in occasional tumors

CLINICAL FEATURES

Plurihormonal adenomas are rare neoplasms, which develop in both genders, although women seem to be younger than men (mean, 30 years). Clinical symptoms are related to hormone production, but are often poorly developed; as a consequence, they are usually macroadenomas at diagnosis with visual disturbances.

PATHOLOGIC FEATURES

The reason for plurihormonality is not well understood, but the morphologies of the tumors are variable, without necessarily corresponding to their differentiation. These tumors are often chromophobic (Figure

---

**PLURIHORMONAL ADENOMA
PATHOLOGIC FEATURES**

Microscopic Findings
▶ Often chromophobic and usually PAS negative
▶ Rare spindled cell type with fibrous stroma

Ultrastructural Features
▶ Two or more distinct cell types
▶ Heterogeneous appearance, but usually with scant granules

Immunohistochemical Results
▶ Monoclonal antibodies identify multiple different hormones
▶ Must be quantitatively increased in frequency

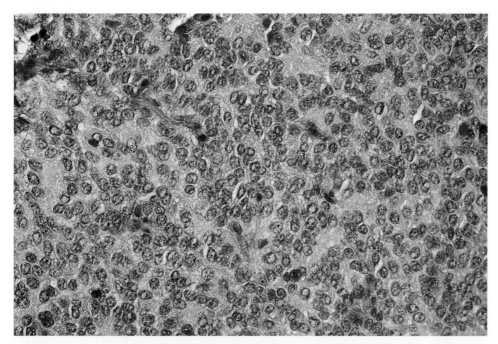

FIGURE 11-26
A chromophobic adenoma is arranged in a solid pattern with indistinct cell borders.

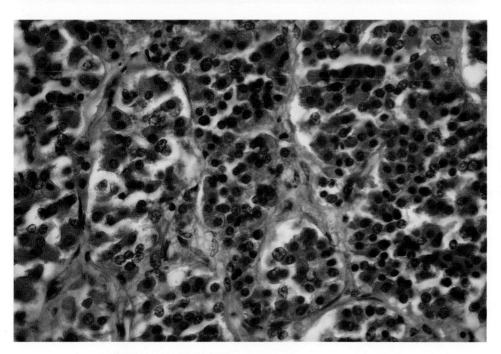

FIGURE 11-27
An acidophilic adenoma is arranged in slightly organoid collections.

11-26), or slightly acidophilic tumors (Figure 11-27) that are usually negative with the PAS stain. Sometimes, spindle shaped cells and fibrous stroma are seen.

ANCILLARY STUDIES

IMMUNOHISTOCHEMICAL RESULTS

By definition, there is immunoreactivity for more than one hormone that is not accounted for by cross reactivity or diffusion artifact. Monoclonal antibodies are recommended as they reduce cross reactivity between hormones of related families. There must be a quantitatively significant proportion of positive cells. A few scattered cells with immunoreactivity for any one hormone is insufficient evidence for true plurihormonality in a tumor, as it often represents entrapped normal pituicytes. The most common patterns include TSH, FSH and GH, or PRL and TSH.

ELECTRON MICROSCOPY

A heterogeneous ultrastructural appearance is common, although some tumors are monomorphous. Most consist of two or more distinct cell types.

PROGNOSIS AND THERAPY

The prognosis and treatment are similar to all other types of pituitary adenomas, although sometimes an invasive tumor may be more biologically aggressive, with an increased frequency of recurrence.

NULL CELL ADENOMA

A pituitary adenoma without clinical, immunohistochemical or ultrastructural evidence of hormone production.

CLINICAL FEATURES

Null cell adenomas represent approximately 25% of non-functioning pituitary adenomas, occur in both genders and are most common in elderly patients (mean, sixth decade). They are usually large, with visual disturbances the chief complaint. Interestingly, hypogonadism and hypothyroidism are frequently associated with this type of tumor as a result of destruction of the pituitary parenchyma. The excellent spatial resolution of MRI shows the tumor, but gives no indication of the type.

**NULL CELL ADENOMA
DISEASE FACT SHEET**

Definition
▶ A pituitary adenoma without clinical, immunohistochemical or ultrastructural evidence of hormone production

Incidence and Location
▶ About 25% of non-functioning adenomas

Morbidity and Mortality
▶ Often are invasive due to large size

Gender, Race and Age Distribution
▶ Equal gender distribution
▶ Elderly patients (mean, sixth decade)

Clinical Features
▶ Visual disturbances
▶ Hypogonadism and hypothyroidism due to pituitary parenchymal destruction (rather than hormone production)

Prognosis and Therapy
▶ Slow growing with invasion yielding frequent recurrences
▶ Surgery

PATHOLOGIC FEATURES

The tumors are yellow and soft with cyst and hemorrhage formation as a result of the long clinical history. Most are either chromophobic or oncocytic, with the round or polyhedral cells arranged in a diffuse or papillary architecture (Figure 11-28). There is generally no PAS reaction. Oncocytomas are more common with increased age and are characterized by the presence of abundant cytoplasmic mitochondria.

ANCILLARY STUDIES

Null cell adenomas are immunonegative (non-reactive) for pituitary hormones and transcription factors, although occasional scattered LH, FSH or TSH cells are encountered. Electron microscopy shows sparse secretory granules, inconspicuous rough endoplasmic reticulum and poorly developed Golgi complexes (Figure 11-29).

DIFFERENTIAL DIAGNOSIS

Null cell adenomas should be separated from clinically 'silent' adenomas, in which there is no endocrine function (silent GH producing adenomas, silent PRL producing adenomas, silent corticotroph adenomas) as these silent adenomas tend to have a more rapid growth rate and demonstrate more frequent recurrence than null cell adenomas.

**NULL CELL ADENOMA
PATHOLOGIC FEATURES**

Gross Findings
▶ Large, yellow, soft and cystic with hemorrhage

Microscopic Findings
▶ Usually chromophobic or oncocytic
▶ Round to polyhedral cells arranged in a diffuse architecture

Immunohistochemical Results
▶ Non-reactive for pituitary hormones and transcription factors
▶ Scattered LH, FSH or TSH positive cells can be seen

Pathologic Differential Diagnosis
▶ Separation of null cell from clinically 'silent' adenomas: the latter tends to be more aggressive with a more rapid clinical growth

---

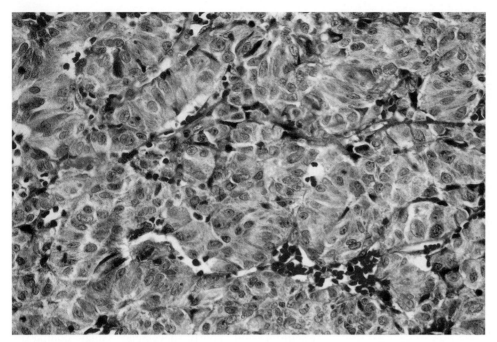

FIGURE 11-28
This null cell adenoma is arranged in a papillary architecture with a few extravasated erythrocytes.

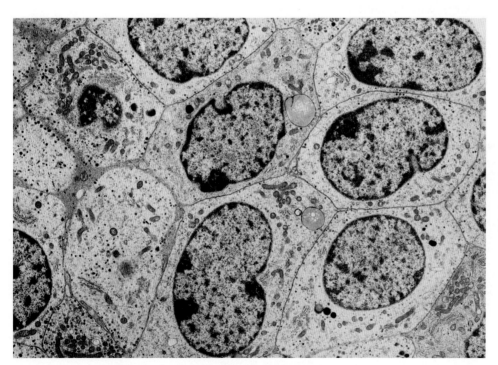

FIGURE 11-29
Null cell adenoma. The small adenoma cells possess sparse and very small secretory granules. The RER and Golgi membranes are poorly developed and there are no signs of functional differentiation into any specific cell line (magnification 4800×). (Courtesy of Dr E Horvath.)

PROGNOSIS AND THERAPY

Most null cell adenomas are slow growing and present at an advanced stage, yielding an increased frequency of recurrences. Surgery yields a good prognosis with complete excision.

INVASIVE ADENOMA

Pituitary adenoma with a tendency to infiltrate or destroy adjacent structures (dura and bones), with a biological behavior intermediate between adenoma and carcinoma.

INVASIVE ADENOMA
DISEASE FACT SHEET

Definition
▸ Infiltration or destruction of adjacent structures (dura and bone)

Incidence and Location
▸ About 35% of adenomas are invasive

Morbidity and Mortality
▸ Increased incidence of recurrence
▸ Dependent upon hormone production

Gender, Race and Age Distribution
▸ Equal gender distribution
▸ Tends to be in younger patients

Clinical Features
▸ Visual disturbances
▸ Headache
▸ Cranial neuropathies and facial neuralgia
▸ Nausea and dizziness
▸ Variable endocrinopathies

Prognosis and Therapy
▸ Increased incidence of recurrence
▸ Surgery, radiation and pharmacotherapy

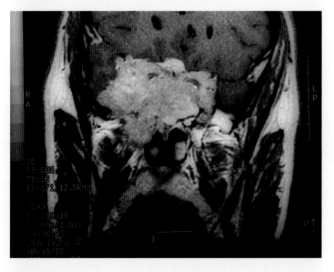

FIGURE 11-30
Separation of invasive adenomas from carcinoma relies on the presence of distant spread. While an extremely large tumor, all of the extrasellar spread, including the dura can still be included within the spectrum of an invasive adenoma.

INVASIVE ADENOMA
PATHOLOGIC FEATURES

Gross Findings
▸ Invasive into surrounding structures, including bone, dura, cavernous sinuses, posterior pituitary stalk, sino-nasal sinuses

Microscopic Findings
▸ Usually chromophobic or sparsely granulated adenomas
▸ Larger tumors are more likely to be invasive

CLINICAL FEATURES

Overall incidence is approximately 35% and is dependent on the adenoma immunophenotype. Invasive tumors tend to occur in younger patients, who present with visual disturbances, headache, cranial neuropathies, facial neuralgia, nausea and dizziness resulting from increased intracranial pressure and endocrine dysfunction. Invasion is best identified by histologic examination, as it is only identified correctly during surgery in 40% of patients and by radiology in 10% of patients.

RADIOLOGIC FEATURES

Radiologic examination shows destruction of the sella, bone erosion, invasion of the dura and cavernous sinus, and cranial nerve involvement (Figure 11-30).

PATHOLOGIC FEATURES

There is no correlation between the histologic appearance of tumors and the clinical behavior, but there is a correlation between size of the tumor and degree of invasion: dural invasion is present in 60% of microadenomas, 80% of intrasellar adenomas and 90% of tumors with suprasellar extension. Most adenomas are chromophobic or sparsely granulated. Invasive adenomas tend to have an increased expression of Ki-67 antigen.

PROGNOSIS AND THERAPY

While recurrence is higher in patients with invasive tumors, metastasis seldom develops. Surgery, radiation and pharmacotherapy are all employed to manage invasive adenomas, with the outcome generally dependent upon the hormone type.

CRANIOPHARYNGIOMA

CLINICAL FEATURES

Craniopharyngioma represents from 3–5% of all intracranial neoplasms, is the most common non-glial intracranial neoplasm in childhood (about 9%), with more than half of craniopharyngiomas occurring in children. There is no gender predilection. Compression of the sellar results in headache (increased intracranial pressure), while optic chiasm involvement yields visual abnormalities. Neurologic and mental changes are occasionally seen. Endocrinopathy due to hormone deficiency is occasionally present and includes delayed puberty, growth failure and obesity.

**CRANIOPHARYNGIOMA
DISEASE FACT SHEET**

Definition
▶ Benign epithelial neoplasm arising from remnants of Rathke's pouch

Incidence and Location
▶ 3–5% of intracranial tumors
▶ Most common non-glial intracranial tumor in children
▶ Over 50% of craniopharyngiomas occur in children

Morbidity and Mortality
▶ Endocrine deficiencies are permanent
▶ Mortality is related to 'invasiveness' of this benign tumor

Gender, Race and Age Distribution
▶ Equal gender distribution
▶ Children and adolescents >> adults

Radiologic Features
▶ Suprasellar calcifications and expanded sella
▶ Cyst with hypo- and hyperintense T1 versus T2 weighted MR images

Clinical Features
▶ Compression of sellar results in headaches
▶ Visual disturbances
▶ Neuropathy, mental changes, endocrinopathies

Prognosis and Treatment
▶ Variable prognosis of 20–80% 5-year survival
▶ Malignant transformation is rare
▶ Papillary type has higher risk of recurrence, although recurrence is common in both types
▶ Surgery is treatment of choice; radiation may result in the development of post-radiation astrocytoma

RADIOLOGIC FEATURES

Skull radiographs showing suprasellar calcification and expansion of the sella in a child are highly suspicious for a craniopharyngioma. CT shows a heterogeneous, partially calcified suprasellar mass with cystic and solid components, while MRI demonstrates a cyst with hypointense T1 weight images (Figure 11-31) and hyperintense T2 weighted images.

PATHOLOGIC FEATURES

GROSS FINDINGS

Most tumors are suprasellar, with about 10% intra-sellar, averaging 3–4 cm in diameter. They are predominately cystic with focal calcifications, showing a microcystic or honeycomb appearance. The cyst wall may have occasional papillae.

MICROSCOPIC FINDINGS

A variable histologic pattern is characteristic, with adamantinomatous and papillary variants the most common. About 90% of tumors are adamantinomatous and consist of islands of epithelial cells, the centers of which are composed of stellate cells loosely arranged with small nuclei and clear cytoplasm. Surrounding the stellate cells and separated by a thin connective tissue membrane, is a row of palisaded, basaloid, columnar cells with polarized nuclei closely resembling

---

**CRANIOPHARYNGIOMA
PATHOLOGIC FEATURES**

Gross Findings
▶ Most are suprasellar (90%)
▶ 3–4 cm in greatest dimension
▶ Cystic with calcifications
▶ Cyst wall may have papillae

Microscopic Findings
▶ *Adamantinomatous*: Islands of basaloid epithelium surrounding stellate cells; rows of palisaded, basaloid columnar cells with polarized nuclei; squamous differentiation is seen; cysts are filled with keratin/cellular debris, cholesterol clefts, psammoma bodies and inflammatory cells; foreign body giant cell reaction
▶ *Papillary*: Papillae have squamous epithelium with little keratin; no calcifications, nuclear palisading, foreign body giant cell reaction or cholesterol clefts

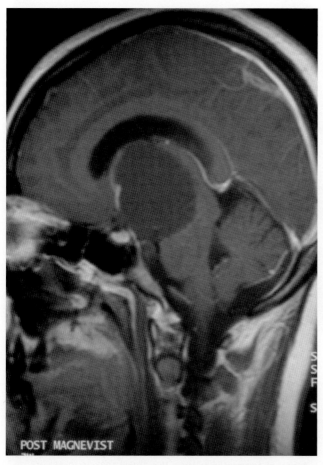

FIGURE 11-31

T1 weighted MRI image demonstrates a hypointense cyst in this cranio-pharyngioma. (Courtesy of Dr A Levy.)

ameloblastomas (Figure 11-32). Areas of squamous differentiation can be seen. The fibrovascular stroma undergoes degenerative changes resulting in cyst formation. The cyst is filled with cellular and keratin debris, colloid-like material, mononuclear inflammatory cells, cholesterol granulomas, gliosis and psammoma bodies with a foreign body giant cell reaction (Figure 11-33).

The papillary type (10% of tumors) occurs predominantly in adults and involves the 3rd ventricle. The papillae are composed of squamous epithelium with little or no keratin. There is no calcification, palisaded nuclei, foreign body giant cells and cholesterol clefts.

PROGNOSIS AND THERAPY

The overall 5-year survival ranges from 20–80%, due to the 'invasive' nature of this benign neoplasm. The papillary type is associated with a higher risk of recurrence, which is high in both types. While complete surgical excision is the treatment of choice, incomplete removal is common and is associated with high incidence of recurrence. Radiation delays recurrence and prolongs survival but is associated with post-radiation astrocytomas. Malignant transformation is rare. The endocrine deficiencies are permanent and hormone substitution therapy is necessary.

FIGURE 11-32

Stellate cells of a craniopharyngioma are surrounded by palisaded, basaloid, columnar cells.

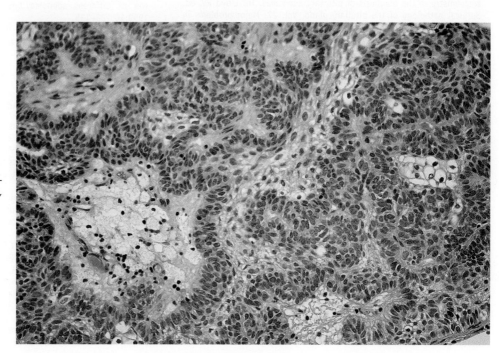

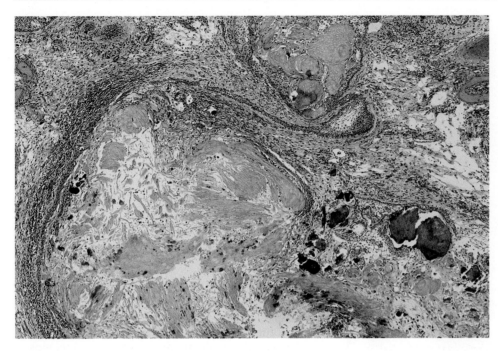

FIGURE 11-33

The cysts of a craniopharyngioma are filled with keratin debris, inflammatory cells and calcifications.

SUGGESTED READING

General Considerations

Asa SL. Tumors of the pituitary gland. Atlas of tumor pathology. Third series. Fascicle 22. Washington, DC: Armed Forces Institute of Pathology, 1998:47–147.

Horvath E. Ultrastructural markers in the pathologic diagnosis of pituitary adenomas. Ultrastruct Pathol 1994;18:171–179.

Kane LA, Leinung MC, Scheithauer BW, et al. Pituitary adenomas in childhood and adolescence. J Clin Endocrinol Metab 1994;79:1135–1140.

Scheithauer BW, Laws ER Jr, Kovacs K, et al. Pituitary adenomas of the multiple endocrine neoplasia type I syndrome. Sem Diagn Pathol 1987;4:205–211.

Stefaneanu L, Kovacs K. Light microscopic, special stains and immunohistochemistry in the diagnosis of pituitary adenomas. In: Lloyd RV, ed. Surgical pathology of the pituitary gland. Vol. 27, Major problems in pathology. Philadelphia: W. B. Saunders Co., 1993;34–51.

Terada T, Kovacs K, Stefaneanu L, Horvath E. Incidence, pathology and recurrence of pituitary adenomas: study of 647 unselected surgical cases. Endoc Pathol 1995;6:301–310.

Prolactin Cell Adenoma

Asa SL. Pituitary adenomas. Tumors of the Pituitary Gland. Atlas of Tumor Pathology, Third Series, Fascicle 22. Washington, DC: Armed Forces Institute of Pathology, 1998:47–148.

Losa M, Mortini P, Barzaghi R, et al. Surgical treatment of prolactin-secreting pituitary adenomas: early results and long-term outcome. J Clin Endocrinol Metab. 2002;87:3180–3186.

Partington MD, Davis DH, Laws ER Jr, Scheithauer BW. Pituitary adenomas in childhood and adolescence. Results of transsphenoidal surgery. J Neurosurg 1994;80:209–216.

Ma W, Ikeda H, Yoshimoto T. Clinicopathologic study of 123 cases of prolactin-secreting pituitary adenomas with special reference to multihormone production and clonality of the adenomas. Cancer 2002;95:258–266.

Saeger W, Horvath E, Kovacs K, et al. Prolactin producing adenoma. In: DeLellis RA, Lloyd RV, Heitz PU, Eng C, eds. Pathology and Genetics of Tumours of Endocrine Organs. World Health Organization Classification of Tumours Series. Lyon, France: IARC, 2004:20–23.

Terada T, Kovacs K, Stefaneanu L, Horvath E. Incidence, pathology, and recurrence of pituitary adenomas: Study of 647 unselected surgical cases. Endocr Pathol 1995;6:301–310.

Growth Hormone-producing Adenoma

Asa SL. Pituitary adenomas. Tumors of the Pituitary Gland. Atlas of Tumor Pathology, Third Series, Fascicle 22. Washington, DC: Armed Forces Institute of Pathology, 1998:47–148.

Furuhata S, Kameya T, Otani M, Toya S. Prolactin presents in all pituitary tumors of acromegalic patients. Hum Pathol 1993;24:10–15.

Kontogeorgos G, Watson RE Jr, Lindell EP, et al. Growth hormone producing adenoma. In: DeLellis of RA, Lloyd RV, Heitz PU, Eng C, eds. Pathology and Genetics of Tumours of Endocrine Organs. World Health Organization Classification of Tumours Series. Lyon, France: IARC, 2004:14–19.

Scheithauer BW, Kovacs K, Stefaneanu L, et al. The pituitary in gigantism. Endoc Pathol 1995;6:173–187.

Voit D, Saeger W, Lüdecke DK. Pituitary adenomas in acromegaly: comparison of different adenoma types with clinical data. Endo Pathol 1999;10:123–135.

Yamada S, Aiba T, Sano T, et al. Growth hormone-producing adenomas: correlations between clinical characteristics and morphology. Neurosurg 1993;33:20–27.

Corticotrophic Cell-producing Adenoma

Asa SL. Pituitary adenomas. Tumors of the Pituitary Gland. Atlas of Tumor Pathology, Third Series, Fascicle 22. Washington, DC: Armed Forces Institute of Pathology, 1998:47–148.

George DH, Scheithauer BW, Kovacs K, et al. Crooke's cell adenoma of the pituitary: an aggressive variant of corticotroph adenoma. Am J Surg Pathol 2003;27:1330–1336.

Meier CA, Biller BM. Clinical and biochemical evaluation of Cushing's syndrome. Endocrinol Metab Clin North Am 1997;26:741–762.

Robert F, Hardy J. Human corticotroph cell adenomas. Semin Diagn Pathol 1986;3:34–41.

Scheithauer BW, Jaap AJ, Horvath E, et al. Clinically silent corticotroph tumors of the pituitary gland. Neurosurgery 2000;47:723–729.

Stadnik T, Stevenaert A, Beckers A, et al. Pituitary microadenomas: diagnosis with two-and three-dimensional MR imaging at 1.5 T before and after injection of gadolinium. Radiology 1990;176:419–428.

Trouillas J, Barkan AL, Watson RE Jr, et al. ACTH producing adenoma. In: DeLellis RA, Lloyd RV, Heitz PU, Eng C, eds. Pathology and Genetics of Tumours of Endocrine Organs. World Health Organization Classification of Tumours Series. Lyon, France: IARC, 2004:26–29.

Glycoprotein Hormone-producing Adenoma

Asa SL, Ezzat S, Watson RE Jr, et al. Gonadotropin producing adenoma. In: DeLellis RA, Lloyd RV, Heitz PU, Eng C, eds. Pathology and Genetics of Tumours of Endocrine Organs. World Health Organization Classification of Tumours Series. Lyon, France: IARC, 2004:30–32.

Asa SL. Pituitary adenomas. Tumors of the Pituitary Gland. Atlas of Tumor Pathology, Third Series, Fascicle 22. Washington, DC: Armed Forces Institute of Pathology, 1998:47–148.

Halliday WC, Asa SL, Kovacs K, Scheithauer BW. Intermediate filaments in the human pituitary gland: an immunohistochemical study. Can J Neurol Sci 1990;17:131–136.

Osamura RY, Sano T, Ezzat S, et al. TSH producing adenoma. In: DeLellis RA, Lloyd RV, Heitz PU, Eng C, eds. Pathology and Genetics Tumours of Endocrine Organs. World Health Organization Classification of Tumours Series. Lyon, France: IARC, 2004:24–25.

Sanno N, Teramoto A, Osamura RY. Long-term surgical outcome in 16 patients with thyrotropin pituitary adenoma. J Neurosurg 2000;93:194–200.

Plurihormonal Pituitary Adenoma

Asa SL. Pituitary adenomas. Tumors of the Pituitary Gland. Atlas of Tumor Pathology, Third Series, Fascicle 22. Washington, DC: Armed Forces Institute of Pathology, 1998:47–148.

Horvath E, Kovacs K, Scheithauer BW, et al. Pituitary adenomas producing growth hormone, prolactin and one or more glycoprotein hormones. Ultrastruct Pathol 1984;5:171–183.

Ho DM, Hsu CY, Ting LT, Chiang H. Plurihormonal pituitary adenomas: immunostaining of all pituitary hormones is mandatory for correct classification. Histopathology 2001;39:310–319.

Horvath E, Lloyd RV, Kovacs K, et al. Plurihormonal adenoma. In: DeLellis RA, Lloyd RV, Heitz PU, Eng C, eds. Pathology and Genetics of Tumours of Endocrine Organs. World Health Organization Classification of Tumours Series. Lyon, France: IARC, 2004:35.

Scheithauer BW, Horvath E, Kovacs K, et al. Plurihormonal pituitary adenomas. Semin Diagn Pathol 1986;3:69–82.

Null Cell Adenoma

Asa SL. Pituitary adenomas. Tumors of the Pituitary Gland. Atlas of Tumor Pathology, Third Series, Fascicle 22. Washington, DC: Armed Forces Institute of Pathology, 1998:47–148.

Sano T, Yamada S, Watson RE Jr, et al. Null cell adenoma. In: DeLellis RA, Lloyd RV, Heitz PU, Eng C, eds. Pathology and Genetics Tumours of Endocrine Organs. World Health Organization Classification of Tumours Series. Lyon, France: IARC, 2004:33–34.

Saeger W, Wilczak W, Ludecke DK, Buchfelder M, Fahlbusch R. Hormone markers in pituitary adenomas: changes within last decade resulting from improved method. Endocr Pathol 2003;14:49–54.

Schmid M, Munscher A, Saeger W, et al. Pituitary hormone mRNA in null cell adenomas and oncocytomas by in situ hybridization comparison with immunohistochemical and clinical data. Pathol Res Pract 2001;197:663–669

Yamada S, Kovacs K, Horvath E, Aiba T. Morphological study of clinically nonsecreting pituitary adenomas in patients under 40 years of age. J Neurosurg 1991;75:902–905.

Invasive Pituitary Adenomas

Cottier JP, Destrieux C, Brunereau L, et al. Cavernous sinus invasion by pituitary adenoma: MR imaging. Radiology 2000;215:463–469.

McKeever PE, Blaivas M, Sima AA. Neoplasms of the sellar region. In: Lloyd R, ed. Surgical pathology of the pituitary gland. Major problems in pathology, Vol. 27. Philadelphia: W. B. Saunders Co., 1993:151–155.

Meij BP, Lopes MB, Ellegala DB, Alden TD, Laws ER Jr. The long-term significance of microscopic dural invasion in 354 patients with pituitary adenomas treated with transsphenoidal surgery. J Neurosurg 2002;96:195–208.

Sautner D, Saeger W. Invasiveness of pituitary adenomas. Pathol Res Pract 1991;187:632–636.

Craniopharyngioma

Asa SL. Craniopharyngioma. Tumors of the Pituitary Gland. Atlas of Tumor Pathology, Third Series, Fascicle 22. Washington, DC: Armed Forces Institute of Pathology, 1998:167–172.

Mincione GP, Mincione F, Mennonna P. Cytological features of craniopharyngioma. Pathologica 1991;83:191–196.

Müller HL, Faldum A, Etavard-Gorris N, et al. Functional capacity, obesity and hypothalamic involvement: cross-sectional study of 212 patients with childhood craniopharyngioma. Klin Padiatr 2003;215:310–314.

Szeifert GT, Sipos L, Horvath M, et al. Pathological characteristics of surgically removed craniopharyngiomas: analysis of 131 cases. Acta Neurochir 1993;124:139–143.

Weiner HL, Wisoff JH, Rosenberg ME, et al. Craniopharyngiomas: a clinicopathological analysis of factors predictive of recurrence and functional outcome. Neurosurgery 1994;35:1001–1011.

Zimmerman RA. Imaging of intrasellar, suprasellar and parasellar tumors. Sem Roentgenol 1990;25:174–197.

12 Malignant Neoplasms of the Pituitary Gland

Lester DR Thompson • Clara S Heffess

PITUITARY CARCINOMA

A malignant neoplasm arising from the adenohypophysial cells with gross central nervous system invasion and/or capable of producing distant metastasis. Whether carcinoma is de novo from the outset or a transformation of an adenoma is unclear, as pituitary carcinoma is a rare tumor, comprising <0.2% of all pituitary neoplasms.

CLINICAL FEATURES

There is equal gender distribution, with most patients presenting in the fifth decade (range, 7–75 years). Most tumors are endocrinologically functional, with prolactin or ACTH producing tumors reported most commonly. The clinical picture is variable, with hormone

---

excess (any of the pituitary peptides), unassociated with hormone excess, and hypopituitarism. There is no increased incidence of pituitary carcinoma in MEN1 or Carney complex patients. However, the diagnosis of carcinoma lies in demonstrating metastatic tumour deposits. Radiographic examination is critical in documenting metastases, usually in a patient with a known pituitary primary. Subarachnoid space, cervical lymph nodes, bone, liver and lungs are the most common sites of metastases.

RADIOLOGIC FEATURES

Sellar enlargement and prominent extrasellar extension is seen in carcinomas with craniospinal metastasis, best demonstrated by computed tomography and magnetic resonance imaging. Carcinomas with extracranial metastasis have little or no sellar expansion, but show evidence of erosion and destruction of the sellar floor. However, there are no radiographically unique features which separate adenoma and carcinoma.

PATHOLOGIC FEATURES

GROSS FINDINGS

Tumors start in the anterior lobe and depending upon the growth rate, spread into the neighboring structures (dura, bone, cranial nerves). Craniospinal space (brain and cerebrospinal fluid) spread and/or systemic spread follows. Discontinuous spread from the primary neoplasm is essential to accurate diagnosis, along with single or multiple metastatic deposits in other organs. Without lymphatic drainage, metastases from the pituitary are thought to be due to soft tissue invasion by the neoplastic cells.

MICROSCOPIC FINDINGS

The diagnosis of pituitary carcinoma *cannot* be based solely on histologic appearance, as invasion, cellular pleomorphism, nuclear abnormalities, mitotic activity, and necrosis can all be seen in adenomas. While these features are seen with increased frequency in carcinoma, there is significant overlap with adenomas,

---

PITUITARY CARCINOMA
DISEASE FACT SHEET

Definition
▶ A malignant neoplasm arising from the adenohypophysial cells with gross central nervous system invasion and/or producing distant metastasis

Incidence and Location
▶ <0.2% of pituitary neoplasms (anterior lobe)

Gender, Race and Age Distribution
▶ Equal gender distribution
▶ Mean, 44 years

Clinical Features
▶ Variable endocrine function: excess, normal, hypofunctional
▶ Metastases to subarachnoid spaces, cervical lymph nodes, bone, lung and liver

Prognosis and Therapy
▶ Poor (70% of patients die from tumor), usually <3 years
▶ Surgery, radiation and/or combination pharmacotherapy

PITUITARY CARCINOMA
PATHOLOGIC FEATURES

Gross Findings

▸ Extension from the sellar into surrounding structures
▸ Discontinuous involvement of the craniospinal spaces
▸ Metastases in distant organs

Microscopic Findings

▸ No histologic features are unique to carcinoma (although increased mitotic figures can suggest the diagnosis)
▸ Brain invasion and/or metastatic deposits

Immunohistochemical Results

▸ Synaptophysin and chromogranin for neuroendocrine type
▸ Specific pituitary hormones (prolactin, ACTH) to suggest pituitary origin

PATHOLOGIC DIFFERENTIAL DIAGNOSIS

▸ Benign pituitary adenoma, metastatic neoplasms, poorly differentiated glial neoplasms

although a remarkably increased number of mitotic figures suggests carcinoma. Confirmation requires the presence of brain invasion and/or metastatic foci (within the cerebrospinal space or extracranial) that either resemble the pituitary tumor, have a similar hormonal phenotype in both the primary tumor and in the metastasis, or show proof of endocrine differentiation by immunohistochemistry and/or electron microscopy.

ANCILLARY STUDIES

Separation of pituitary adenoma from carcinoma cannot be conclusively made by immunohistochemistry alone. However, synaptophysin (and chromogranin) will confirm the neuroendocrine differentiation of the neoplasm. Specific pituitary hormone immunoreactivity (prolactin, ACTH) may help to establish that the carcinoma is pituitary based. Expression of *TP53* seems to be highest in carcinomas, while generally lacking in adenomas.

DIFFERENTIAL DIAGNOSIS

The differential diagnosis of pituitary carcinoma lies with benign adenomas and other metastatic neoplasms. A good clinical history and immunohistochemical studies can usually reliably separate pituitary carcinoma from other lesions. It bears repeating that in *pituitary pathology*, invasion does not equate with proof of malignancy; malignancy must be proved by cerebrospinal and/or systemic metastasis.

PROGNOSIS AND THERAPY

By definition, metastasis is present when the diagnosis is rendered; consequently, patients with pituitary carcinoma have a poor prognosis, with approximately 70% of patients dying in <3 years. Interestingly, patients with cerebrospinal metastases have a longer survival (mean, 8 years) than patients with extracranial metastases (mean, 2.5 years). Treatment options include surgery followed by radiation or pharmacotherapy in combination with surgery or radiotherapy. However, pharmacotherapy seems to be less effective controlling pituitary carcinoma.

METASTATIC NEOPLASMS

The evidence of metastasis to the pituitary gland varies and mainly depends on the aggressive search for their presence, with up to about 25% in autopsy series.

CLINICAL FEATURES

If the neurohypophysis is involved diabetes insipidus may develop, but most patients do not have overt pituitary symptomatology. While the genders are equally

METASTATIC NEOPLASMS
DISEASE FACT SHEET

Definition

▸ Secondary tumors which metastasize to or directly invade into the pituitary gland

Incidence and Location

▸ Up to 25% in autopsy series

Morbidity and Mortality

▸ Usually associated with widely disseminated deposits in the terminal phase of the malignancy

Gender, Race and Age Distribution

▸ Equal gender distribution, although tumor origin specific (see microscopic)
▸ Middle aged to older patients

Clinical Features

▸ Asymptomatic usually
▸ Diabetes insipidus when the posterior lobe is affected

Prognosis and Therapy

▸ Poor (usually <1 year), but related to underlying primary

affected, women are affected with breast, lung and stomach cancer most frequently, while men are affected by lung, prostate and stomach cancer. When breast carcinoma is identified within the pituitary, other endocrine organs are also commonly affected. Hematopoietic neoplasms may involve the pituitary in about 20% of cases. Radiographic studies are non-specific, except if there is a known primary, and a metastatic work-up is being pursued. In this context, bone destruction, cavernous sinus invasion (especially when associated with cranial neuropathies), and infundibular stalk invasion suggest metastatic tumor.

PATHOLOGIC FEATURES

GROSS FINDINGS

Metastases occur predominantly in normal glands, although metastasis to pituitary adenomas are reported. The posterior pituitary is affected nearly two times as commonly by metastatic tumors as a result of the extensive vascular supply versus the anterior lobe, which is more commonly affected by direct extension. Histologic examination is required to confirm metastatic deposits or direct invasion, although firm, difficult to resect lesions suggest metastatic disease.

MICROSCOPIC FINDINGS

The histology is dependent upon the primary site, although carcinomas are most common (Figure 12-1). Occasionally, the histologic appearance is undifferentiated, necessitating immunohistochemical analysis.

METASTATIC NEOPLASMS
PATHOLOGIC FEATURES

Gross Findings
▸ Usually metastases are to a normal gland
▸ Posterior lobe affected twice as frequently as anterior

Microscopic Findings
▸ Dependent upon primary site, with carcinomas most frequent

Immunohistochemical Results
▸ Similar to primary site

Pathologic Differential Diagnosis
▸ Pituitary adenoma

DIFFERENTIAL DIAGNOSIS

The diagnosis of a metastatic neoplasm is usually quite straight forward, although distinction from a pituitary adenoma may sometimes be a challenge. However, immunohistochemical or ultrastructural examination will help with the diverse morphologic appearance of primary pituitary neoplasms.

PROGNOSIS AND THERAPY

The survival time of patients with metastasis to the pituitary gland is usually short with death occurring

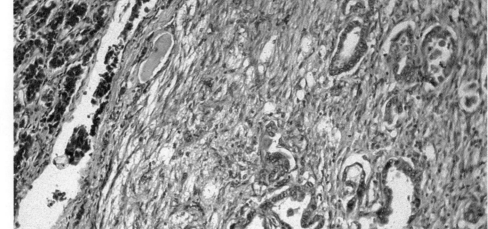

FIGURE 12-1
A metastatic adenocarcinoma is identified within the posterior lobe of the pituitary parenchyma.

in less than 1 year due to the extent of carcinomatosis at the time of diagnosis. Treatment is limited to palliation and includes surgery and radiotherapy.

SUGGESTED READING

Pituitary Carcinoma

Asa SL. Pituitary carcinoma. Tumors of the Pituitary Gland. Atlas of Tumor Pathology, Third Series, Fascicle 22. Washington, DC: Armed Forces Institute of Pathology, 1998:149–150.

Pernicone PJ, Scheithauer BW, Sebo TJ, et al. Pituitary carcinoma: a clinicopathologic study of 15 cases. Cancer 1997;79:804–812.

Popovic EA, Vatuone JR, Siu KH, et al. Malignant prolactinomas. Neurosurgery 1991;29:127–30.

Scheithauer BW, Kovacs K, Horvath E, et al. Pituitary carcinoma. In: DeLellis RA, Lloyd RV, Heitz PU, Eng C, eds. Pathology and Genetics Tumours of Endocrine Organs. World Health Organization Classification of Tumours Series. Lyon, France: IARC, 2004:36–39.

Scheithauer BW, Fereidooni F, Horvath E, et al. Pituitary carcinoma: an ultrastructural study of eleven cases. Ultrastruct Pathol 2001;25: 227–242.

Metastatic Neoplasms

Aaberg TM Jr, Kay M, Sternau L. Metastatic tumor to the pituitary. Am J Ophthalmol 1995;119:779–785.

Asa SL. Metastatic neoplasms of the sella turcica. Tumors of the Pituitary Gland. Atlas of Tumor Pathology, Third Series, Fascicle 22. Washington, DC: Armed Forces Institute of Pathology, 1998:187–190.

Heshmati HM, Scheithauer BW, Young WF Jr. Metastases to the pituitary gland. Endocrinologist 2002;12:45–49.

Kovacs K, Horvath E, Ruibal V, et al. Secondary tumours. In: DeLellis RA, Lloyd RV, Heitz PU, Eng C, eds. Pathology and Genetics Tumours of Endocrine Organs. World Health Organization Classification of Tumours Series. Lyon, France: IARC, 2004:45–47.

Max MB, Deck MD, Rottenberg DA. Pituitary metastasis: incidence in cancer patients and clinical differentiation from pituitary adenoma. Neurology 1981;31:998–1002.

Teears RJ, Silverman EM. Clinicopathologic review of 88 cases of carcinoma metastatic to the pituitary gland. Cancer 1975;36:216–220.

13

Diseases of the Paraganglia System

Jennifer Hunt

PARAGANGLIOMA

Extra-adrenal paragangliomas arise from paraganglia distributed along the paravertebral sympathetic and

PARAGANGLIOMA
DISEASE FACT SHEET

Definition
▸ Tumors arising from the paraganglia along the parasympathetic or sympathetic nerves

Incidence and Location
▸ Rare (incidence estimate of 0.2–1/100 000 population)
▸ Carotid body, vagal body, middle ear (jugulotympanic), organ of Zuckerkandl, aortico-pulmonary, larynx,

Morbidity and Mortality
▸ Infiltrative growth and local recurrence can lead to death
▸ <10% are malignant

Gender, Race and Age Distribution
▸ Equal gender distribution (F > M in high altitude for carotid body tumors)
▸ Fifth and sixth decades

Clinical Features
▸ Slow growing, painless mass
▸ Ear lesions may produce tinnitus, hearing loss and nerve dysfunction
▸ Occasionally may be a pulsatile lesion
▸ Headache, perspiration, palpitation, pallor and hypertension for abdominal cavity lesions
▸ About 10% are bilateral, multiple, familial, pediatric, and malignant

Radiographic Findings
▸ CT shows enhancing mass in characteristic location
▸ Hyperintense T2 weighted MRI
▸ Angiography shows splaying of the internal and external carotid arteries with a tumor blush
▸ ^{123}I-MIBG localizes tumor(s)

Prognosis and Therapy
▸ Good prognosis if completely resected, although may be indolent and recur/metastasize years later
▸ Surgery with preoperative adrenergic blockage and/or embolization

parasympathetic chains, and include carotid body, jugulotympanic, orbital, nasopharynx, vagal, laryngeal, paraspinal (aortico-sympathetic and visceral-autonomic), urinary bladder, and the organ of Zuckerkandl tumors. While the most common site of paraganglioma development is within the adrenal gland (referred to as pheochromocytoma), discussion will be limited to head and neck and abdominal sites (see adrenal chapter for pheochromocytoma).

The pathogenesis of paraganglioma is not entirely understood. The best-studied tumor is the carotid body tumor, which is derived from the oxygen sensing chemoreceptive organ at the bifurcation of the carotid artery. In people who live at high altitudes, this organ can become hyperplastic, presumably secondary to chronic hypoxia. The oxygen sensing activity in the carotid body led investigators to the germline mutations associated with hereditary paragangliomatosis. These mutations are located in several genes encoding the various subunits of the succinate-ubiquinone oxidoreductase gene (SDH), which is an enzyme in the mitochondrial respiratory chain complex II. These genes include *PGL*1, which encodes SDH subunit D (on 11q23), *PGL*2 mapping to 11q13; *PGL*3, which encodes SDH subunit C (on 1q21), and *PLG*4, which encodes the SDH subunit B (on 1p36). Interestingly, point mutations and/or deletion mutations in these genes can also be identified in up to 20% of patients with presumed spontaneous paragangliomas.

CLINICAL FEATURES

Normal paraganglia are located throughout the body, and consequently paragangliomas have been described in nearly every anatomical location. The head and neck are the most common locations for extra-adrenal paragangliomas, accounting for up to 70% of these tumors, with the most common sub-sites being carotid body tumors at the bifurcation of the internal and external carotid arteries, glomus tympanicum or glomus jugulare in the middle ear, and glomus vagale. In the head and neck, the normal paraganglia are associated with the parasympathetic nervous system, adjacent to cranial nerves or to the arterial vasculature. It must be stressed that cervical or thoracic sympathetic paragangliomas are separated from parasympathetic paragangliomas arising in nearby locations. Cervical sympathetic para-

TABLE 13-1

Genetic Syndromes Associated with Paraganglioma and Pheochromocytoma

Syndrome	Gene Locus	Gene	Paraganglia Tumor	Other Abnormalities
Von Hippel Lindau	3p26	VHL	Pheochromocytoma in 10–20%	Renal cysts and renal cell carcinoma Visceral organ cysts Hemangioblastomas
Hereditary Paragangliomatosis	11q23 11q13 1q21 1p36	PGL1 PGL2 PGL3 PGL4	Multiple paragangliomas (100%)	
Neurofibromatosis Type 1 (von Recklinghausen disease)	17q11.2	Neurofibroma	Pheochromocytoma in 1–5%	Neurofibromas Schwannomas CNS gliomas
MEN 2A	10q11.2	RET	Pheochromocytoma in 50–70%	Parathyroid hyperplasia Medullary thyroid carcinoma
MEN 2B	10q11.2	RET	Pheochromocytoma in 50–70%	Medullary thyroid carcinoma Mucosal neuromas Skeletal abnormalities

gangliomas are separate from the carotid body and other structures, and are vanishingly rare.

Most patients with head and neck paragangliomas are in the fourth and fifth decades without any gender differences (although females predominate in patients living at high altitude). Patients present with a slow growing, painless mass and may have related symptoms. These symptoms commonly include tinnitus, hearing loss, or cranial nerve dysfunction depending on the location of the tumor. Only rare head and neck paragangliomas are biochemically active (up to 4%). In superficial locations, paragangliomas may be described clinically as a pulsatile mass. In the middle ear, examination of the ear may demonstrate a reddish-purple mass behind the tympanic membrane. About 10–15% of tumors are bilateral, multiple, familial, in pediatric patients, and malignant.

In the abdomen (non-adrenal), the neoplasms are most often associated with the sympathetic nervous system. Tumors in the abdomen are more often functional, and patients can present with clinical symptoms secondary to the secretion of catecholamines, such as headache, perspiration, palpitations, pallor, and hypertension. Abdominal paraganglioma (organ of Zuckerkandl accounts for the majority of extra-adrenal sympathetic paragangliomas) may be discovered incidentally when radiologic surveys are performed for other reasons. Paragangliomas can be associated with hereditary paragangliomatosis. Tumors arising in patients with a genetic syndrome are more likely to be multiple and bilateral (Table 13-1). Pheochromocytomas are more commonly syndrome associated.

RADIOLOGIC FEATURES

The most common studies used to assess paragangliomas are angiography, computed tomography (CT), magnetic resonance imaging (MRI) and iodinated metaiodobenzylguanidine (^{123}I-MIBG) scans. Contrast-enhanced CT scans will demonstrate an enhancing mass in characteristic locations (Figure 13-1). Contrast-enhanced MRI is also characteristic; showing a hyperintense T2 weighted image, and a salt and pepper vascularity within the tumor.

Angiography is often used for patients who are undergoing operative resection and this type of imaging will demonstrate the characteristic pronounced tumor vascularity. In carotid body paragangliomas, the tumor will splay the internal and external carotid arteries, which is a diagnostic feature of paraganglioma (Figure 13-2). In some cases, ultrasound may be helpful in localizing superficial paragangliomas. ^{123}I-MIBG scans have been reported to aid in localization of paragangliomas.

PATHOLOGIC FEATURES

GROSS FINDINGS

Most paragangliomas are resected en bloc, although the surgery is often bloody and difficult. The resected specimen will consist of a round to oval mass lesion with a

---

PARAGANGLIOMA
PATHOLOGIC FEATURES

Gross Findings

▸ Gray to hemorrhagic mass with fibrous pseudocapsule

Microscopic Findings

▸ Nests of various sizes
▸ Polygonal cells with granular, basophilic to eosinophilic cytoplasm
▸ Hyperchromatic nuclei with possible pleomorphism
▸ Network of fibrovascular septae

Immunohistochemical Results

▸ Chief cells positive with chromogranin, synaptophysin, NSE, CD56
▸ S-100 protein positive sustentacular cells

Pathologic Differential Diagnosis

▸ Neuroendocrine adenoma of the middle ear, ceruminous adenoma, meningioma, schwannoma, hyalinizing trabecular adenoma of thyroid, metastatic renal cell carcinoma, carcinoid, atypical carcinoid, medullary thyroid carcinoma

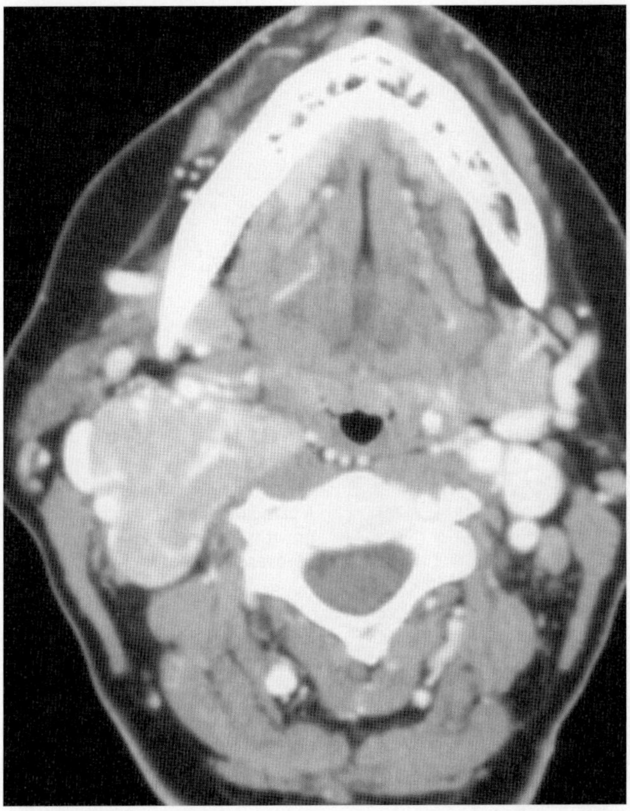

---

smooth, encapsulated or well circumscribed periphery (Figure 13-3). Carotid body tumors average about 4 cm, but can grow to 10 cm. Tumors of the middle ear tend to be small. The tumors are firm and vary from light tan to dark reddish-brown, the latter correlating with the hemorrhage or congestion within these highly vas-

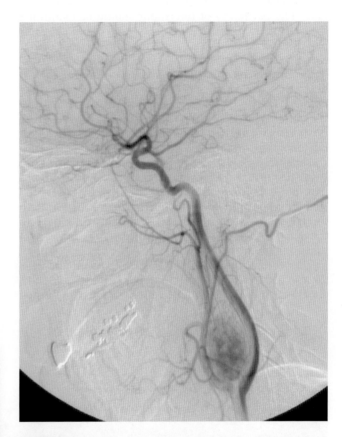

FIGURE 13-2

Angiography demonstrates splaying of the internal and external carotid arteries by a well-vascularized paraganglioma.

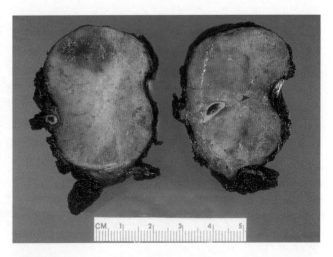

FIGURE 13-3

Gross image of a carotid body paraganglioma with a pseudocapsule and congested cut surface. (Courtesy of Dr JA Ohara.)

FIGURE 13-1

Contrast enhanced CT demonstrates a large enhancing mass at the bifurcation of the carotid artery on the left.

cular tumors. The risk of recurrence due to incompletely resected tumors makes a comment about inked margins vital in the final report.

MICROSCOPIC FINDINGS

A fibrous pseudocapsule that can be incomplete on histologic sections will most often surround paragangliomas. The periphery of the tumor should be examined for clear margins of resection. In some cases, capsular penetration and vascular invasion may be found, but these features are not indicative of malignancy. Architecturally, the tumor cells are arranged in round to oval nests that can vary in size, the so-called 'zellballen' pattern (Figure 13-4). Sometimes, fibrosis may obscure the classic nested pattern (Figure 13-5). Rarely, other types of patterns can predominate, such as trabecular, angioma-like, or spindled growth.

Hemorrhage may be present in these tumors, but frank necrosis is not a common feature. Paragangliomas may be embolized before surgery. In these cases, the tumor may be infracted or hemorrhagic, and may contain foreign material in the vascular channels secondary to the embolization (Figure 13-6). This should not be mistaken for tumor necrosis.

The cytomorphology of paraganglioma tumor cells varies. The main cell type is the chief cell (type I cells, chemoreceptive cells). These cells are neuroectodermal in origin. The cytoplasm can vary from a finely granular eosinophilic appearance, to deeply eosinophilic, or even clear cytoplasm in some cases (Figure 13-7). Similarly, the nuclear features can vary from small and round to large and vesicular with bizarre random pleomorphism. Mitoses are sparse and they should not be atypical.

A characteristic feature in paragangliomas is the supporting network of stromal cells and vessels that surround the nests of neoplastic cells. These supporting cells are called sustentacular cells. They are histologically and ultrastructurally non-distinct, but are highlighted with S-100 protein immunohistochemistry.

Middle ear and laryngeal paraganglioma deserve special mention, as their histologic features can be somewhat confusing in these locations. Jugulotympanic paragangliomas are often fragmented and tend to be comprised of smaller nests of cells and higher vascularity (Figure 13-8), which can lead to confusion with other tumors in the middle ear. Laryngeal paragangliomas are extremely rare and must not be confused with neuroendocrine tumors of the larynx (atypical carcinoid and neuroendocrine carcinoma). Occasionally, paragangliomas can be pigmented (postulated to be neuromelanin), may contain amyloid, and may occasionally have eosinophilic cytoplasmic globules (Figure 13-9). None of these features alter prognosis, but may be a pitfall for appropriate diagnosis.

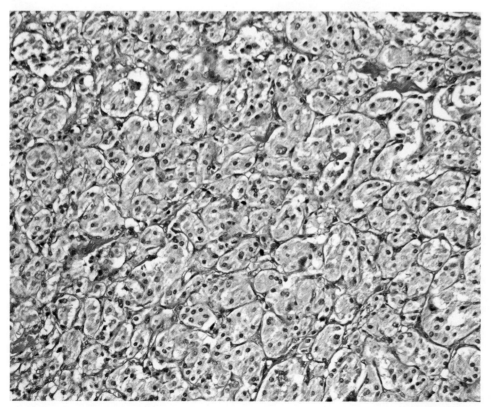

FIGURE 13-4

A paraganglioma showing the nested growth ('zellballen') with delicate fibrovascular septae.

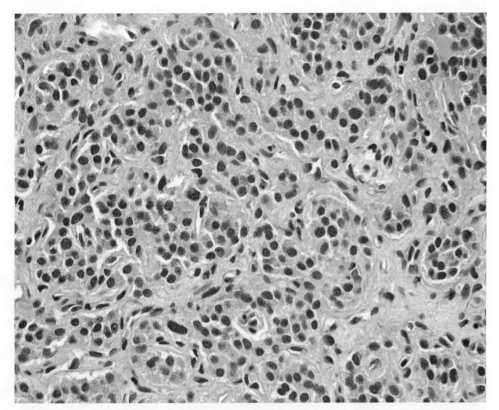

FIGURE 13-5

Fibrosis separates the islands of tumor cells which have eosinophilic cytoplasm and the centrally placed round, hyperchromatic nuclei.

FIGURE 13-6

Portions of the tumor show the characteristic nested pattern (left), while embolic material associated with foreign-body giant cells is noted in this embolized neoplasm (right).

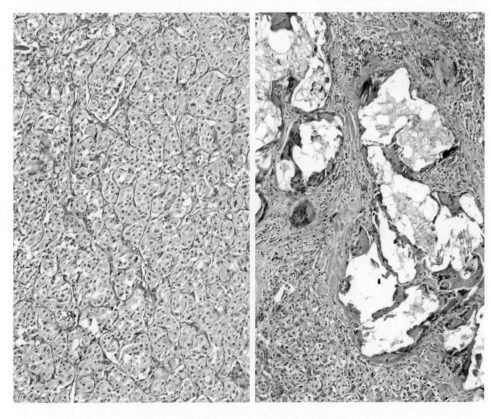

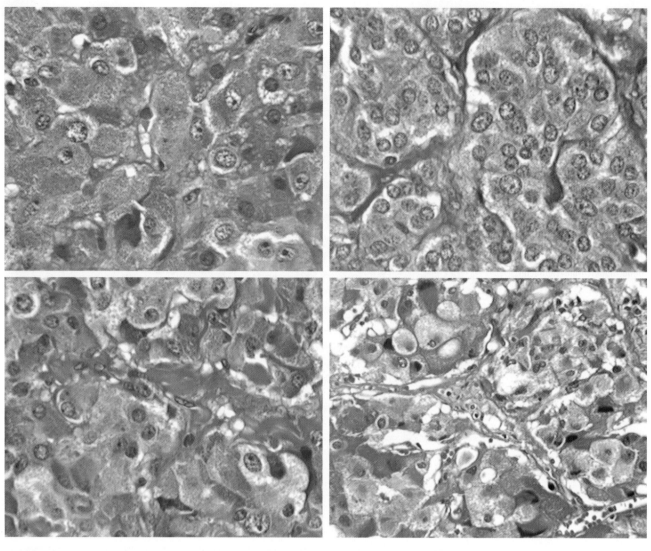

FIGURE 13-7

The various cytomorphologic features include basophilic cytoplasm (left upper), granular cytoplasm with fibrosis (left lower), a syncytial architecture (right upper), and focal clearing in cells that are moderately pleomorphic (right lower).

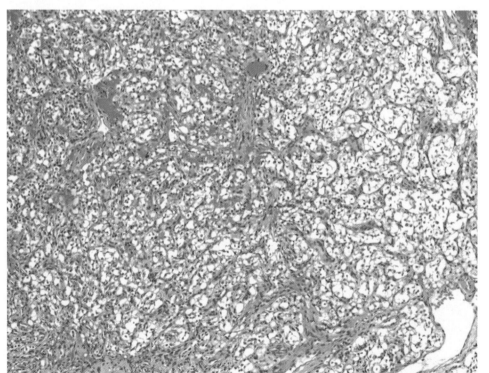

FIGURE 13-8

A jugulotympanic paraganglioma showing small nests and increased vascularity.

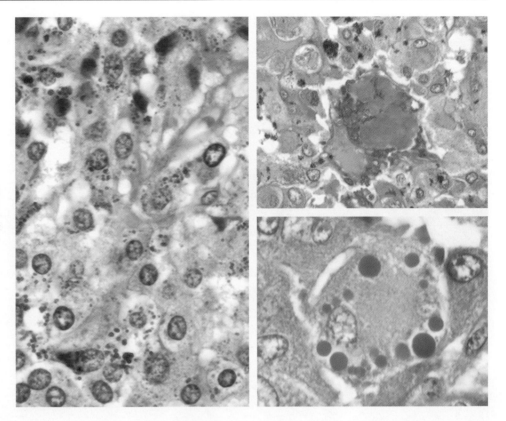

FIGURE 13-9
Left: Melanin pigment may be found in paraganglioma. Right upper: Amyloid deposition in a paraganglioma. Right lower: Eosinophilic cytoplasmic globules in a paraganglioma.

ANCILLARY STUDIES

ULTRASTRUCTURAL FEATURES

Electron microscopy is not used often, but shows characteristic dense-core neurosecretory granules. The granules can vary in number and in morphology, often correlating with the secretory characteristics.

IMMUNOHISTOCHEMICAL RESULTS

The 'non-chromaffin' cells of paragangliomas will invariably stain for neuroendocrine immunohistochemical markers, including chromogranin, synaptophysin, neuron specific enolase (NSE), CD56, Leu-7, S-100 protein, and a variety of specialized neuropeptides in a smaller subset of tumors (i.e., somatostatin, substance P, ACTC, and calcitonin). The supporting sustentacular cells have a unique staining pattern in that they are uniformly S-100 protein positive, highlighting the periphery of the tumor (Figure 13-10).

FINE NEEDLE ASPIRATION

Fine needle aspiration of paraganglioma is generally not recommended as it may result in significant hemorrhage and manipulation of a functional tumor can produce hypertensive crisis. However, in unsuspected cases, the FNA specimens are usually hypercellular, demonstrating single cells or small groups arranged in a 'pseudorosette' pattern (Figure 13-11). Small to moder-

ate sized polygonal cells have wispy, pale cytoplasm with variably sized and shaped nuclei. Binucleated or multinucleated cells are noted (Figure 13-12).

DIFFERENTIAL DIAGNOSIS

The differential diagnosis for paraganglioma depends upon the location of the tumor.

JUGULOTYMPANIC PARAGANGLIOMA

Paraganglioma may be difficult to separate from other tumors when biopsies are small and may be crushed. Tumors include middle ear adenoma, ceruminous adenoma, meningioma, schwannoma, metastatic renal cell carcinoma. Morphologic overlap can usually be resolved with a pertinent panel of immunohistochemistry studies (Table 13-2). Paraganglioma is not reactive with keratin or EMA, which will help separate a number of these tumors.

LARYNGEAL PARAGANGLIOMA

Laryngeal paraganglioma are very uncommon. Carcinoid, atypical carcinoid, small cell neuroendocrine carcinomas, and other neuroendocrine tumors that can secondarily involve the larynx, such as medullary thyroid carcinoma or metastases from other locations are raised in the differential. However, different

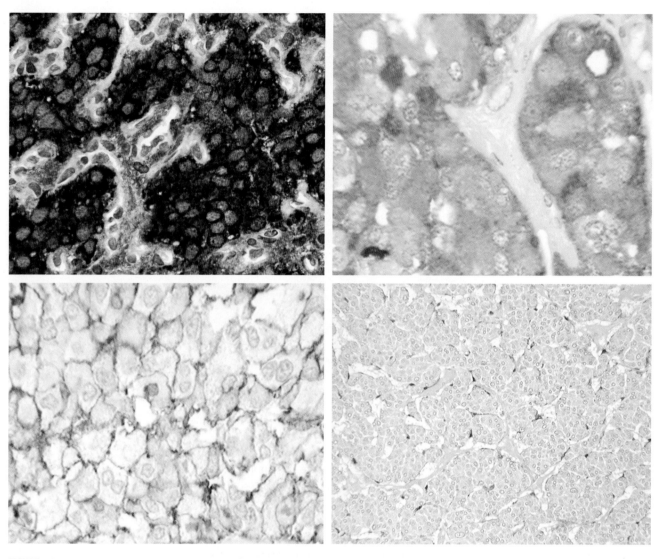

FIGURE 13-10

The paraganglia cells will be positive with chromogranin (upper left, 150×), CD56 (lower left, 300×), and synaptophysin (right upper, 300×); S-100 protein highlights the sustentacular cells (right lower, 50×).

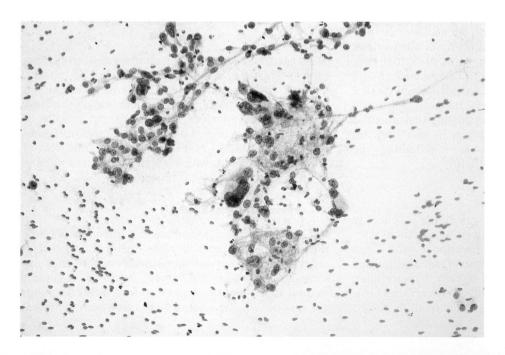

FIGURE 13-11

A Papanicolau stained, alcohol fixed smear of a paraganglioma showing small 'rosette' of cells with variable, hyperchromatic nuclei. Focal spindling is noted.

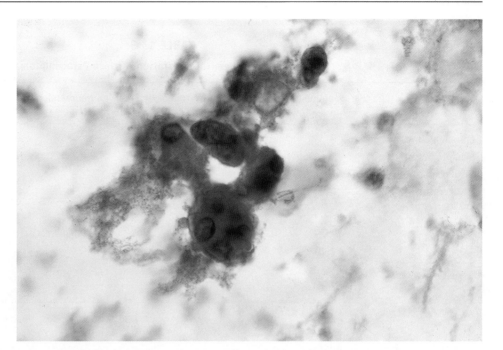

FIGURE 13-12

An alcohol fixed, H&E stained smear shows a multinucleated cell with wispy cytoplasm and nuclear variability in this paraganglioma.

TABLE 13-2

Immunohistochemical Separation of Ear Tumors

Stain	Paraganglioma	Neuroendocrine Adenoma of the Middle Ear	Metastatic Renal Cell Carcinoma	Meningioma
Chromogranin	+	+	−	−
Synaptophysin	+	+	−	−
S-100 protein	+ (s)	−	−	−/+ (rare)
Cytokeratin	−	+	+	−/+ (rare)
EMA	−	+	+	+
CD10	Unknown	Unknown	+	Unknown

s, sustentacular

VAGAL AND CAROTID BODY TUMORS

In this location, paraganglioma must be differentiated from other neuroendocrine tumors, including medullary thyroid carcinoma, hyalinizing trabecular tumor of the thyroid, and neuroendocrine carcinoma. Medullary thyroid carcinoma will be positive for calcitonin, TTF-1, and CEA. Neuroendocrine carcinomas will be positive for cytokeratins, as well as the typical neuroendocrine markers (Table 13-3). Clinical and radiographic correlation will also be of use in separating these tumors.

patterns of growth, increased nuclear pleomorphism, necrosis, increased mitoses, and a carefully selected immunohistochemistry panel will help in this differential.

PROGNOSIS AND THERAPY

Paragangliomas are indolent tumors, without very well-established histologic criteria for malignancy. Therefore, even though the tumors are histologically benign in appearance, life-long clinical (including biochemical and/or radiographic studies) follow-up is necessary to exclude potential recurrence or metastasis (regional lymph node or distant sites). Local symptoms may persist due to mass effect, or if the tumor was functional, catecholamine excess can be debilitating and dangerous. For the most part, if recurrence or metastasis does develop, an overall >90% 5-year survival will decrease substantially (10% 5-year survival).

TABLE 13-3

Immunohistochemical Separation of Neck Paraganglioma

Stain	Paraganglioma	Medullary Thyroid Carcinoma	Larynx Neuroendocrine Carcinoma	Metastatic Neuroendocrine Carcinoma
Chromogranin	+	+	+	+
Synaptophysin	+	+	+	+
S-100 protein	+ (s)	–	–	–
Cytokeratin	–	+	+	+
CEA	–	+	+	+
Calcitonin	–	+	+/–	+/–
TTF-1	–	+	–	+/–

s, sustentacular

Surgery is the treatment of choice, with pre-operative treatment with alpha and beta-blockers and/or embolization. Gamma knife radiation has been used with mixed results.

MALIGNANT PARAGANGLIOMA

Malignant paragangliomas are relatively uncommon, although in some studies of extra-adrenal paragangliomas, malignancy rates are 50%. Regrettably, the pathologist is rarely able to make the diagnosis of malignancy in the primary tumor, as there are no reproducible, reliable and well accepted histologic criteria for malignancy. Multifocal, multiple, and bilateral tumors can make the determination of metastatic disease a challenge. Therefore, malignancy is narrowly defined as the presence of metastatic disease in sites not normally known to have chromaffin tissue. The most common sites for diagnosis of true metastatic disease are regional lymph nodes, bone, and lungs. The clinical course is indolent and prolonged in many patients, despite known metastatic disease. Functional tumors may make the determination of recurrence a little easier.

CLINICAL FEATURES

The clinical parameters are indistinguishable from benign tumors, although patients tend to be slightly older and are more likely to be symptomatic than patients with benign tumors.

**MALIGNANT PARAGANGLIOMA
DISEASE FACT SHEET**

Definition
▸ Malignant tumor arising from the paraganglia along the parasympathetic or sympathetic nerves

Incidence and Location
▸ Very rare
▸ Most malignant paragangliomas are abdominal

Morbidity and Mortality
▸ Protracted clinical course with late recurrences
▸ Functional tumors have symptomatic recurrences

Gender, Race and Age Distribution
▸ Equal gender distribution
▸ Fifth to seventh decades

Clinical Features
▸ Identical symptoms and signs as benign tumors
▸ May be larger than benign counterparts
▸ More likely to be functional (catecholamine secretion) than benign tumors

Prognosis and Therapy
▸ <50% 10-year survival
▸ Recurrences and metastases in about 50%, often late
▸ Surgery (debulking) with catecholamine blockade
▸ Radiolabeled analogues show promise

RADIOLOGIC FEATURES

The principle role of radiographic studies is to define the extent of disease and presence of multifocal or metastatic deposits pre-operatively to allow for appropriate intervention. Metastatic deposits can be FDG-avid, suggesting PET scanning may be useful. ^{123}I-MIBG studies or a labeled dopamine analog tracer may be useful for imaging as well as therapy.

PATHOLOGIC FEATURES

GROSS FINDINGS

Malignant paragangliomas tend to be large, demonstrating areas of confluent necrosis and hemorrhage. Extensive and significant gross capsular and/or vascular invasion may be noted.

MICROSCOPIC FINDINGS

While no features are absolute, a few histologic features are correlated with metastatic potential: extensive capsular or vascular invasion, confluent necrosis, increased cellularity, large nests or diffuse growth, profound pleomorphism, increased mitoses (>3/10 high power fields), and atypical mitotic figures. These features are uncommon in head and neck locations, making it difficult to prospectively predict outcome.

ANCILLARY STUDIES

There are no currently available histochemical, immunohistochemical, ploidy, or molecular/genetic markers which accurately predict a malignant paraganglioma. However, malignancy is suggested when there is a *loss* of S-100 protein positive sustentacular cells, correlating

with a diffuse growth or large nest pattern; and if there is an increased proliferation index (Ki-67). Additional techniques show promise, but require validation.

DIFFERENTIAL DIAGNOSIS

Separation between benign and malignant paraganglioma causes the most difficulty and may be impossible to accurately diagnose. Paragangliomatosis may sometimes be mistaken for metastatic tumor. Malignant paraganglioma may mimic other neuroendocrine tumors, medullary thyroid carcinoma, adrenal cortical carcinoma and renal cell carcinoma. These tumors can usually be eliminated with immunohistochemistry studies.

PROGNOSIS AND THERAPY

The tumors are indolent, but progressive, resulting in <50% 10-year survival for malignant paraganglioma overall. When metastasis develops, lymph node, bone, liver and lung are the most common sites. Without accepted histologic criteria for malignancy, all patients with paraganglioma will need life-long clinical follow-up for any evidence of metastatic or recurrent disease. Surgery, especially debulking procedures, is the treatment of choice, with symptomatic management resulting from excess catecholamines (α-blockade and β-blockade). Radio-labeled analogues may be used in functional tumors, but chemotherapy and radiation do not seem to impact survival.

MALIGNANT PARAGANGLIOMA PATHOLOGIC FEATURES

Gross Findings
▸ Usually large tumors with hemorrhage and necrosis

Microscopic Findings
▸ Widely invasive lesions (capsule, vessel, into surrounding parenchyma/soft tissue)
▸ Confluent necrosis
▸ Large nests or diffuse growth
▸ Profound pleomorphism
▸ Increased mitotic figures and atypical forms

Immunohistochemical Results
▸ *Decreased* S-100 protein positive sustentacular cells suggests malignancy
▸ *Increased* Ki-67 labeling index suggests malignancy

Pathologic Differential Diagnosis
▸ Benign paraganglioma, atypical carcinoid, neuroendocrine carcinoma, medullary thyroid carcinoma, adrenal cortical carcinoma, renal cell carcinoma

---

SUGGESTED READING

Paraganglioma

Ali-el-Dein B, el-Sobky E, el-Baz M, Shaaban AA. Abdominal and pelvic extra-adrenal paraganglioma: a review of literature and a report on 7 cases. In Vivo 2002;16:249–254.

Bauters C, Vantyghem MC, Leteurtre E, et al. Hereditary phaeochromocytomas and paragangliomas: a study of five susceptibility genes. J Med Genet 2003;40:e75.

Baysal BE, Myers EN. Etiopathogenesis and clinical presentation of carotid body tumors. Microsc Res Tech 2002;59:256–261.

Bikhazi PH, Messina L, Mhatre AN, et al. Molecular pathogenesis in sporadic head and neck paraganglioma. Laryngoscope 2000;110: 1346–1348.

Edstrom Elder E, Hjelm Skog AL, Hoog A, Hamberger B. The management of benign and malignant pheochromocytoma and abdominal paraganglioma. Eur J Surg Oncol 2003;29:278–283.

Erickson D, Kudva YC, Ebersold MJ, et al. Benign paragangliomas: clinical presentation and treatment outcomes in 236 patients. J Clin Endo Metabol 2001;86:5210–5216.

Ferlito A, Barnes L, Wenig BM. Identification, classification, treatment, and prognosis of laryngeal paraganglioma. Review of the literature and eight new cases. Ann Otol Rhinol Laryngol 1994;103:525–536.

Kimura N, Capella C, De Krijger RR, et al. Extra-adrenal sympathetic paraganglioma: Superior and inferior paraaortic paraganglioma. In: DeLellis RA, Lloyd RV, Heitz PU, Eng C, eds. Pathology and Genetics of Tumours of the Endocrine Organs. Kliehues P, Sobin LH, series eds. World Health Organization Classification of Tumours. Lyon, France: IARC Press, 2004:164–165.

Kimura N, Chetty R, Capella C, et al. Extra-adrenal paraganglioma: Carotid body, jugulotympanic, vagal, laryngeal, aortico-pulmonary. In: DeLellis RA, Lloyd RV, Heitz PU, Eng C, eds. Pathology and Genetics of Tumours of the Endocrine Organs. Kliehues P, Sobin LH, series eds. World Health Organization Classification of Tumours. Lyon, France: IARC Press, 2004:159–161.

Koch CA, Vortmeyer AO, Zhuang Z, et al. New insights into the genetics of familial chromaffin cell tumors. Ann New York Acad Sci 2002;970:11–28.

Lack EE, Lloyd RV, Carney JA, Woodruff JM. Association of Directors of Anatomic and Surgical Pathology: Recommendations for reporting of extra-adrenal paragangliomas. Mod Pathol 2003;16:833–835.

Maher ER, Eng C. The pressure rises: update on the genetics of phaeochromocytoma. Hum Mol Genet 2002;11:2347–2354.

McCaffrey TV, Meyer FB, Michels VV, et al. Familial paragangliomas of the head and neck. Arch Otolaryngol Head Neck Surg. 1994;120:1211–1216.

McNichol AM. Differential diagnosis of pheochromocytomas and paragangliomas. Endocr Pathol. 2001;12:407–415.

Milroy CM, Ferlito A. Immunohistochemical markers in the diagnosis of neuroendocrine neoplasms of the head and neck. Ann Otol Rhinol Laryngol 1995;104:413–418.

Moran CA, Albores-Saavedra J, Wenig BM, Mena H. Pigmented extraadrenal paragangliomas: A clinicopathology and immunohistochemical study of five cases. Cancer. 1997;79:398–402.

Pellitteri PK, Rinaldo A, Myssiorek D, et al. Paragangliomas of the head and neck. Oral Oncol 2004;40:563–575.

Plukker JT, Brongers EP, Vermey A, et al. Outcome of surgical treatment for carotid body paraganglioma. Br J Surg 2001;88:1382–1386.

Rao AB, Koeller KK, Adair CF. From the archives of the AFIP. Paragangliomas of the head and neck: radiologic-pathologic correlation. Radiographics 1999;19:1605–1632.

Tischler AS, Komminoth P. Extra-adrenal sympathetic paraganglioma: Cervical paravertebral, intrathoracic and urinoary bladder. In: DeLellis RA, Lloyd RV, Heitz PU, Eng C, eds. Pathology and Genetics of Tumours of the Endocrine Organs. Kliehues P, Sobin LH, series eds. World Health Organization Classification of Tumours. Lyon, France: IARC Press, 2004:165–166.

van der Mey AG, Jansen JC, van Baalen JM. Management of carotid body tumors. Otolaryngol Clin North Am 2001;34:907–924.

Wasserman PG, Savargaonkar P. Paragangliomas: classification, pathology, and differential diagnosis. Otolaryngol Clin North Am 2001;34:845–862, v–vi.

Weber PC, Patel S. Jugulotympanic paragangliomas. Otolaryngol Clin North Am 2001;34:1231–1240.

Whiteman ML, Serafini AN, Telischi FF, et al. [111]In octreotide scintigraphy in the evaluation of head and neck lesions. AJNR 1073;18:1073–1080.

Malignant Paraganglioma

Argiris A, Mellott A, Spies S. PET scan assessment of chemotherapy response in metastatic paraganglioma. Am J Clin Oncol 2003;26:563–566.

Brown HM, Komorowski RA, Wilson SD, et al. Predicting metastasis of pheochromocytomas using DNA flow cytometry and immunohistochemical markers of cell proliferation: A positive correlation between MIB-1 staining and malignant tumor behavior. Cancer. 1999;86:1583–1589.

Edstrom Elder E, Hjelm Skog AL, Hoog A, Hamberger B. The management of benign and malignant pheochromocytoma and abdominal paraganglioma. Eur J Surg Oncol 2003;29:278–283.

Shah MJ, Karelia NH, Patel SM, et al. Flow cytometric DNA analysis for determination of malignant potential in adrenal pheochromocytoma or paraganglioma: an Indian experience. Ann Surg Oncol 2003;10:426–431.

Thompson LD. Pheochromocytoma of the Adrenal gland Scaled Score (PASS) to separate benign from malignant neoplasms: a clinicopathologic and immunophenotypic study of 100 cases. Am J Surg Pathol 2002;26:551–566.

Anatomy, Embryology and Histology

Jason C Fowler • Lester DR Thompson

INTRODUCTION

Nowhere in the human body is the embryology and anatomy more complex than in the head and neck and endocrine organs. The purpose of this appendix is to provide a reference to the major anatomic sites that are often encountered in routine surgical pathology of endocrine organs. This section will serve as a beginning reference only, with the interested reader referred to the suggested reading for a more comprehensive discussion on the anatomy, embryology and histology. The following anatomic sites will be discussed: neck, thyroid gland, parathyroid gland, adrenal gland, and pituitary gland with a specific presentation of the embryology, anatomy, and histology.

NECK

Much of head and neck embryology centers around the pharyngeal (branchial) arches, pouches and clefts. The branchial apparatus is responsible for a vast majority of the development of structures in the head and neck (Figure A-1). The branchial arches arise as swellings of mesenchyme along the sidewalls of the developing gut tube. There are five arches that arise, although the 5th arch is vestigial and eventually disappears, but not before giving rise to the ultimobranchial body. Each branchial arch is supplied by its own cranial nerve and blood supply. Each of the arches are separated by depressions on the inside of the pharynx known as pouches and depressions on the outside known as clefts. There are total of four pouches and four clefts between the five arches. Each arch gives rise to specific anatomic structures in the head and neck (Tables A-1 and A-2), with the interplay of the ectoderm, mesoderm and endoderm layers too complicated to describe in detail here.

THYROID

The thyroid gland derives from the foregut as the median anlage (endodermal derivation), a bilobed diverticulum attaching to the tongue by the thyroglossal duct and opening at the foramen cecum (Figure A-2). The thyroglossal duct provides the route for descent in front of the pharyngeal gut, to a point where the thyroid gland ultimately lies below the thyroid cartilage and below the hyoid bone as a midline structure by the 7th week of development; the isthmus and two lobes are identified by this time. Thyroid function begins at about the 10–12th week, when follicles containing colloid first become visible (Figure A-3). Residua of the thyroglossal duct may form a cyst or a fistula, while remnants of thyroid gland tissue may be identified along this path of decent. Additionally, thyroid tissue may be intertwined in the skeletal muscle in the region of the isthmus.

The thyroid gland contains two lobes and an isthmus, wrapped around the anterior portion of the larynx and trachea, usually just below the level of the cricoid cartilage (Figure A-4). A pyramidal lobe may extend upward from the isthmus towards the hyoid bone. The adult gland weighs about 15 to 25 grams, obviously variable based on gender or pathologic state. The lateral thyroid lobes are somewhat conical, measuring about 5 cm in height and 3 cm wide. The gland is invested by a fibrous connective tissue capsule, with extensions into the gland forming septa which divide the gland into lobules. The lobules contain a rich vascular plexus and nerve supply, which surrounds the functional unit – the follicle. The follicles are variable in shape, although usually rounded, lined by a single layer of flattened to cuboidal epithelial cells (Figure A-5). The center of each follicle is filled with proteinaceous, eosinophilic material (colloid), which has been secreted from the follicular cells. Follicular cells have eosinophilic cytoplasm surrounding small nuclei which are round to oval, displaying evenly distributed nuclear chromatin. Nucleoli are small. Follicular cells are strongly and diffusely immunoreactive with keratin,

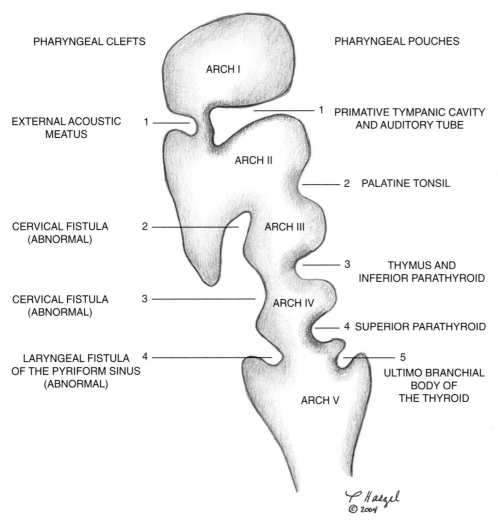

PHARYNGEAL CLEFTS

PHARYNGEAL POUCHES

ARCH I

EXTERNAL ACOUSTIC
MEATUS

1 — 1 PRIMATIVE TYMPANIC CAVITY
AND AUDITORY TUBE

ARCH II

2 PALATINE TONSIL

CERVICAL FISTULA
(ABNORMAL)

2 — ARCH III

3 THYMUS AND
INFERIOR PARATHYROID

CERVICAL FISTULA
(ABNORMAL)

3 — ARCH IV

4 SUPERIOR PARATHYROID

LARYNGEAL FISTULA
OF THE PYRIFORM SINUS
(ABNORMAL)

4 — 5
ULTIMO BRANCHIAL
BODY OF
THE THYROID

ARCH V

FIGURE A-1

The five pharyngeal arches and the anatomic structures (or abnormalities) resulting from the pouches (internal) and clefts (external). Virtually all structures in the head and neck are derived from the pharyngeal (branchial) arches and pouches. (Reprinted by permission of Trisha Haszel, Des Moines, IA.)

TABLE A-1

Anatomic Derivatives of the Pharyngeal (Branchial) Arches

Pharyngeal Arch	Cranial Nerve	Anatomic Structures Derived from Arch
1	V (Trigeminal)	Muscles of mastication, tensor veli palatini muscle, tensor tympani muscle, anterior belly of digastric muscle, mylohyoid muscle, mandibular process, malleus, sphenomandibular ligament, incus
2	VII (Facial)	Muscles of the face, stapedius muscle, stylohyoid muscle, posterior belly of digastric muscle, stapes, styloid process, stylohyoid ligament, hyoid bone (portion of body)
3	IX (Glossopharyngeal)	Stylopharyngeus muscle, greater cornu and body of hyoid bone
4	X (Vagus)	Cricothyroid and constrictor muscles of the pharynx, laryngeal cartilages
5	X (Vagus)	Laryngeal muscles, laryngeal cartilages

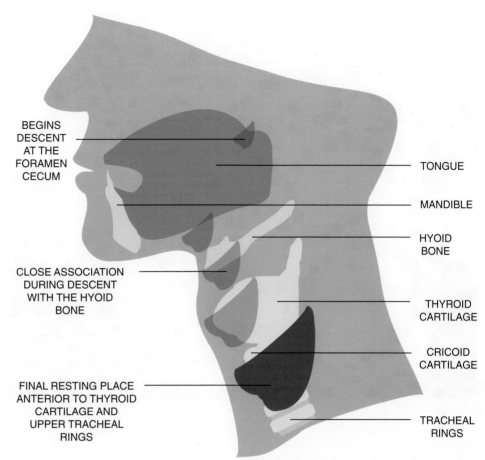

FIGURE A-2

Embryologic development of the thyroid from the base of the tongue to the anterior neck.

BEGINS DESCENT AT THE FORAMEN CECUM

TONGUE

MANDIBLE

HYOID BONE

CLOSE ASSOCIATION DURING DESCENT WITH THE HYOID BONE

THYROID CARTILAGE

CRICOID CARTILAGE

FINAL RESTING PLACE ANTERIOR TO THYROID CARTILAGE AND UPPER TRACHEAL RINGS

TRACHEAL RINGS

TABLE A-2

Anatomic Derivatives of the Pharyngeal (Branchial) Pouches (Clefts)

Cleft (Pouch)	Cleft Derivative (External)	Pouch Derivative (Internal)
1	External acoustic meatus (Work Type I & II Fistulas)	Middle ear cavity and auditory tube
2	Cervical fistula (abnormal)	Palatine tonsil
3	Cervical fistula (abnormal)	Thymus, inferior parathyroid gland
4	Pyriform sinus fistula (abnormal)	Superior parathyroid gland
5	N/A	Ultimobranchial body of the thyroid

TTF-1 and, to a lesser degree with thyroglobulin and vimentin. Thyroglobulin must be interpreted with caution, as it tends to have diffusion artifact and may have high background staining. TTF-1 tends to show strong, diffuse nuclear staining in > 99 % of the cells.

Usually identified in the middle to upper third of the lateral lobes, C-cells are derived from the ultimobranchial body, a derivative of the 5th pharyngeal pouch. These cells are located in a parafollicular distribution (occasionally called 'parafollicular cells'), and are larger than thyroid follicular cells. They are polyhedral with larger nuclei surrounded by finely granular, clear to slightly basophilic cytoplasm (Figure A-6). They are difficult to identify in routinely processed tissue in adults. However, the cells are strongly and diffusely immunoreactive with calcitonin, chromogranin, synaptophysin, p-carcinoembryonic antigen (p-CEA), somatostatin and serotonin.

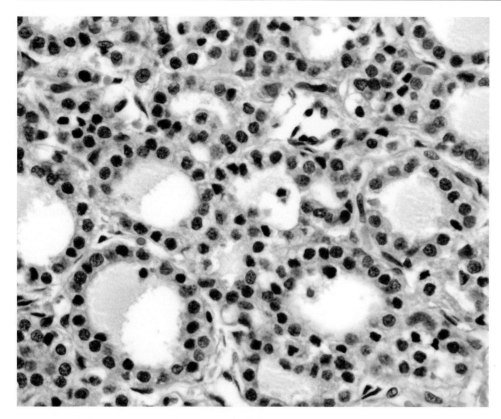

FIGURE A-3
Thyroid follicles are small and tight in this 24 week fetus. Colloid is present, but it is thin.

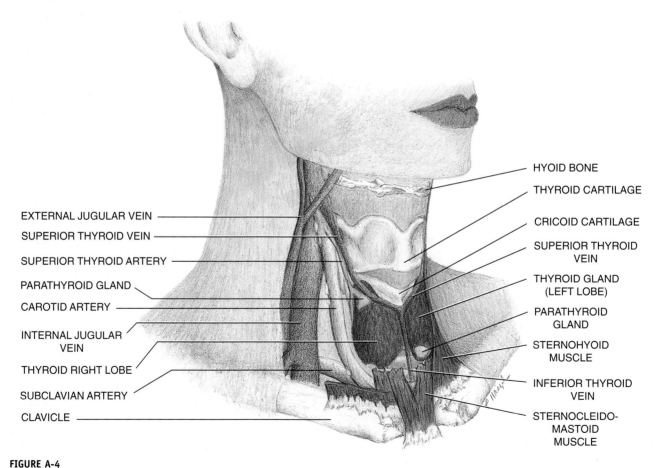

HYOID BONE

THYROID CARTILAGE

CRICOID CARTILAGE

SUPERIOR THYROID VEIN

THYROID GLAND (LEFT LOBE)

PARATHYROID GLAND

STERNOHYOID MUSCLE

INFERIOR THYROID VEIN

STERNOCLEIDO-MASTOID MUSCLE

EXTERNAL JUGULAR VEIN

SUPERIOR THYROID VEIN

SUPERIOR THYROID ARTERY

PARATHYROID GLAND

CAROTID ARTERY

INTERNAL JUGULAR VEIN

THYROID RIGHT LOBE

SUBCLAVIAN ARTERY

CLAVICLE

FIGURE A-4
The complex anatomy of the neck must be considered during interventions of the thyroid gland.

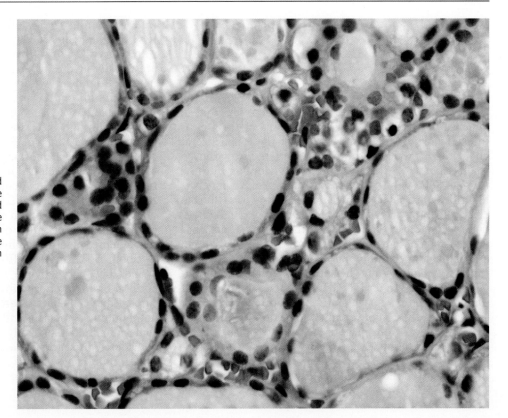

FIGURE A-5

A high power of normal thyroid parenchyma demonstrating the low cuboidal cells arranged around eosinophilic colloid. Cracks in the colloid are a result of their high protein content. The nuclei are round to slightly elongated with heavy chromatin distribution.

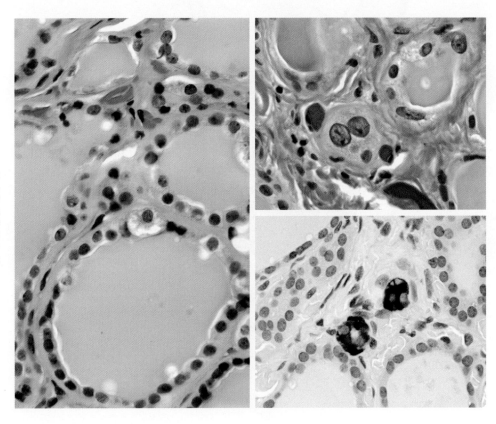

FIGURE A-6

Left: C-cells are often located in a parafollicular distribution. However, they are often difficult to identify on routine H&E material. Right upper: These C-cells have slightly basophilic, granular cytoplasm with round nuclei. Right lower: Calcitonin strongly reacts in the cytoplasm of these C-cells.

PARATHYROID GLAND

As already suggested in the section on the neck, the third and fourth endodermally derived pharyngeal pouches have a dorsal and ventral wing at their most inferior portion. The dorsal wing of these pouches at about the 5th week begin to differentiate into parathyroid tissue, while the ventral portions develop into the thymus. The parathyroid tissue from the 3rd pouch is identified on the posteromedial aspect of the thyroid gland, forming the inferior parathyroid gland. The 4th pouch tissue loses contact with the pharynx, attaches to the cephalad portion of the migrating thyroid gland, and is usually found along the superior border of the thyroid gland, forming the superior parathyroid gland.

Four glands are usually identified, but about 10% of the population may have more than four glands (Figure A-7). Given the complex embryologic development, the final anatomic resting place of the parathyroid is remarkably variable, although predicted by known routes of migration. The superior gland tends to be found at the intersection of the recurrent laryngeal nerve and the inferior thyroid artery, although it is not uncommon to have the gland identified within the thyroid parenchyma, retropharyngeal or retroesophageal. The inferior glands are usually at the lower pole of the thyroid gland, but may be found anywhere from the hyoid bone to the mediastinum, and even within the pericardium. Parathyroid glands weigh about 120 mg in aggregate, although variable through life. Most glands are about 0.5 cm in greatest dimension. The glands are brown, ovoid structures, often appearing somewhat flattened in their long axis. They are enveloped by a delicate, thin fibrous connective tissue capsule. A complex vascular network surrounds the parenchymal tissue. The gland is composed of stromal adipocytes with chief cells and oxyphilic cells (Figure A-8). The ratio of parenchyma to fat varies through life, usually high in children, and then changing to about 50% in the fifth decade, where it remains stable. The parenchymal cells are arranged in nests, cords and solid groups with occasionally follicular structures. Chief cells have cleared to slightly eosinophilic or amphophilic cytoplasm with intracellular lipid. Intracytoplasmic lipid is usually absent in cells which are considered 'hormonally active.' The nuclei are round and contain heavy, coarse nuclear chromatin. Oxyphilic cells are usually only present in adults. They may form

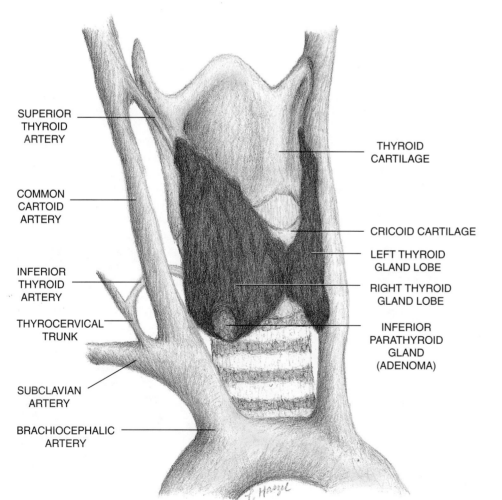

SUPERIOR THYROID ARTERY

COMMON CARTOID ARTERY

INFERIOR THYROID ARTERY

THYROCERVICAL TRUNK

SUBCLAVIAN ARTERY

BRACHIOCEPHALIC ARTERY

THYROID CARTILAGE

CRICOID CARTILAGE

LEFT THYROID GLAND LOBE

RIGHT THYROID GLAND LOBE

INFERIOR PARATHYROID GLAND (ADENOMA)

FIGURE A-7

The anatomy of the parathyroid glands in relationship to the anatomic structures of the neck.

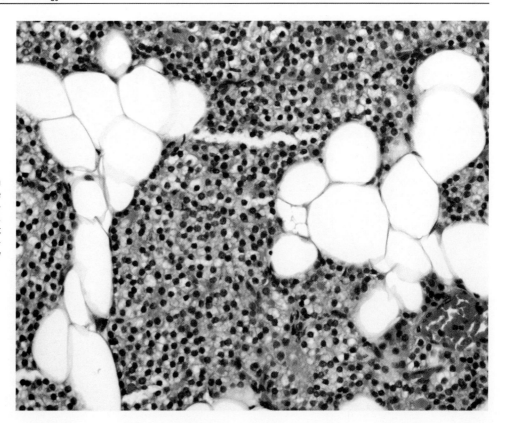

FIGURE A-8

A normal parathyroid gland with chief cells and adipose connective tissue. Note a few oncocytes, suggesting the sample is from an adult. The proportion of each constituent varies with age, with this illustration demonstrating approximately 50 % parenchyma.

small nodules or collections, and will increase in number as patient age. The cells contain eosinophilic, granular cytoplasm, the granularity conveyed by the increased number of mitochondria in the cytoplasm.

ADRENAL GLAND

Similar to the pituitary gland, the adrenal gland has a dual origin: the cortex derived from mesoderm and the medulla from ectoderm. The complex development of the adrenal gland occurs about the 6th week in the region of the root of the mesentery, the mesonephric duct and the developing gonad. The cortex proliferates from mesodermal cells which are surrounded by connective tissue from the mesonephric tissues (Figure A-9). The medulla forms when tissue from the sympathetic ganglionic tissue separates the developing cortex. The initial adrenal cortical tissue undergoes involution before the development of the permanent cortex, which does not reach full differentiation until about the 12th year of life. The medulla develops from neural crest primitive cells, which ultimately form pheochromocytes. The chromaffin tissue is predominantly extraadrenal during development, but will involute after birth. Interestingly, the fetal adrenal gland is proportionately much larger than adult adrenal gland.

The adrenal glands are usually located above the kidney, measuring about $5 \times 3 \times 1$ cm in dimension with an overall pyramidal shape and weighing up to 10 grams in adults (Figure A-10). The right gland is posterior to the vena cava and the right lobe of the liver, while the left gland is associated with the tail of the pancreas. There is a very rich vascular supply, along with extensive innervation, although the latter is only present in the medullary tissues. The gland is histologically separated into the cortex and the medulla (Figure A-11), with the cortex comprised of three concentrically layered zones: a subcapsular zona glomerulosa, a middle zona fasciculata and an innermost zona reticularis. Each of these zones is responsible for different hormone production, with aldosterone, glucocorticoids and sex hormones, respectively. The zona glomerulosa is a discontinuous layer composed of compact, polyhedral cells. The zona fasciculata contains larger cells arranged in columns with distinct cell borders and foamy, vacuolated cytoplasm. The nuclei are somewhat open and vesicular. The zone reticularis has small cells arranged in anastomosing cords, containing a more compact, eosinophilic cytoplasm. Accurate histologic separation of these zones is not always possible on routine microscopy. The medulla contains groups of cells in nests. The cells have a syncytial quality with abundant, granular, basophilic cytoplasm surrounding slightly eccentric nuclei. The nuclei often contain prominent nucleoli.

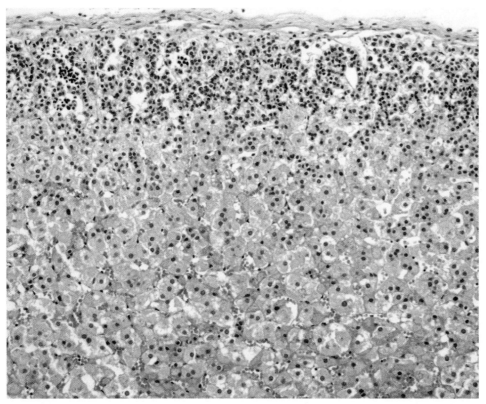

FIGURE A-9

A fetal adrenal gland (approximately 24 weeks gestation) demonstrates a cord-like distribution of the zona glomerulosa as it interfaces with the more column-like eosinophilic cells of the zona fasciculata.

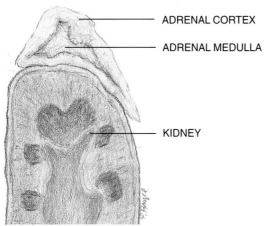

ADRENAL CORTEX

ADRENAL MEDULLA

KIDNEY

FIGURE A-10

The anatomic relationships around the adrenal gland.

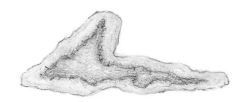

FIGURE A-11

The adrenal gland is divided into the cortex and medulla.

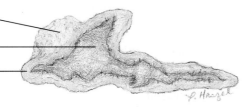

ADRENAL CORTICAL ADENOMA

ADRENAL MEDULLA

ADRENAL CORTEX

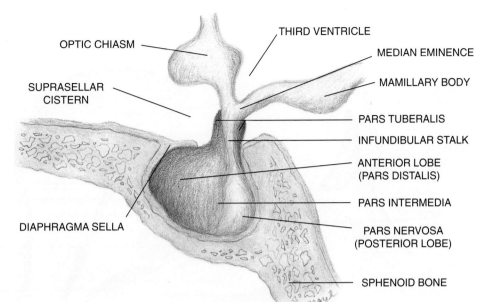

OPTIC CHIASM

THIRD VENTRICLE

MEDIAN EMINENCE

MAMILLARY BODY

SUPRASELLAR
CISTERN

PARS TUBERALIS

INFUNDIBULAR STALK

ANTERIOR LOBE
(PARS DISTALIS)

PARS INTERMEDIA

PARS NERVOSA
(POSTERIOR LOBE)

DIAPHRAGMA SELLA

SPHENOID BONE

FIGURE A-12

The embryologic development of the pituitary gland from Rathke's pouch and from the infundibulum.

PITUITARY GLAND

The hypophysis (pituitary) is formed from two completely separate parts: one is an ectodermal pouch from the stomodeum immediately anterior to the buccopharyngeal membrane called Rathke's pouch, and the second is a downward extension from the diencephalon called the infundibulum. At about 3 weeks gestation, Rathke's pouch grows dorsally towards the infundibulum through the developing sphenoid bone, loosing the connection to the oral cavity/pharynx by about the 8th week of development (Figure A-12). Cells within the anterior portion of Rathke's pouch proliferate and differentiate to form the anterior lobe (adenohypophysis; pars distalis), while a small cephalic extension of this lobe (pars tuberalis) grows along the stalk of the infundibulum, eventually surrounding it. The pars intermedia develops from the posterior portion of Rathke's pouch, but does not seem to play a significant role in later life in humans. Meanwhile, the infundibulum grows to form the stalk and the posterior lobe (pars nervosa or neurohypophysis). The nerve fibers within the posterior lobe extend from the hypothalamic area and play a critical role in hormone secretion. The pituitary gland is well developed by the 3rd month of gestation. Each of the parts of the pituitary gland secrete a particular hormone, with the adenohypophysis secreting growth hormone, adrenocorticotropic hormone, prolactin, thyrotropin, and gonadotropins (follicle-stimulating hormone and luteinizing hormone). The neurohypophysis contains pituicytes, nerve fibers and neurosecretory material involved in the transportation and release of oxytocin and vasopressin.

The pituitary is seldom removed intact in surgical material; however, it is about 1 cm in greatest dimension, weighing approximately 0.5 g. The anterior lobe accounts for about 80% of the overall weight of the gland. The pituitary gland in the sella turcica is completely surrounded by dura mater, with only a small opening (diaphragm sella) for its stalk attachment to the hypothalamus (Figure A-13). The pituitary is immediately adjacent to the internal carotid arteries, the optic nerves (optic chiasm), and the cavernous sinuses. Given the 'master-gland' control function, there is an extensive vascular supply, critical to the hormone secretory activity of the gland (Figures A-14 and A-15). Considered beyond the scope of this description, the specific histologic, immunohistochemical, and ultrastructural findings of the various hormone secreting cells will not be presented in detail. Suffice it to say, the small nests of cells are surrounded by a delicate, arborizing vascular plexus, and contain acidophilic (usually lateral), basophilic (usually median), and chromophobe (seen throughout) cells, the separation depending upon their affinity for acid or basic dyes.

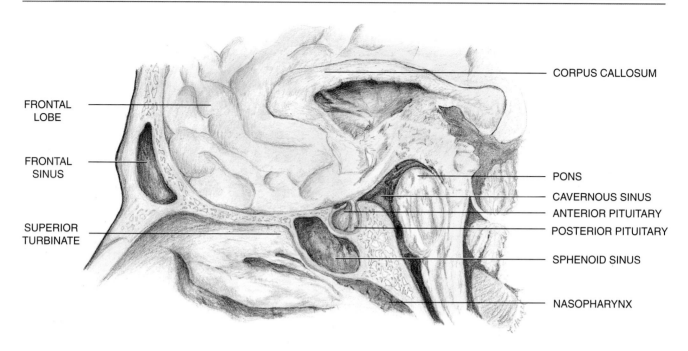

FIGURE A-13

The anatomic relations of the pituitary gland to the surrounding structures.

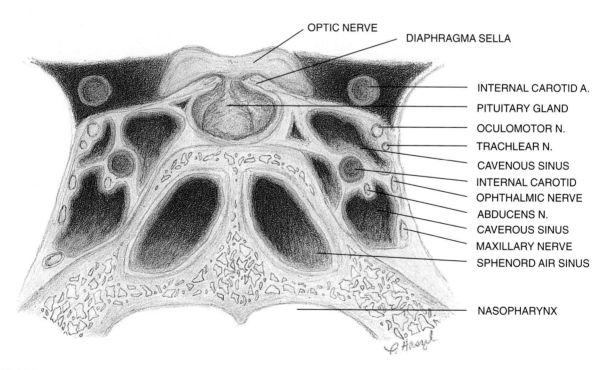

FIGURE A-14

An anterior (coronal) view of the pituitary gland and its relationships to the surrounding vessels and nerves.

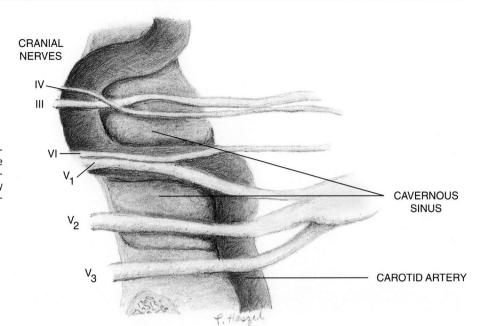

CRANIAL
NERVES

IV

III

VI

V₁

V₂

V₃

CAVERNOUS
SINUS

CAROTID ARTERY

FIGURE A-15

This lateral (sagittal) view of the pituitary gland and its relationships to the
surrounding vessels and nerves (specifically the carotid artery). The pituitary
gland is not shown, but the lateral structures are shown.

ACKNOWLEDGMENT

The authors would like to express their sincerest gratitude to Ms. Trisha Haszel of Des Moines, Iowa for her
superb artwork and illustrations.

SUGGESTED READING

Agur AM, Lee MJ. Grant's Atlas of Anatomy, 10th edition. Baltimore, MD:
    Lippincott, Williams and Wilkins, 1999.
Cochard LR. Netter's Atlas of Human Embryology. Teterboro, NJ: Icon
    Learning Systems LLC, 2002.
Dalley AF, Moore KL. Clinically Oriented Anatomy, 4th edition. Baltimore,
    MD: Lippincott, Williams and Wilkins, 1999.
Heath JW, Young B. Wheater's Functional Histology: A Text and Color Atlas,
    4th edition. London: Churchill Livingstone, 2000.
Langman J. Medical embryology. 4ᵗʰ ed. Baltimore: Williams & Wilkins,
    1981.
Larsen WJ. Human Embryology, 3rd edition. Philadelphia: Churchill-
    Livingstone, 2001.
Moore KL. The Developing Human: Clinically Oriented Embryology
    (Developing Human: Clinically Oriented Embryology), 7th edition. Phila-
    delphia: W.B. Saunders Co, 2003.
Netter F. Atlas of Human Anatomy, 2nd edition. Philadelphia: Rittenhouse
    Book Publishers, 1997.
Sadler TW. Langman's Medical Embryology, 7th edition. Baltimore, MD:
    Williams and Wilkins, 1995
Sternberg SS. Histology for Pathologists, 2nd edition. Philadelphia:
    Lippincott-Raven, 1997.
Wenig BM, Heffess CS, Adair CF. Atlas of endocrine pathology. Philadelphia:
    WB Saunders Co, 1997.

Intraoperative Consultation and Grossing Techniques

Jason C Fowler • Lester DR Thompson

INTRAOPERATIVE CONSULTATION

Intraoperative consultations (whether frozen sections, crush preparations, smears, touch preparations or gross examinations) are widely accepted as an efficient tool for patient management. The pathologist often plays a crucial role in determining the surgical outcome of patients undergoing resections for diseases of the endocrine organs. There are a number of scenarios for which surgeons will request an intraoperative consultation, but most of the time the aim is to obtain accurate diagnostic information that will either determine or alter the course of surgical treatment. Five areas result in possible errors: inaccurate communication, indications for intraoperative assessment, inadequate sampling (by surgeon or pathologist), incorrect interpretation, and technical difficulties.

COMMUNICATION

It is imperative that clear, open and effective communication is achieved between all parties during intraoperative consultation: surgeons, pathologists, operating room (OR) staff and pathologist's assistants. Physical presence in either the operating room or the gross laboratory by the pathologist and/or surgeon respectively, is often critical to achieve proper orientation and to identify specific areas of interest or concern. Furthermore, interaction is necessary for building confidence and teamwork. While axiomatic, the pathologist is ultimately responsible for appropriate specimen handling.

Specimens submitted for intraoperative consultation should be received fresh, but kept moist with a small amount of saline, optimally wrapped in a portion of sterile, saline-soaked gauze. Specimens for intraoperative consultation should never be submitted in formalin or other fixatives. Ideally, specimens should be submitted to the frozen section suite as they are removed to facilitate decision making in real time. Education and training of operating room and grossing room staff in correct specimen handling, labeling and transportation is essential to achieve error free specimen processing.

INDICATIONS AND CONTRAINDICATIONS FOR INTRAOPERATIVE CONSULTATION

There are only a selected number of instances in which samples in endocrine pathology need to have a frozen section performed. These include:
- Determination of specimen adequacy for special procedures such as cultures, immunophenotypic analysis, molecular studies, ultrastructural examination, or flow cytometry;
- A different definitive therapy would be conducted based upon the diagnosis (extent of disease determinations);
- Numerous previous attempts at diagnosis have been unsuccessful; and
- Assessment of adequate surgical margins of resection, although uncommon in endocrine organs.

In specimen adequacy determinations, only a portion of the tissue should be initially evaluated in order to triage the material and maintain tissue integrity for the specific studies chosen.

When assessing margins of resection, specimens should be taken (after appropriate inking and orientation) to include the closest margin, ideally on the main specimen, rather than small biopsies sent separately. However, if sent separately, no more than 2 cm of margin should be submitted to reduce sampling errors. The number and location of frozen sections depends on the confidence level and skill of the surgeon. A tumor is usually removed en-bloc with a rim of normal and supporting tissue. A shave (en face) margin or a radial (perpendicular) margin can be performed depending upon whether a distance to the closest margin is to be assessed (radial) or if a large surface is to be assessed (en face) (Figures B-01 and B-02).

While intraoperative consultations are an invaluable tool, they are also frequently misused. An intraoperative consultation, specifically frozen section, should *never* be performed just for intellectual or academic curiosity, gamesmanship, family reassurance, financial gain or rote examination, and should be discouraged when the tissue is heavily calcified, predominantly fat, if the specimen is exceptionally small, and for lesions suspected of being unique or unusual, requiring a number of additional studies (such as cultures, flow cytometry, immunofluorescence, ultrastructural examination). Levelheaded, direct communication with the surgeons on a regular basis, particularly during tumor board confer-

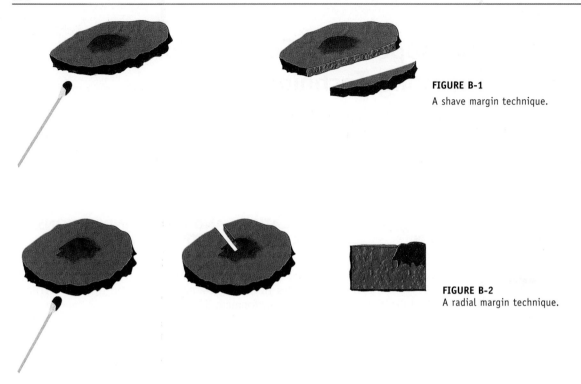

FIGURE B-1
A shave margin technique.

FIGURE B-2
A radial margin technique.

ences, should help to avoid unnecessary requests for intraoperative consultation.

SAMPLING

While sampling errors cannot be completely eliminated, they can be avoided to an extent by thoroughly examining the specimen(s) submitted for intraoperative consultation while communicating directly with the surgeon about specific area(s) in question. The use of sutures or a tissue pen to orient the margins of the specimen is crucial. Sampling errors may also be avoided by taking multiple sections from the main specimen, particularly the case with thyroid neoplasms. Proper orientation is extremely important, especially when trying to assess mucosal margins, although this is uncommon in endocrine organs. These samples should be placed in frozen section media such that both the epithelium and submucosal soft tissues are seen on the slide. Margins submitted by the surgeon should be marked with either ink or cautery so that the 'true margin' is the one represented on the slide for diagnosis.

INTERPRETATION

There are a number of factors that can lead to a pathologist misinterpreting an intraoperative consultation.

The most problematic area of histopathologic interpretation on frozen section diagnosis rests with thyroid lesions, and especially with the separation of follicular neoplasms. Mesenchymal and inflammatory lesions usually present with the problem of insufficient sampling, as there are often multiple different patterns of growth within a single tumor which can cause diagnostic difficulty. Of particular importance is the clinical history, as previous radiation, chemotherapy and/or surgery can alter the tissue architecture. Of course, communication errors are often only realized after the fact. While a personal bias, it is better to err on the side of benignancy and delay definitive therapy rather than perform a radical surgery for a benign disease. According to Dr Lauren Ackerman, frozen section should be performed by a person 'rich in experience, conservative in attitude, and most important, he [she] must have judgment'.

TECHNIQUES AND TECHNICAL PROBLEMS

A variety of commercial preparations are available for preparing and cutting the specimens, without a specific technique or product better than another. However, technical problems can result from cryostat difficulties to poor staining quality. Any type of technical problem can affect interpretation and the subsequent diagnosis. It is the pathologist's responsibility to correct any technical issues as they arise. Although diagnoses may occasionally be deferred, there is a high degree of accuracy with frozen section techniques.

The wide array of equipment and stains available precludes recommending a particular protocol by which intraoperative consultations be performed. However, a few points are considered universal in achieving technically high quality frozen sections. Assign a unique identifier to the specimen after delivery time stamp. A thorough macroscopic examination will determine the proper sample for evaluation. If a frozen section is to be performed, make certain the sample is taken perpendicular to the capsule which has been inked appropriately, and that it is oriented correctly in the mounting media. The optimal freezing temperature is at least −20°C, with sections cut at 5–6 μm intervals. Multiple levels (ribbons) should be obtained during the initial evaluation. Results should be orally communicated to the surgeon in a timely fashion; the College of American Pathologists recommends that 90 % or greater of all frozen sections be reported within 20 minutes. A permanent record of the frozen section request and diagnosis should be maintained in the patient's record and in the pathology suite (electronically as allowed by governing bodies), with the slide retained indefinitely along with the permanent H&E sections.

GROSSING TECHNIQUES

INITIAL EVALUATION

Every specimen prior to evaluation must have accurate patient identification and a unique identifier associated with it. Pertinent clinical history is imperative, including symptoms, past treatment, radiographic findings, and clinical suspicion. Specific specimen identification, including exact anatomic site is essential, including laterality (right or left). The latter is most important with parathyroid gland sampling, especially if multiple samples are to be evaluated. Any specific or special requests should be noted, including cultures, ultrastructural examination, immunofluorescence, immunohistochemistry, flow cytometry, molecular/genetic studies and/or chain of custody requirements.

ORIENTATION

The complexity of many endocrine organ samples is further compounded by lack of distinct anatomic landmarks. Orientation is easily maintained and preserved through the use of suture and tissue marking pens, although ideally direct communication with the surgeon to orient the sample is paramount. Sometimes, a small drawing on the requisition can serve to orient the specimen.

GROSSING PROCEDURES AND TECHNIQUES

The importance of a thorough gross description cannot be stressed enough! The aim of each dissection is to answer questions that will lead to an accurate pathologic diagnosis and pathologic staging if a tumor is present. The macroscopic description must include the patient name and identifier, surgeon, specific specimen(s), and procedure performed (biopsy, lymph node dissection, thyroid lobectomy, adrenalectomy, radical resection, etc.). It is also important to note whether the specimen was received fresh, in formalin or in another fixative.

All anatomic structures present must be measured and described, specifically paying attention to recognized landmarks which will later aid in staging. Measuring the whole specimen (in centimeters), along with including measurements of specific structures included in the sample are important, to say nothing of measuring the lesion (tumor) itself. Giving distances from the tumor to margins or extent of involvement into adjacent structures is imperative. Weights are usually included for parathyroid, thyroid, pituitary, and adrenal gland samples, using an ultra sensitive scale for parathyroid and pituitary gland specifically.

The application of indelible (permanent) inks as an aid to recognizing specimen margins on histologic slides is vital for margin assessment. In most cases, a single color is sufficient; however there are many instances when multiple colors are necessary to accurately identify specific margins of resection. While pedantic, I use blue – superior (the sky is up); green – inferior (the grass is down); yellow – lateral (two 'l's' in yellow and lateral); orange – medial; anterior – red; posterior – black (Figure B-03). The ink should be 'fixed' to the tissue by the use of a mordant such as 95 % ethyl alcohol, 10 % glacial acetic acid, or Bouin's. It is imperative that the ink is completely dry before sectioning to prevent ink tracking, seepage, and spilling from creating a false positive margin.

The main lesion/tumor must be accurately described in terms of size, location, appearance, growth pattern, color, structures involved and distance from margins. Prior to any sectioning, the margins must be assessed and submitted as necessary. For the vast majority of endocrine organ specimens, there are not usually numerous margins, with margin assessments generally limited to the final reporting. Decalcification may be required for some thyroid specimens if the tumor has been present for a long duration, but inking will preserve histologic orientation.

Most specimens will need to be sectioned in order to determine the extent of disease and routes of infiltration. If the sample is a biopsy, the description should include the number and size of the fragments, all of which should be completely embedded. If the sample of tissue is greater than 4 mm, the specimen should be bisected. When the tissue is smaller than 4 mm, multiple serial cuts should be requested at the time of the initial sectioning to avoid loss of diagnostic material in subsequent recut requests. If

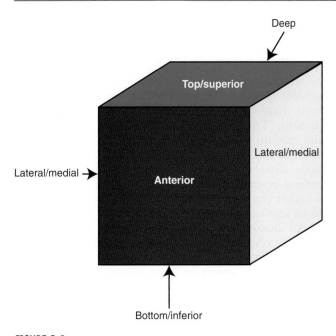

FIGURE B-3
Margin and inking diagram.

needed, alternate levels can be stained with hematoxylin and eosin (H&E), with the unstained (or charged) slides held for additional studies as needed. Developing a routine or standard approach is suggested, with minor alterations implemented for each unique specimen/sample as necessary to try to demonstrate the relationship of the 'lesion' or 'tumor' to the surrounding structures histologically.

Although perhaps slightly out of sequential order, proper and adequate fixation of all specimens is unconditionally required to obtain high quality histologic sections. Depending on tissue type and size of the resection, 6–8 hours of fixation in 10% formalin is minimum, with 24 hours considered ideal. Specimens which contain a substantial component of bone should be fixed with a mixture of formalin and decalcifying solution for at least 48 hours. Clearing agents may aid in lymph node dissections by removing the fat. When faced with turn-around time constraints, I routinely suggest that a correct diagnosis made in three days on a well fixed and grossed specimen is always superior to an inaccurate diagnosis rendered the following day on hastily grossed and insufficiently fixed or sampled material.

The histologic sections submitted depend upon the anatomic site and the lesion in question. Trying to demonstrate normal or uninvolved in relation to the lesion/tumor is vital in making an accurate diagnosis. Thin sections (<2 mm thick) which are well fixed will yield the best histologic slides.

GROSSING TECHNIQUES FOR SPECIFIC ENDOCRINE ORGANS

NECK DISSECTIONS

Neck dissections are performed to either evaluate a patient's lymph node status or to resect obvious clinical disease. For clinical and pathologic staging purposes, the neck is broken down in lymphatic zones. With the exception of zone Ia (submental), each zone is paired on either side of the neck. Specific zones are identified, with particular attention to the jugular chain (Figure B-04).

Neck dissections can be done on a limited basis where only the lymph nodes and soft tissue are removed (selective neck dissection), or they can be quite extensive and involve removal of many structures within the neck (modified-radical neck dissection). Selective neck dissections generally tend to include levels 2–4, although level 1 and level 5 nodes may also be removed. Removal of the submandibular gland (level 1b) is also quite frequent. A truly radical neck dissection involves removal of the internal jugular vein, the SCM, and the spinal accessory nerve in addition to the lymph nodes and associated soft tissue. A modified-radical dissection would include preservation of any one of the three aforementioned structures. Extended neck dissections would include any structures not previously mentioned (paratracheal nodes, carotid artery, etc).

Lymph nodes should be separated out from their respective levels or zones, and sections submitted accordingly for histology. All identified lymph nodes must be submitted. For larger lymph nodes, if the entire node is submitted, it is imperative to note in your gross dictation if a single cassette contains multiple sections of a single lymph node. Otherwise, the total lymph node count could be affected and possibly have an adverse impact on the patient's adjuvant therapy.

THYROID

Requests for intraoperative assessment of thyroid lesions have decreased remarkably with the increased use of fine needle aspiration as a screening tool. Debate exists as to the necessity for frozen section. While frozen sections have a high specificity (>90%), they have a sensitivity of only about 60%. Therefore, if a preoperative fine needle aspiration has yielded a diagnosis of 'thyroid follicular epithelial proliferation,' whether accompanied by a 'favor adenomatoid nodule' or 'favor follicular neoplasm,' frozen section assessment will not change the management. Separation of cellular adenomatoid nodules, follicular adenomas and follicular carcinoma relies on the presence of a well formed capsule and on the presence of invasion (capsular or vascular). Even when multiple different sites

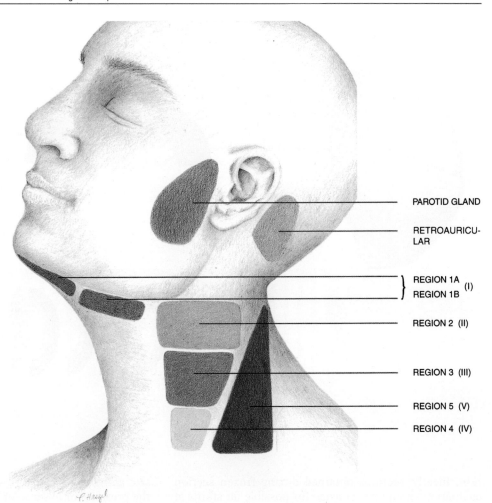

FIGURE B-4

Neck dissection lymph node compartments. With the exception of level Ia (submental), there are two corresponding zones, one for each side of the neck. Level Ib (submandibular); levels II–IV (jugular chain); and level V (posterior triangle).

PAROTID GLAND

RETROAURICU-LAR

REGION 1A
REGION 1B   (I)

REGION 2 (II)

REGION 3 (III)

REGION 5 (V)

REGION 4 (IV)

of a nodule in question are sampled, it is still extremely difficult to render a definitive diagnosis. Therefore, frozen section diagnosis of 'follicular neoplasm, deferred to permanent sections' does not guide the surgeon nor does it alter the management intraoperatively. Therefore, since most authors have reported influencing the intraoperative management of a patient in < 1% of cases, the time commitment to perform the procedure, the unnecessary loss of tissue to perform the frozen section, and the increased cost, all combine to make this procedure unnecessary. Occasionally, assessment of an adjacent 'nodule' may be needed to exclude invasion or metastatic disease to a lymph node.

Having said thus, if an intraoperative assessment is still necessary, touch preparations, scrape preparations and frozen section examination will yield the best overall interpretation. Touch preparations and scrape preparations (smears) allow for an assessment of the fine nuclear details which may help diagnose a papillary carcinoma. The frozen section (often multiple) should be taken from the tumor-to-capsule-to-parenchymal interface in order to attempt documenting invasion (Figure B-05). After sectioning, the material should be re-submitted as a frozen section control. The controversy about whether a completion thyroidectomy should be performed immediately if there is papillary carcinoma, is still up for debate. In light of the excellent long term clinical prognosis for papillary carcinoma, especially in patients < 45 years of age, it is my bias to manage these patients with lobectomy alone, rather than obligating them to life-long replacement therapy and the attendant risks of another surgery.

PARATHYROID

Hyperparathyroidism can be caused by a number of disorders, with adenoma and hyperplasia the two principle contenders. Although advances have been made in radiolabelled studies and in intraoperative rapid hormone analysis, intraoperative assessment of parathyroid gland tissue is still necessary. Knowing if the gland sampled has been biopsied or if the tissue is from an enlarged or normal gland is paramount in initial evaluation. The gland must be labeled, measured and weighed after removing any excess adipose tissue. Whereas, touch preparations can be performed to confirm parathyroid tissue, frozen section is much more sensitive and specific in parathyroid *disease* determina-

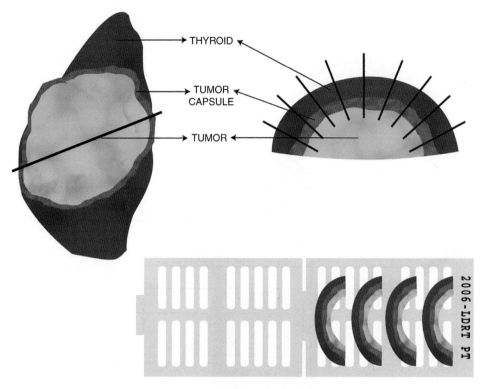

The sectioning of a tumor mass in the thyroid gland.

tion. Ideally, sections obtained during frozen section evaluation should be set aside for possible fat stains at a later time.

Although axiomatic, it is first important to document parathyroid tissue before continuing the valuation of the underlying process. Lymph nodes, thyroid, thymus and fat may all be inadvertently sampled during neck exploration. Frozen section will help to confirm that parathyroid tissue is present. If only one gland is sampled, it may be wise to limit the amount of tissue frozen so as not to adversely affect the tissue in permanent sections. However, practically speaking, one is seldom able to predict with any degree of certainty the number of samples obtained. Separation between a sample of thyroid and parathyroid may occasionally be quite difficult. The clear to microvacuolated cytoplasm and a more pronounced intercellular border may help to confirm a parathyroid gland.

It is my practice to state 'parathyroid tissue identified' without any qualification if only one parathyroid gland is sampled or if no additional clinical, laboratory or radiographic information is provided. To separate uneven nodular parathyroid hyperplasia from parathyroid adenoma on a single sample without additional information is asking for trouble. Knowing the number of glands which have been assessed, whether in-situ by the surgeon or to be sent to pathology, will make a difference in how the diagnosis is phrased. Adenoma involves a single gland while hyperplasia involves multiple glands. Usually, the largest and most clinically obvious gland is removed. However, one cannot rely on size alone, nor on the presence of a normal rim, or on the presence or absence of stromal adipose tissue. Many times, if only a single gland is sampled, 'cellular parathyroid gland tissue' or 'parathyroid proliferative disease' is the most that can be stated with confidence. However, if a second gland is sampled, then perhaps a more definitive diagnosis can be rendered based on a comparison between the size, cellularity, and stromal fat content. Suffice it to say, definitive diagnoses on intraoperative frozen section material on parathyroid diseases is difficult, often requiring examination of the permanent sections and an evaluation of the serum calcium and/or parathyroid hormone levels post-operatively.

Developments in imaging, biochemical studies, intraoperative parathyroid hormone analysis, and surgical techniques may supercede intraoperative frozen section or touch preparation cytology in a number of patients. Technetium-99m sestamibi scanning has a good positive predictive value, but is better for single gland rather than multi-gland disease. It has a false negative rate of up to 20%. Combination radiographic techniques (subtraction scintigraphy; CT-sestamibi image fusion; positron emission tomography [PET] scanning) may compliment the sestamibi result. Intraoperative quick assay of intact parathyroid hormone before and after excision with a fall of at least 50%, will help to predict accuracy of the surgery. This technique is also most accurate for single gland disease. Further utilization of these newer techniques, especially in combination, will yield a degree of comfort in making a more specific diagnosis in the future.

ADRENAL

Intraoperative assessment is seldom requested for adrenal gland pathology, although computed tomography guided core needle biopsies may be performed. In general these samples are requested to rule out metastatic disease or an infectious etiology, rather than assessing a primary lesion. Clinical symptoms, laboratory results, and radiographic images are usually sufficiently able to determine if a resection is necessary. Adrenalectomy is the treatment for most adrenal gland tumors, and partial adrenaclectomies are generally not performed.

Sections through the adrenal gland should be perpendicular to the long axis, such that the cortex to medulla can be assessed, along with the relationship of any lesion or tumor to the cortex and/or medulla. Touch preparations can be a useful screening technique to determine what additional studies may be useful in yielding a diagnosis. Frozen sections are generally not useful, as separation between adrenal cortical adenoma and carcinoma cannot usually be achieved on a small sample.

PITUITARY

Intraoperative assessment is usually limited to the adequacy of the tissue for ultimate diagnostic determination. Pituitary tumors are seldom removed whole, and so the sample will contain multiple fragments of tissue. Touch preparations, squash or smear preparations, and or frozen sections can be performed to confirm the pituitary origin of the tissue, and may also be used to give an idea about the neoplastic nature of the lesion. Material can then be separated for ultrastructural examination and routine histologic evaluation. Immunohistochemistry analysis may be necessary for the ultimate determination of the lesion, although in many patients the serologic hormone or protein assessment may already guide in the determination of the type of tumor.

ACKNOWLEDGMENT

The authors express their sincerest gratitude to Ms Trisha Haszel of Des Moines, Iowa for her superb artwork and illustrations.

SUGGESTED READING

Ackerman LV, Ramirez GA. The indications for and limitations of frozen section diagnosis. A review of 1269 consecutive frozen section diagnoses. Br J Surg 1959;46:336–350.

Barnes EL. Surgical pathology of the Head and Neck. 2nd ed. New York: Marcel Dekker, 2001.

Barnes L, Johnson JT. Pathologic and clinical considerations in the evaluation of major head and neck specimens resected for cancer. Part 1. In: Sommers SC, Rosen PP, Fechner RE, eds. Pathology Annual. Vol. 21, part 1. Norwalk: Appleton-Century-Crofts, 1986.

Fu Y, Wenig BM, Abemayor E, Wenig B. Head and Neck Pathology with Clinical Correlations. Philadelphia: Churchill-Livingstone, 2001.

Gandour-Edwards RF, Donald PJ, Lie JT. Clinical utility of intraoperative frozen section diagnosis in head and neck surgery: a quality assurance perspective. Head Neck 1993;15:373–376.

Holaday WJ, Assor D. Ten thousand consecutive frozen sections. A retrospective study focusing on accuracy and quality control. Am J Clin Pathol 1974;61:769–777.

Lester S. Manual of Surgical Pathology 2nd ed. Philadelphia: Churchill-Livingstone, 2006.

Saltzstein SL, Nahum AM. Frozen section diagnosis: accuracy and errors; uses and abuses. Laryngoscope 1973;83:1128–1143.

Westra WH, Hruban RH, Phelps TH, Isacson C. Surgical Pathology Dissection: An Illustrated Guide. 2nd ed. London: Springer-Verlag, 2003.

TNM Classification and Consensus Reporting of Head and Neck and Endocrine Organ Tumors

Leslie H Sobin • Lester DR Thompson

INTRODUCTION

The current UICC/AJCC TNM classification only recognize staging for thyroid gland tumors. Although the UICC/AJCC does not classify a number of unique entities in the endocrine organs, a proposed staging systems has been presented. The following introduction contains a general discussion of TNM principles and a summary of the major changes in the TNM classifications that occurred from the previous (5th) to the present (6th) edition.

The TNM Classification describes the anatomic extent of cancer. It is based on the fact that the choice of treatment and the chance of survival are related to the extent of the tumor at the primary site (T), the presence or absence of tumor in regional lymph nodes (N), and the presence or absence of metastasis beyond the regional lymph nodes (M). Tumors are classified prior to treatment, i.e., clinical or cTNM, and after resection, i.e., pathological or pTNM. T is usually divided into four major parts (T1–T4), expressing increasing size or spread of the primary tumor. N and M comprise at least two categories each (0 and 1 – absence or presence of tumor). A number of sites have subcategories. The criteria for cTNM and pTNM are identical for head and neck tumors. Note: A help desk for specific questions about the TNM classification is available at http://www.uicc.org.

STAGE GROUPING

Classification by TNM achieves a reasonably precise description of and system for recording the apparent anatomical extent of disease. However, a tumor with four T, three N, and two M categories will have 24 possible TNM categories. For purposes of tabulation and analysis, except in very large series, it is necessary to condense these categories into a more convenient number of TNM stages. This aims to ensure that each stage group is more or less homogeneous in respect to survival and management, and that the survival rates of these groups for each cancer site are distinctive, e.g., patients with stage I tumors usually survive their disease; those with stage IV usually succumb to the disease.

OBJECTIVES

The objective of TNM staging is to:
- Aid the clinician in the planning of treatment;
- Give some indication of prognosis;
- Assist in the evaluation of the results of treatment;
- Facilitate the exchange of information; and
- TNM can also serve as a means of assessing the management of patients and as a yardstick to measure early detection (screening) efforts.

The 6th edition TNM classification of the International Union Against Cancer (UICC) and American Joint Committee on Cancer (AJCC) was introduced in January 2003. Although relatively unchanged for most cancer sites, the head and neck and endocrine organ sections of the classification underwent substantial revision in the 6th edition. The major changes that occurred between the 5th and 6th TNM editions are summarized below.

T4

The fundamental composition and content of the head and neck TNM classification has not changed in decades. However, with evolution in treatment approaches over the past decade, a simple description of the primary tumor beyond the site of origin to characterize locally 'advanced' disease is no longer adequate for this group of patients. Therefore, the 6th edition introduced a subdivision of T4 across all sites into T4a and T4b based on the principle of a reasonable opportunity for disease control in T4a, compared to the virtual certainty of poor outcome in T4b.

GENERAL ISSUES

- Stage IVA is classified as T4a N0-N1, or any N2 lesion without T4b.
- T-category and N-category allocation remains the same for stages I, II, III and IVC as in the 5th edition.
- T4 lesions have been divided into T4a (lower risk) and T4b (higher risk), facilitating a division of stage IV into stage IVA, stage IVB, and stage IVC.

SPECIAL SYMBOLS

Developments in multimodality therapy have increased the importance of the "y" symbol, designating tumors that are classified after radiation or chemotherapy, and the "R" (residual tumor) classification. New surgical techniques have resulted in the elaboration of the "sn" (sentinel node) symbol. Immunohistochemistry has brought about the classification of "itc" (isolated tumor cells) and their distinction from micrometastasis.

TUMOR REPORTING IN GENERAL

THYROID GLAND

Many parameters can be considered for inclusion in the final pathology report. The following are considered to be most helpful, although not always necessary, a modification of the recommendations of the Directors of Anatomic and Surgical Pathology:
- Clinical data and demographics
- Organ and type of specimen (nodulectomy, lobectomy, thyroidectomy, etc.)
- Gross description (including tumor location and largest dimension)
- Results of intraoperative consultations (if any)
- Tumor histologic type and/or subtype
- Presence of invasion (capsular, vascular, and extra-thyroidal extension)
- Surgical margin status
- Presence of tumor multifocality
- Remaining gland pathology
- Parathyroid gland appearance and pathology (if any)
- Number and status of the lymph nodes (if any; if metastatic disease, give the size of the largest lymph node and presence or absence of perinodal tumor extension).

PAPILLARY, FOLLICULAR AND MEDULLARY HISTOLOGIC SUBTYPES

No convincing evidence of a break point at the 1 cm (present in the 5th edition) and 2 cm size points is available for differentiated thyroid carcinoma. Hence an adoption of a demarcation at 2 cm and 4 cm provides consistency with other head and neck size break points. Disease limited to the thyroid gland has favorable prognosis, including tumor invading the first strap muscle layer (sterno-thyroid muscle), common when the disease has extend beyond the parenchyma (a situation analogous to salivary gland where such disease is also T3) and represents a change from the 5th edition TNM. In contrast more extensive disease invading sterno-hyoid muscle, trachea, larynx or esophagus and beyond has an adverse prognosis and should be T4 (a or b), together with other adverse features.

Level VI lymph nodes are regarded separately from other nodes. The rational for the separation is based on clinical management (i.e., surgical techniques used) and not on prognosis. Indeed there is little evidence that different types of nodal involvement have different prognosis in differentiated thyroid carcinoma or even that lymph node involvement itself is prognostic, at least in young patients with this disease. Therefore the N1 category is retained but separates level VI and other nodes into sub-categories (N1a vs. N1b). The N1b category is allocated to stage IVA in the older patients since nodal metastases do have an adverse impact on prognosis in patients over the age of 45 years.

T-categories have been revised (see Table C-1):
- Size demarcations altered to be the same as other head and neck sites.
- T3: Tumor more than 4 cm in greatest dimension limited to the thyroid or any tumor with minimal extrathyroidal extension (e.g. extension to sterno-thyroid muscle or perithyroidal soft tissues).

N-categories revisions are different to other head and neck sites:
- N1a – Metastasis to Level IV (pretracheal, paratracheal, and prelaryngeal/Delphian lymph nodes).
- N1b – Metastasis to unilateral, bilateral, or contralateral cervical or superior mediastinal lymph nodes.
- T3N0 allocated to Stage III (in 5th edition, T3N0 was Stage II).
- T1–3N1a is Stage III.
- All T4 lesions are allocated to the Stage IV groups (e.g., in the 5th edition, T4N0 papillary and follicular were stage III and T3-T4N0 medullary carcinoma were stage II).
- Stage IV is now classified as IVA and IVB depending on T4a or T4b or presence of N1b (IVA).

TABLE C-1

TNM Classification of Carcinomas of the Thyroid Gland

T – Primary Tumor

TX	Primary tumor cannot be assessed
T0	No evidence of primary tumor
T1	Tumor 2 cm or less in greatest dimension, limited to the thyroid
T2	Tumor more than 2 cm but not more than 4 cm in greatest dimension, limited to the thyroid
T3	Tumor more than 4 cm in greatest dimension, limited to the thyroid or any tumor with minimal extrathyroidal extension (e.g., extension to sternothyroid muscle or perithyroidal soft tissues)
T4a	Tumor extends beyond the thyroid capsule and invades any of the following: subcutaneous soft tissues, larynx, trachea, esophagus, recurrent laryngeal nerve
T4b	Tumour invades prevertebral fascia, mediastinal vessels, or encases carotid artery
T4a (anaplastic)*	Tumor (any size) limited to the thyroid (considered surgically resectable)
T4b (anaplastic)*	Tumor (any size) extends beyond the thyroid capsule (considered surgically unresectable)

N – Regional Lymph Nodes (the Regional Lymph Nodes are the Cervical and Upper/Superior Mediastinal Nodes)

NX	Regional lymph nodes cannot be assessed
N0	No regional lymph node metastasis
N1	Regional lymph node metastasis
N1a	Metastasis in level VI (pretracheal and paratracheal, including prelarnygeal and Delphian lymph nodes)
N1b	Metastasis in other unilateral, bilateral or contralateral cervical or upper/superior mediastinal lymph nodes

M – Distant Metastasis

MX	Distant metastasis cannot be assessed
M0	No distant metastasis
M1	Distant metastasis

Stage Definitions

Papillary or follicular – under 45 years			
Stage I	Any T	Any N	M0
Stage II	Any T	Any N	M1
Papillary or follicular – 45 years and older and medullary			
Stage I	T1	N0	M0
Stage II	T2	N0	M0
Stage III	T3	N0	M0
	T1, T2, T3	N1a	M0
Stage IVA	T1, T2, T3	N1b	M0
	T4a	N0, N1	M0
Stage IVB	T4b	Any N	M0
Stage IVC	Any T	Any N	M1
Anaplastic/undifferentiated (all cases are stage IV)			
Stage IVA	T4a	Any N	M0
Stage IVB	T4b	Any N	M0
Stage IVC	Any T	Any N	M1

*All anaplastic/undifferentiated thyroid carcinomas are considered T4.
Note: Multifocal tumors of all histological types should be designated (m) (the largest determines the classification), e.g., T2(m).

ANAPLASTIC THYROID CARCINOMA

Anaplastic thyroid carcinoma has extremely adverse prognosis and death invariably results from uncontrolled local disease. This occurs irrespective of local disease presentation (i.e. intrathyroidal and extrathyroidal) as it uniformally behaves in a very adverse way. This is deemed to merit the most adverse T-category designation (i.e., T4a/T4b) based on prognostic assessment. Therefore, in the 6th edition TNM there is no T1-T3 categories; all anaplastic carcinomas are considered T4a or T4b. An occasional small anaplastic lesion confined to the thyroid gland may be a candidate for long term cure. Such lesions are exceedingly rare and may represent transformation from a previous well differentiated tumor with foci of anaplastic transformation but merit complete resection by thyroidectomy. In practice, the extremely adverse prognosis means that the principle of separating T4 in T4a and T4b is more directed at a treatment rationale rather than outcome prediction.

ADRENAL GLAND

Many parameters can be considered for inclusion in the final pathology report. The following are considered to be most helpful, although not always necessary, a modification of the recommendations of the Directors of Anatomic and Surgical Pathology:
- Clinical data and demographics (including endocrinologic data)
- Organ and type of specimen (biopsy, adrenalectomy, radical resection, etc.)
- Macroscopic description (including exact site, size in three dimensions, weight, description of tumor, appearance of adjacent uninvolved adrenal gland, and any other attached organs)
- Tumor location and largest dimension
- Results of intraoperative consultations (if any)
- Tumor histologic type and/or subtype
- Histologic grade (if pertinent)
- Surgical margin status
- Remaining gland pathology (if hyperplastic, atrophic, etc.)
- If neuroblastoma, include cytogenetic and molecular markers used in prognostic assessment
- Number and status of the lymph nodes (if any)
- Comment or descriptive features (correlation between intraoperative assessment, fine needle aspiration or other diagnostic studies, special studies performed, if staging is known).

TABLE C-2
Proposed TNM Classification of Adrenal Cortical Carcinoma

T – Primary Tumor

TX	Primary tumor cannot be assessed
T0	No evidence of primary tumor
T1	Tumor ≤ 5 cm, no local invasion
T2	Tumor ≥ 5 cm, no local invasion
T3	Tumor of any size with local invasion but without invasion of adjacent organs
T4	Tumor of any size with invasion of adjacent organs

N – Regional Lymph Nodes (the Regional Lymph Nodes are the Cervical Nodes)

NX	Regional lymph nodes cannot be assessed
N0	No regional lymph node metastasis
N1	Regional lymph node metastasis

M – Distant Metastasis

MX	Distant metastasis cannot be assessed
M0	No distant metastasis
M1	Distant metastasis

Stage Definitions

Stage	T	N	M
Stage I	T1	N0	M0
Stage II	T2	N0	M0
Stage III	T1	N1	M0
	T2	N1	M0
	T3	N0	M0
Stage IV	T3	N1	M0
	T4	N0	M0
	Any T	Any N	M1

This classification is not an official TNM classification, i.e., not approved by the UICC and AJCC. It is a proposal published in the TNM Supplement for classification of adrenal cortical carcinoma and is based on data from Henley et al., Sullivan et al., Wooten et al., and Wachenberg et al. It is also included in the 'Recommendations for reporting of tumours of the adrenal cortex and medulla' by the Association of Directors of Anatomy and Surgical Pathology. It is presented here for testing. Publication of results is encouraged.

SUGGESTED READING

AJCC Cancer Staging Manual. Greene FL, Page D, Morrow M, Balch C, Haller D, Fritz A, Fleming I, eds. 6th ed. New York: Springer, 2002.

Henley DJ, van Heerden JA, Grant CS, et al. Adrenocortical carcinoma – A continuing challenge. Surgery 1983;94:926–931.

Hughes CJ, Shaha AR, Shah JP, Loree TR. Impact of lymph node metastasis in differentiated carcinoma of the thyroid: a matched-pair analysis. Head Neck 1996;18:127–132.

International Union Against Cancer (UICC). TNM classification of malignant tumors. Sobin LH, Wittekind Ch, eds. 6th ed. New York: Wiley, 2002.

Johnson SJ, Sheffield EA, McNicol AM. Best Practice No 183: Examination of parathyroid gland specimens. J Clin Pathol. 2005;58:338–342.

Lack EE, Askin FB, Dehner LP, et al. Recommendations for reporting of tumors of the adrenal cortex and medulla. Hum Pathol 1999;30: 887–890.

Recommendations for reporting of tumors of the adrenal cortex and medulla. Association of Directors of Anatomic and Surgical Pathology. Mod Pathol. 1999 Aug;12(8):835–839.

Rosai J, Carcangiu ML, DeLellis RA, Simoes MS. Recommendations for the reporting of thyroid carcinomas. Association of Directors of Anatomic and Surgical Pathology. Hum Pathol. 2000;31:1199–1201.

Sullivan M, Boileau M, Hodges CV. Adrenal cortical carcinoma. J Urol 1978; 120:660–665.

Wachenberg BL, Arbergaria Pereira MA, Modona BB et al. Adrenocortical carcinoma. Clinical and laboratory observations. Cancer 2000;88: 711–736.

Wittekind Ch, Henson DE, Hutter RVP, Sobin LH (editors). TNM Supplement: a commentary on uniform use. 3rd ed. Wiley, New York 2003:130–131.

Wooten MD, King DK. Adrenal cortical carcinoma. Epidemiology and treatment with mitotane and a review of the literature. Cancer 1993;72:3145–3155.

Subject Index

Notes: Page numbers suffixed by 'f' indicate figures: page numbers suffixed by 't' indicate tables.